Books are to be returned on or before
the last date below.

7–DAY LOAN

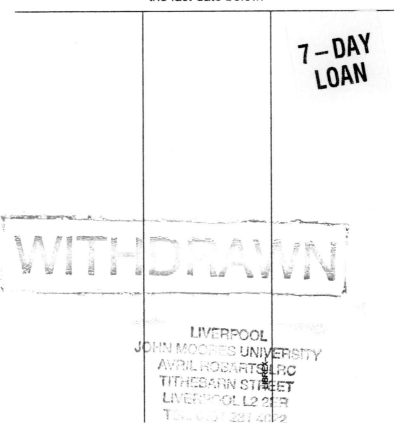

Clinical Gait Analysis

For Elsevier:

Commissioning Editor: Robert Edwards
Project Manager: Gail Wright
Senior Designers: George Ajayi and Stewart Larking
Illustration Manager: Bruce Hogarth
Illustrators: AntBits Illustration and Lee Hulteng

Clinical Gait Analysis
Theory and Practice

Chris Kirtley MD PhD
Associate Professor, Department of Biomedical
Engineering, The Catholic University of America,
Washington, DC, USA

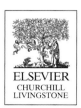

ELSEVIER
CHURCHILL
LIVINGSTONE

EDINBURGH LONDON NEW YORK OXFORD PHILADELPHIA ST LOUIS SYDNEY TORONTO 2006

ELSEVIER
CHURCHILL
LIVINGSTONE

First published 2006

ISBN 0 4431 0009 8

British Library Cataloguing in Publication Data
A catalogue record for this book is available from the British Library

Library of Congress Cataloging in Publication Data
A catalog record for this book is available from the Library of Congress

Notice
Knowledge and best practice in this field are constantly changing. As new research and experience broaden our knowledge, changes in practice, treatment and drug therapy may become necessary or appropriate. Readers are advised to check the most current information provided (i) on procedures featured or (ii) by the manufacturer of each product to be administered, to verify the recommended dose or formula, the method and duration of administration, and contraindications. It is the responsibility of the practitioner, relying on their own experience and knowledge of the patient, to make diagnoses, to determine dosages and the best treatment for each individual patient, and to take all appropriate safety precautions. To the fullest extent of the law, neither the publisher nor the author assumes any liability for any injury and/or damage.

The Publisher

 ELSEVIER
**your source for books,
journals and multimedia
in the health sciences**

www.elsevierhealth.com
Printed in China

The
Publisher's
policy is to use
**paper manufactured
from sustainable forests**

Contents

Preface

In 1996, while in Perth, Australia, Ray Smith and I started a website called 'Clinical Gait Analysis' http://www.univie.ac.at/cga with a companion email list for the discussion of walking disorders. Shortly afterwards, I moved to Vienna, Austria, where Andreas Kranzl helped develop the site further with 'Case of the Week'. Eight years later, the list has over 1200 subscribers from around the world; more than 40 clinical cases have been presented and a multitude of technical issues debated. This book is an attempt at collecting together some of the material contributed over that time.

Gait is undoubtedly complex, making its understanding a daunting challenge for the beginner. In this endeavour, many insights can be gained from looking not only at normal level gait, but also at the compensations that are made for age, speed, inclines, stairs, etc. The effects of abnormalities such as weakness, spasticity, deformity and pain can greatly enlighten the study of normal function. Moreover, the ways in which function is improved or restored by the therapist and surgeon, or substituted by the prosthetist and orthotist, can reinforce the theoretical knowledge learned. For this reason, although this book is not intended as a treatment manual for gait disorders, relevant clinical interventions and prosthetic or orthotic designs are included wherever possible, with the aim of consolidating the biomechanical theory.

Some areas of gait analysis excite great controversy and debate. Rather than hide these issues from the student, I think it best to highlight them when they arise. A useful way to do this is to encourage a debate between students, each arguing for a particular position. Doing this stimulates critical thinking and provides a useful incentive for background reading and literature searches.

There is no doubt that the greatest challenge in biomechanics is also its greatest strength: mathematics. Being able to express concepts in equations and figures (even if they are approximate) elevates understanding greatly. As Lord Kelvin pointed out[1], you never really understand something until you can put numbers to it. Very often, insight can be gleaned merely from the act of calculating something. I have therefore sprinkled occasional multiple-choice questions through the text in order to provide opportunities for testing your grasp of the more tricky sections.

The book is broadly divided into Theory and Practice. This is partly for practical necessity, in that theoretical foundations need to be laid down before a biomechanical understanding of gait can proceed; yet it is also meant as a separation between the science of measurement, which is imperfect but ought to be objective, and the clinical interpretation of the results, which inevitably is contaminated by opinion, past experience and even prejudices. It is

---

[1] When you measure what you are speaking about and express it in numbers, you know something about it, but when you cannot express it in numbers your knowledge about it is of a meagre and unsatisfactory kind (Popular lectures and addresses [1883]).

important to realize that the clinical application of biomechanics is still relatively new and subject to winds of change as research proceeds. This can sometimes make gait analysis frustrating and inconsistent but is also the source of much of the excitement that accompanies any pursuit on the edge of our understanding. There is still much to know about normal gait, let alone that affected by pathology.

Finally, it has to be said that biomechanics can be tough going, with all this emphasis on mathematics and physics. With this in mind, I have included a number of boxes addressing interesting but slightly peripheral aspects of gait. I hope you enjoy this miscellany of art, history and philosophical rumination!

Washington, D.C.   *Chris Kirtley*
2004

Introduction: Theory and practice in gait analysis

There are two modes of knowledge, through argument and experience. Argument brings conclusions and compels us to concede them, but it does not cause certainty nor remove doubts in order that the mind may remain at rest in truth, unless this is provided by experience.

Roger Bacon, *Opus Maius*

In theory there is no difference between theory and practice. In practice there is.

Yogi Berra

Many a new clinical graduate is disappointed to discover that their many years of study seem a frustratingly inadequate preparation for diagnosing the seemingly endless variety of ailments that come their way. With time, the relevance of at least some of the theory becomes clear, but a better integration of theory and practice is surely needed. This book is designed to do just that for the study of gait, combining an understanding of physical concepts and engineering tools with clinical applications.

WHAT IS GAIT ANALYSIS?

The term *gait analysis* can mean many things to different people, from a brief observation to sophisticated computerized measurements. Surprisingly (given the amount of research done in the field over the last 30 years), no single unifying concept has emerged to explain the motion of the body during gait. Instead, each approach to gait analysis tends to rely on its own paradigm. For example, in podiatric biomechanics, the theories propounded by Root are still influential, although a 'new biomechanics' is growing in popularity. In physiotherapy, approaches such as Bobath are current. Prosthetics uses a classification largely derived from Northwestern University in Chicago. In cerebral palsy, the pioneering ideas of Perry, Sutherland and Gage have provided a standard terminology and approach. Physiologists and zoologists, who attempt to boil locomotion down to its fundamentals, focus on body centre of mass and total body energy. Exercise physiologists too are interested in energy, but usually measure metabolic work via oxygen consumption rather than physical work. Some approaches are intimately bound up with a treatment philosophy (e.g. Bobath or Root). This often leads to a circular logic, in which measurements are used to confirm the theory, which is then used to explain the measurements.

All of this can be very confusing, and underlines the important interplay between theory and practice. A good understanding of theoretical principles is essential to both astute observation and discrimination between useful and bogus treatments. The range of treatments for locomotor disorders is fast changing and beyond the scope of this book. Nevertheless, it is to be hoped that it will equip the clinician with the skills needed to better judge the relative merits of the various options available.

It is worth considering the factors that characterize the differences in style between the scientific and clinical practice.

OBJECTIVITY AND SUBJECTIVITY

Like any other branch of science, clinical biomechanics is built on three foundations:

- Objective theoretical principles (laws)
- Data collection (measurements)
- Subjective interpretations (hypotheses).

Ideally, all of these would be objective – free from error, prejudice or opinion. In reality, however, the practice of science is rarely completely objective. While the fundamental biomechanical principles are now reasonably well understood, clinical hypotheses are much more dynamic – evolving with new knowledge, but also prone to changing fashions, parochial bias and even to commercial interests. Moreover, due to practical constraints in the clinical environment, data collection is often imperfect and inadequate. It should therefore be no surprise to learn that the clinical interpretation of biomechanical data can be a very subjective process indeed.

QUALITATIVE VERSUS QUANTITATIVE MEASURES

Objective assessment implies quantitative measurement, in which some sort of tool is used to put a number to a certain measured quantity. On the other hand, subjective assessments are usually qualitative, lacking numerical measurement. They can sometimes be made semi-quantitative, e.g. by the use of clinical scales such as the visual analogue scale.

ANALYSIS AND SYNTHESIS

The word *science* is derived from the Latin verb 'to know'. In general, science proceeds in two ways:

1. *Inductive reasoning* (synthesis) involves making conclusions on the basis of careful observation, e.g. Darwin's theory of evolution by natural selection.
2. *Hypothetico-deductive reasoning* (analysis), in which hypotheses (possible causes) are proposed, based on past experience with similar questions. Multiple alternative hypotheses should be proposed whenever possible. They must be testable, but it is important to note that although they can be eliminated, they cannot be proved with absolute certainty. A very robust hypothesis that survives repeated rigorous testing may finally be called a 'law'.

While most fundamental biomechanical principles have been derived through analytic reasoning, many clinical ideas arose by synthesis. This difference in approach is often the cause of misunderstandings between the two disciplines.

LABORATORY SCIENCE VERSUS COMMERCIAL IMPLEMENTATION

Very often in the field of gait analysis, commercial developments have been adopted even as discussion continues as to the merits of the underlying biomechanics. For example, in 1981 sportswear companies introduced shock-absorbing running shoes. However, controversy still continues about whether shock is harmful to the body. Similarly, the classification of people into pronators and supinators has stimulated a huge industry in prescription functional foot orthoses despite the lack of solid biomechanical foundation. Meanwhile, several findings have focused attention on the role of the foot–ankle complex in gait. Since it was recognized some 15 years ago, the function of ankle push-off is still hotly debated, even as energy-storing feet have gained popularity in prosthetics. Similarly, the development of much gait theory has been influenced by commercial developments in measurement systems. This is not necessarily wrong, but should always be borne in mind. For this reason, the main products on the market for gait analysis are extensively discussed.

OUTLINE OF THE BOOK

Part I addresses the theoretical aspects, focusing on the biomechanical tools used for analysing movement:

- Temporal–spatial parameters
- Kinematics
- Centre of mass and whole body energetics
- Joint kinetics
- Electromyography
- Joint power.

These chapters form a fairly logical sequence with a steadily increasing level of difficulty – each one providing a deeper understanding of the neuromuscular processes underlying gait. It therefore makes good sense to read the chapters in the order in which they are presented.

Part II aims at applying these principles and techniques to an understanding of normal and pathological gait. A systematic framework is provided for this by dividing the gait cycle into three functional subtasks: loading, support/progression and propulsion/swing. Disorders affecting each of these tasks are used to reinforce an understanding of normal function. Although it is normally the first procedure used, observational analysis has been left until the very last chapter of Part II. This is because it requires a comprehensive understanding of biomechanics as well as a familiarity with common gait abnormalities and compensations.

It is difficult to address the relative merits of various theories of disease causation, pathophysiology and biomechanical compensations adopted by the patient. Any attempt will inevitably mislead the reader since new data will often render many conclusions invalid. This book therefore concentrates on those principles and techniques that are by now well studied and tested. It is to be hoped that this will provide a sufficiently solid foundation to facilitate gait analysis in the most objective and illuminating way possible. With this in mind, some current controversial issues and interpretations are introduced (marked by the symbol) in an attempt to show how biomechanical data can be used to bolster or refute a clinical hypothesis. It must be stressed that there is presently no right answer to these conundrums, but they form fertile ground for debate.

PART I

Theory

Part I Theory

Introduction

People seem to think there is something inherently noble and virtuous in the desire to go for a walk.

Max Beerbohm, 'Going Out for a Walk'

Gait can be defined as any method of locomotion characterized by periods of loading and unloading of the limbs. While this includes running, hopping, skipping and perhaps even swimming and cycling, walking is the most frequently used gait, providing independence and used for many of the activities of daily living (ADLs). It also facilitates many social activities and is required in many occupations.

A BRIEF HISTORY OF GAIT ANALYSIS

If thou examinest a man having a smash of his skull, ... while his eye is askew because of it, on the side of him having that injury which is in his skull [and] he walks shuffling with his sole ... with his sole dragging, so that it is not easy for him to walk, when it [the sole] is feeble and turned over, while the tips of his toes are contracted to the ball of his sole, and they [the toes] walk fumbling the ground.

This is possibly the first ever gait analysis report, from case number 8 of the 4000-year-old *Edwin Smith Surgical Papyrus* (Wilkins & Wilkins 2000). Gait has been a recurring preoccupation throughout history, often reflecting the technology and preoccupations of the age. Aristotle ruminated on the differences between human and animal gait. In *On the Gait of Animals* (384–322 BC), he astutely observed that:

If a man were to walk on the ground alongside a wall with a reed dipped in ink attached to his head, the line traced by the reed would not be straight but zigzag, because it goes lower when he bends and higher when he stands upright.

In his *De Motu Animalum* (On the Motion of Animals, 1680), the renaissance scientist Giovani Borelli saw parallels with the machinery of his day. The Franco-Prussian wars stimulated the German Weber brothers and the engineers Braune and Fischer to develop theories of marching based on efficiency of movement. Meanwhile, the astute observations made by James Parkinson and Trendelenberg made the gaits they described eponymous. In the 19th century the Frenchman Étienne-Jules Marey and Englishman Eadweard Muybridge adapted the newly invented technique of photography to capture the first motion pictures (coincidentally spawning the film industry). Marey, and later Dudley Morton, also designed ingenious apparatus for measuring the forces under the foot.

Warfare has been a recurring stimulant for biomechanical advances. Prosthetic needs following the two World Wars drove research by Bernstein in Russia and the remarkably productive collaboration of Herbert Elftman (anatomist), Verne Inman (surgeon), Howard Eberhardt (engineer and amputee) and Henry Ralston (physiologist) at Berkeley, California. In the 1960s the introduction of hip replacement arthroplasty by John Charnley in Manchester, UK, motivated attempts to measure joint forces at the hip by John Paul in Glasgow. By the early 1980s, the pioneers of video technology began to replace cine film with many of the commercial systems used today, such as *Vicon* and *Coda* in the UK, *Motion Analysis Corporation* in the US, *Selspot* in Sweden, WATSMART (now *Optotrak*) in Canada and *Elite* in Italy.

For several years, poliomyelitis and spina bifida made orthotic design and assessment a major focus of attention in California (Jacqueline Perry and David Sutherland) and Oswestry (ORLAU) in the UK (Gordon Rose). In their place, the treatment of problems caused by cerebral palsy has become the major driving force behind gait analysis development, advocated by enthusiastic surgeons such as James Gage in St Paul, Minnesota. Currently, the computer games industry is stimulating a lot of motion capture refinements and providing novel visualization and animation techniques which are enabling complex mathematical models and simulations to be built and refined (Felix Zajac).

NUMBER OF STEPS IN A YEAR

Part of the problem with understanding walking is that because we do so much of it so effortlessly and subconsciously, it is difficult to appreciate the immense complexities involved.

The average person takes between 5000 and 15,000 steps per day – that's about 2–5 million per year – on average 27,000 km, or a complete circuit of the earth! Of course, the actual number depends on the activity level (Schmalzried et al 1998, Silva et al 2002), with some people regularly taking up to 30,000 steps a day (Seedhom & Wallbridge 1985). In a study of 265 men and 228 women, the average number of steps per day taken by men decreased from 11,900 to 6700, and by women from 9300 to 7300, as age increased from 25 to 74 years (Sequeira et al 1995).

People are generally not walking as much as they used to, however (Fig. A1). The 10–19 age group, in particular, now walks 25% less than their predecessors did just a decade ago, and this may be one of the factors behind increased levels of teenage obesity.

Figure A1   Average distance walked per year in the community by age (data from the National Travel Survey, Department for Transport, UK).

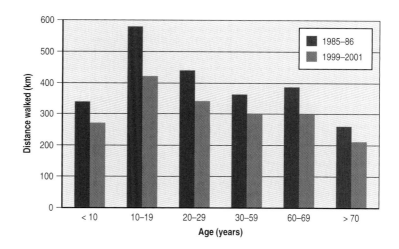

She cursed the weaver and the walker,
The cloth that they had wrought.

Thomas Percy, *Reliques*

The word *walk* is an interesting one. It comes from the Anglo-Saxon *wealcan* (to roll); whence *wealcere*, a roll of cloth (Brewer 1894). To walk, therefore, is to roll along.

Walking is so uniquely human that it has often been used as a metaphor in speech and literature. Indeed, some idea of its importance can be had from noting just how many words describe various types of gait: e.g. amble, dawdle, hike, hobble, limp, lope, lumber, lurch, march, meander, prance, promenade, saunter, scamper, scramble, scurry, shuffle, slink, slouch, stagger, step, stride, stroll, strut, swagger, tread, trot, trudge, wander (and many more!). St Augustine exclaimed '*Solvitur ambulando*' (it is solved by walking), while Spanish-speakers greet each other by asking '*¿Como andas?*' (literally, how do you walk?), and the Japanese have a word, *tekoteko*, for the *sound* of walking. The name of a famous German tavern and beer, *Schlenkerla*, comes from the Franconian word for the strange limp of its 19th century owner.

On July 20, 1969, Neil Armstrong announced '*One small step for (a) man, one giant leap for mankind*' as he stepped onto the moon (the '*a*' was unfortunately cut out by radio static, which slightly spoiled the poetic impact of his words). Barring a chance meteorite impact, his and Buzz Aldrin's footprints (Fig. A2) will last for millions of years, but the boots that made them were jettisoned to save weight for the return to earth.

Figure A2

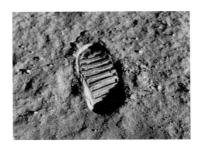

Brewer E C 1894 The Dictionary of Phrase and Fable. Henry Altemus, Philadelphia

ALTERNATIVES TO GAIT

It should always be borne in mind that *reciprocal gait*, in which the legs swing forwards alternately, is not the only method of locomotion available to humans. The metabolic cost of many pathological gaits may be so high that using a wheelchair becomes an attractive alternative. Wheelchairs use about half the energy required for gait over the same distance, and most people with gait problems opt for a wheelchair when the cost per distance of their gait exceeds three times that of normal healthy gait. Wheeled mobility also becomes a preferred option when gait speed falls below a critical level. For example, social interaction becomes difficult if you can't keep up with other people.

MEASUREMENT THEORY

Analysing gait often requires making and interpreting a lot of measurements, so it's worth acquainting yourself with some basic concepts. Every measurement is uncertain to some extent. These uncertainties, or errors, are of two kinds: *random* and *systematic*.

RANDOM ERROR

Random errors occur when, for example, an observer starts a stopwatch at the instant someone walks past a finishing line. Due to difficulty in deciding the precise moment that this happens, the stopwatch may be pressed slightly too early or too late. Thus, repeated measurements will vary randomly around the actual, or correct, value. If the time axis is divided up into small intervals (e.g. 5.40–5.45 s, 5.45–5.50 s etc.) and a token placed in each interval whenever the time recorded falls within that interval, a *normal distribution* develops (Fig. A3).

It's pretty obvious that the interval in which the measured time most frequently falls is the 5.55–5.60 s one. Nevertheless, there are lots of other measurements that don't fall within this interval – even a few way out to each side (meaning that the time recorded was much lower or higher than usual). The overall shape is that of a bell, with most of the tokens in the centre and fewer out at the edges.

Figure A3   Normal distribution constructed by measuring the time required to walk a certain distance.

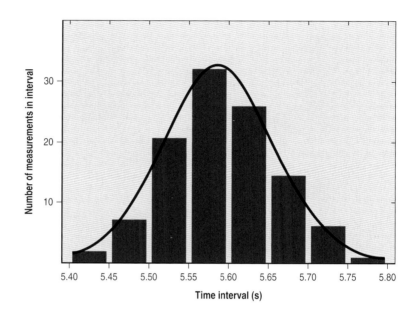

The SI system of measurement

The *Système International d'Unités*, or International System of Units, or simply the 'SI System', was inaugurated at the Treaty of the Metre (*Convention du Mètre*), in Paris on May 20, 1875. There are currently only three countries in the world that have not adopted the SI system: Burma, Liberia and the United States of America. Although the USA was one of the original signers of the Treaty (Thomas Jefferson was an early enthusiast), congressional legislation on metrification was defeated by a single vote in 1902, and consequently the old English (now called 'US customary units') are still in use.

There are three basic units: the metre (m), kilogram (kg) and second (s). Other units are derived from these – e.g. the newton is defined as the force that accelerates a mass of one kilogram at the rate of one metre per second per second, or 1 kg m/s^2 (it's also, curiously, the force that caused a typical 102 g apple to hit Sir Isaac Newton's head! – Fig. A4). A kilogram is the mass of a litre of water.

Each unit can be subdivided or grouped into multiples of 1000: e.g. 1 mm (1/1000 m) or 1 km (1000 m). The *centi*metre (cm) is, strictly speaking, part of the former CGS (cm-gram-second) system, and not an SI acceptable unit (because it is 1/100th of a metre), but is a useful clinical measure. Let's hope nobody at the *Bureau International des Poids et Mesures* (the Paris office

Figure A4

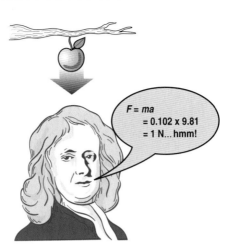

which keeps an eye on such things) is reading this! Here are some conversion factors for common units used in movement analysis:

To convert from	to	multiply by (divide to go the other way)
inch	centimetre (cm)	2.54
foot	centimetre (cm)	30
miles per hour (mph)	metres per second (m/s)	0.45
pound (lb)	kilogram (kg)	0.45
pound-force (lbf)	newton (N)	4.45
foot pound-force (ft lbf)	newton-metre (N m)	1.35
pounds per square inch (psi)	kilopascal (kPa)	6.9
horsepower (hp)	watt (W)	746
calorie (cal)	joule (J)	4.2

The best estimate of the 'correct' value for the measured time is, of course, the *average* or *mean*, which can be calculated by adding all the measurements together and dividing by the number of measurements taken. This doesn't tell the whole story, though. The width, or *spread*, of the distribution indicates how much confidence should be placed in this mean value. This parameter is called the *standard deviation* (SD), and is calculated as follows:

1. Find the difference between each measurement and the mean
2. Square this difference (to make them all positive)
3. Average the squares
4. Take the square root of the average.

The SD represents the *statistical uncertainty* of a measurement, and is very important in interpreting gait analysis data. Notice that it is really a combination of two factors:

- Variation in the quantity being measured – in this case, the time
- Variation or imprecision in the instrument – in this case, the observer pressing the stopwatch.

In practice, almost all gait measurements are affected by these two factors, so SD is an important concept to understand. A very useful property of normal distributions is that it is known that 67% of all the measurements fall within ± 1 SD of the mean, 95% fall within ± 2 SD, and 99.7% within ± 3 SD (Fig. A5).

Since most biological measurements seem to be normally distributed, this provides a way to define normative data ranges. If a measurement falls outside these limits, it could still be normal, but relatively high or low due to natural biological variation or instrument imprecision. Classifying such a result as *abnormal* would constitute making what is known as a *false positive* mistake. The likelihood of this happening can be estimated quite simply (Table A1).

Figure A5   If a population is normally distributed, 67% of measurements will be contained within a range defined by mean ± 1 SD; 95% within 2 SDs and 99.7% within 3 SDs. This principle is the basis of clinical definitions of normality and normative ranges for biomechanical variables.

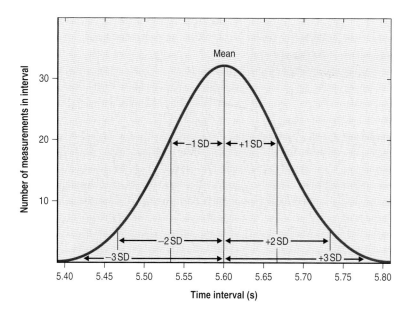

Table A1   Likelihood of making a false positive error decreases as the normative range is widened

Normative range definition	Likelihood of false positive
Mean ± 1 SD	33%
Mean ± 2 SD	5%
Mean ± 3 SD	0.3%

Clearly, a normative range based on mean ± 1 SD is a bit risky, because 33% of truly normal measurements will be wrongly classified as being abnormal. For this reason, most medical diagnostics (e.g. blood tests) use a range defined by mean ± 2 SD or even 3 SD.

Gait measurements often have large SDs due to the two sources of variability (biological and instrument). This makes normative ranges based on mean ± 2 or 3 SD rather wide, meaning that many abnormal measurements would be considered normal – a mistake known as a *false negative*. As of this time, this problem remains unsolved, and most gait laboratories routinely use normative ranges based on mean ± 1 SD. This is unsatisfactory, and it is to be hoped that as data collection procedures and motion analysis equipment improve, the normative ranges will be tightened.

It is often desirable to compare the SD of different types of measurement. This makes no sense if the means of each measurement are different, because the size of the SD is often related to the size of the mean. To get around this, another measure is commonly used, called the *coefficient of variation*. This is simply the ratio of the SD to the mean, expressed as a percentage:

$$\text{Coefficient of Variation (\%)} = (\text{SD} \times 100)/\text{Mean}$$

The magical talus and the beginnings of statistics	*God does not play dice* Albert Einstein Hermes (an adaptation of the Egyptian messenger god Thoth, called Mercury by the Romans) brought the arts of writing, arithmetic, and masonry to ancient Greece, along with a magical cube: the die. Made from the *astragaloi* (talus bones) of sheep or goats (Fig. A6), these *tali* (hence also the term *talisman*) were rounded on two sides with the other four marked *supinum*, *pronum*, *planum*, and *tortuosum*, corresponding to the numbers 3, 4, 1 and 6. The nearly cubic talus of the Libyan antelope, *boibalis*, was used for divination and prophesy. The talus is mystically and practically suited to its role in divination. It is the only bone in the body with no muscle attachments and functions in the ankle as a pivot, responding to the vicissitudes and irregularities of the ground surface. The god Talus was lame (see chapter 6) and was identified with Janus, the 'guardian of the door', after which the month of January is named – a god who looks both ways. Games of chance of any kind were forbidden in Rome, except during the Saturnalia festival in December.

Figure A6

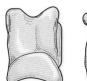

In 49 BC Julius Caesar crossed the Rubicon and declared war on Rome with the phrase *Iacta alea est!* ('Let the die be cast!'). The *alea* of the phrase was the Latin word for a die – the same root is *aleatory* (depending on chance). Die and dice come from the Latin *datum*, from which the word *data* is derived.

SYSTEMATIC ERROR

One good property of random error is that, though it adds variability to the data (increasing the spread of the distribution), it does not affect the mean (Fig. A7). This is because each separate measurement is just as likely to be low as to be high.

Unfortunately, there is another type of error: systematic error (Fig. A8), which causes the mean to deviate from its true value, introducing a *bias* into the measurement. This is usually a much more difficult error to deal with, because it can't be removed by averaging. The only solution would be to predict or determine the amount of bias and subtract it from all the measurements. For example, in our example of timing a person walking past a finishing line, there will be a certain time delay (about 100 ms, or 0.1 s) in pressing the stopwatch due to the time it takes for nerve impulses to travel from the observer's eye to their brain and from brain to hand in order to operate the stop watch. This sensorimotor delay is likely to make each timing measurement slightly longer than it should be. The time delay of the observer could be estimated and then subtracted from each measurement, but clearly this might be difficult and will require another experiment to be performed.

There are many examples of systematic error in gait measurements – sometimes they can be reduced or eliminated by careful design of methodology and equipment, but some errors remain and many researchers are working to try to tackle them. Meanwhile, the most

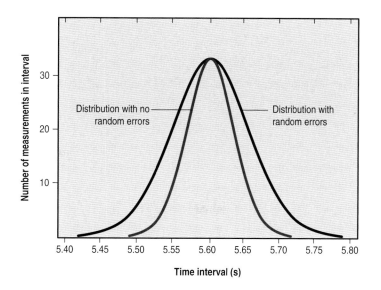

Figure A7 The effect of purely random error is to increase the spread (SD) of the distribution, but the mean is unaffected.

Figure A8 The effect of a systematic error is to move the distribution laterally, with a different mean.

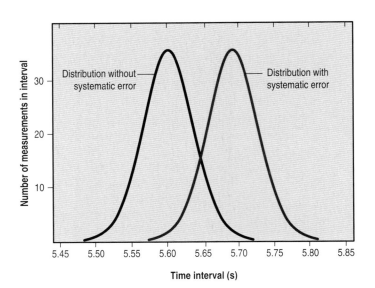

sensible approach is to take advantage of the fact that different measures rarely share the same systematic errors, so by using multiple measures and instruments a more accurate sense of what's going on can be achieved. This *triangulation* strategy is especially useful in gait analysis, and essential in preventing misdiagnosis.

References

Schmalzried T P, Szuszczewicz E S, Northfield M R et al 1998 Quantitative assessment of walking activity after total hip or knee replacement. Journal of Bone and Joint Surgery 80A:54–59

Seedhom B, Wallbridge N 1985 Walking activities and wear of prostheses. Annals of the Rheumatic Diseases 44(12):838–843

Sequeira M M, Rickenbach M, Wietlisbach V et al 1995 Physical activity assessment using a pedometer and its comparison with a questionnaire in a large population survey. American Journal of Epidemiology 142:989–999

Silva M, Shepherd E F, Jackson W O et al 2002 Average patient walking activity approaches 2 million cycles per year: pedometers under-record walking activity. Journal of Arthroplasty 17(6):693–697

Wilkins R H, Wilkins G K 2000 Neurosurgical classics II. American Association of Neurological Surgeons, Chicago

Chapter 1

The temporal-spatial parameters

I am a slow walker, but I never walk backwards.

Abraham Lincoln

OBJECTIVES

- Learn the basic terminology of the gait cycle
- Define the temporal-spatial parameters of gait and be able to measure them clinically
- Awareness of the equipment available for measurement of the temporal-spatial parameters
- Appreciation of the effects of age and speed on the temporal-spatial parameters
- Appreciation of the use of normalization in reducing the variation caused by stature
- Know how to interpret the temporal-spatial parameters in healthy and pathological gait

THE GAIT CYCLE: STEPS & STRIDES

Each time a leg goes forward, it makes a step. For example, when the right leg goes forward, it makes a right step, when the left swings forward it makes a left step. *Step length* is the distance from the heel of the trailing limb to the heel of the leading one.

When one of each (right and left) has occurred, the person has taken a *stride*, or performed one *gait cycle*, and the time it takes for this to occur is called the gait cycle duration, or *stride time* (Fig. 1.1).

KEY EVENTS IN THE GAIT CYCLE

It's usual to start the cycle (0%) with the first contact (*initial contact*, often called heel contact in normal gait) of one foot, so that the end of the cycle (100%) occurs with the *next* contact of the same (*ipsilateral*) foot, which will be the initial contact of the next cycle.

In normal symmetrical walking, toe-off occurs at about 60–62%, dividing the cycle into *stance* (when the foot is on the ground) and *swing* phases (Fig. 1.2).

Since there are two lower-limbs, the events on the opposite (*contralateral*) limb are offset by 50%, so contralateral initial contact occurs at 50% cycle. When one limb is in swing phase, the other is in stance (Fig. 1.3).

Figure 1.1 One gait cycle, or *stride*, is completed when two *steps* have been taken. Stride length is usually measured between two successive contacts of the same foot.

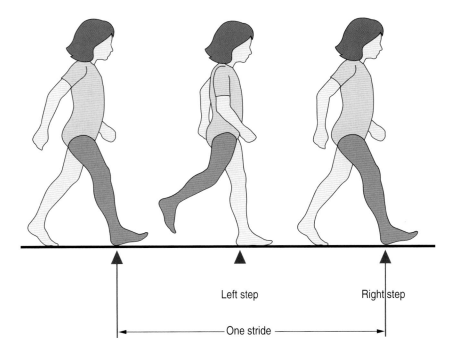

Left step   Right step

|← ——————— One stride ——————— →|

Figure 1.2 Toe-off divides the gait cycle into stance and swing phases.

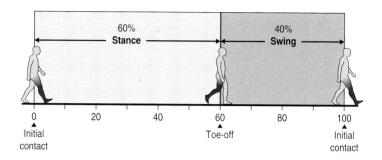

Figure 1.3 Left initial contact occurs when the right side is at 50% cycle.

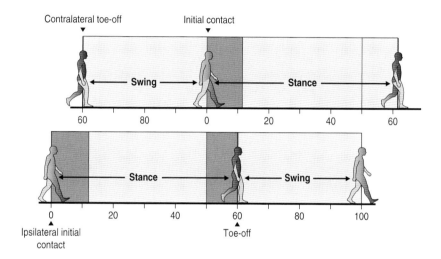

DOUBLE SUPPORT

Since each stance phase is 60%, and $2 \times 60 = 120$, it follows that for 20% of the cycle both feet are on the ground. This time period is called *double support,* and is, in fact, the definition of walking: as speed increases, double support time falls (Kirtley et al 1985), and running begins when it becomes 0% (i.e. when stance duration is 50%). The double support time is divided into two parts, which can be termed *initial* (in which weight is being transferred from contralateral to ipsilateral) and *terminal* (in which weight is being transferred from ipsilateral to contralateral limb). Of course, the initial double support of one limb is the same as the terminal double support of the opposite one (Fig. 1.4).

Knowing the stance duration, the double support can be calculated, and vice versa:

Total double support time, DS = Stance – Swing
But, Swing = 100% – Stance, so DS = Stance – (100 – Stance)
i.e. Stance = (DS + 100)/2

Figure 1.4 There are two periods of overlap (double support), when both feet are on the ground.

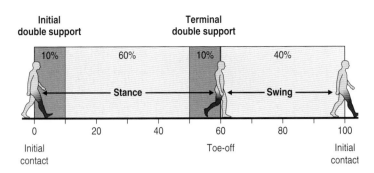

The part of stance phase between the double support phases (when only one foot is on the ground) is called single limb support (SLS).

 MCQ 1.1

What would be the stance duration for a gait with a total double support of 30%?
(a) 50%
(b) 60%
(c) 65%
(d) 70%

WALKING SPEED

Walking speed can be calculated from the equation:

$$\text{Speed} = \text{Distance}/\text{Time}$$

Although everyone has a *natural* (free or self-selected) walking speed, the actual speed is continuously adjusted according to the conditions. Speed must be quickly slowed or increased to avoid collisions with other pedestrians or vehicles, and is consciously or subconsciously varied according to mood and schedule. When two people walk together, they rapidly adopt a mutually acceptable speed in order to walk together. It almost goes without saying that most walking problems result in a reduction of speed.

MCQ 1.2

How long would it take to walk 30 m at a speed of 1.5 m/s?
(a) 5 s
(b) 10 s
(c) 15 s
(d) 20 s

Central pattern generators

Since there is no mechanical coupling between the lower-limbs, the coordination responsible for the alternating motion of the legs must arise somewhere within the nervous system. In cats, rhythmic locomotor patterns are generated in the spinal cord by self-sustaining circuits called *central pattern generators* (CPGs). As every parent knows, newborn babies will make stepping movements when their feet are touched alternately onto a surface. Similarly, cats will walk on a motorized treadmill even if the whole brain is removed (or if the thoracic spinal cord is transected). This observation has given rise to a new approach to gait rehabilitation called *body weight support therapy*. The appropriate sensory feedback needs to be synchronized to events in the gait cycle, e.g. when one limb is loaded the contralateral limb must be unloaded. Robotic exoskeletons (Fig. 1.5), such as *Lokomat*™ (Hocoma AG, Zürich, Switzerland), have been devised to automate the therapy, which is now being used for patients who have had a spinal cord injury (SCI) or stroke.

Figure 1.5 (Reproduced by permission of Dr J Hidler, National Rehabilitation Hospital, Washington, DC.)

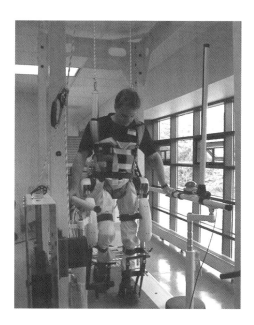

Dietz V 2003 Spinal cord pattern generators for locomotion. Clinical Neurophysiology 114(8):1379–1389

Jezernik S, Scharer R, Colombo G, Morari M 2003 Adaptive robotic rehabilitation of locomotion: a clinical study in spinally injured individuals. Spinal Cord 41:657–666

CADENCE

The number of steps per minute is called the cadence. Really, it would be more logical to express this as strides (or gait cycles) per second. However, cadence is an old concept that originated in the military, and steps are easier to count than strides (try it!). Since there are two steps (left and right) in every stride, and 60 seconds in one minute, steps per minute can be converted to strides per second by dividing by 120. Note also that the stride time is simply 120/Cadence. Natural cadence is a little less than 120 steps/minute (i.e. about one gait cycle per second). Similarly, the cadence (in strides/s) is the reciprocal of the stride time, so a cadence of 120 steps/min is equivalent to a stride time of 120/120 = 1 s.

? MCQ 1.3

? MCQ 1.3

What is a cadence of 80 steps per minute expressed in strides/s?
(a) 0.3
(b) 0.5
(c) 0.67
(d) 0.8

Cadence is related to the length of the lower-limb in a similar fashion to a pendulum in a grandfather clock: longer legs have a slower cadence (Fig. 1.6). Consequently, most people seem to maintain a constant 'walk ratio' (stride length divided by cadence) throughout life (Sekiya & Nagasaki 1998). Since women are, on average, a little shorter than men, they tend to have a slightly higher cadence. Small children have an even more rapid cadence (up to 180 steps/min), which gradually falls as they grow taller (Rose-Jacobs 1983).

Figure 1.6 Cadence decreases as limb length increases, in a similar way to the pendulum of a clock (data from Sutherland 1994).

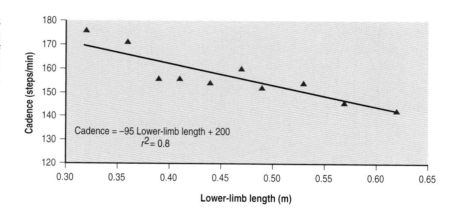

Cadence = −95 Lower-limb length + 200
$r^2 = 0.8$

STRIDE LENGTH

Walking speed is the product of cadence and stride length. Since cadence is usually measured in steps/minute, it needs to be divided by 120, so the final equation is:

$$\text{Speed} = (\text{Cadence} \times \text{Stride Length})/120$$

This is a very useful equation, because it enables any one of the three variables to be calculated, given the other two. Speed is easily measured from the time taken to walk a known distance, and by watching carefully the number of steps taken in that time can be counted. Stride length can be determined by dividing the distance travelled by the number of steps and doubling the result (1 stride = 2 steps), or by rearranging the above equation:

$$\text{Stride Length} = (120 \times \text{Speed})/\text{Cadence}$$

e.g. given a cadence of 120 steps/min and walking speed = 1.5 m/s, we can calculate:

$$\text{Stride Length} = (120 \times 1.5)/120 = 1.5 \text{ m}$$

Since stride time is the reciprocal of cadence (in strides per second), the equation can also be written:

$$\text{Stride Length} = \text{Speed} \times \text{Stride Time}$$

Note that, like walking speed, stride length has to be constantly adjusted in order to negotiate kerbs, potholes, corners, steps, etc. The dependence of speed on both variables allows a flexible range of combinations of cadence and stride length to be used to maintain speed under a variety of circumstances.

Together, the walking speed, cadence and stride length are called the *temporal-spatial parameters* (TSPs) of gait, and their measurement forms the basis of any gait assessment.

? MCQ 1.4

What is the stride *length* of a person walking at 1 m/s and 120 steps/min?
(a) 0.5 m
(b) 1 m
(c) 1.2 m
(d) 1.5 m

? MCQ 1.5

What is the stride *time* of a person with stride length 1.2 m and speed 0.8 m/s?
(a) 0.5 s
(b) 0.67 s
(c) 1.2 s
(d) 1.5 s

USES OF THE TSPs

The TSPs are important functional measures – the *vital signs* of gait. The main applications for them are:

- *Screening* (e.g. to detect elderly people at risk of falling)
- As a *performance* measure (e.g. to grade a patient's level of disability)
- *Monitoring* the efficacy of therapy (i.e. as an *outcome measure*)
- *Normalization* of other gait measurements (in order to compare results from people walking at different speeds).

CLINICAL POINTER – MEASUREMENT OF THE TSPs

Although a stopwatch and a measured distance are all that is needed to measure the TSPs, there are also several commercial systems available for automated measurement. The simplest of these is an optical or *infrared detector* (e.g. the *Speedlight* Timing System, SWIFT Performance Equipment, Alstonville, Australia, cost US$3,390; *Powertimer*, Newtest, Oulu, Finland, cost US$4300), which turns a timer on and off when the subject breaks two light beams placed a known distance apart (Mitchell & Sanders 2000). This is fine for measuring walking speed, but an observer is still needed to count the number of steps taken in order to calculate cadence and stride length.

To count the number of steps, a *pedometer* can be used. These are inexpensive devices (ca. US$20) that can be attached to the subject's belt, and they count each time they detect a step (Sequeira et al 1995). Unfortunately, they are prone to over- and underestimating (Schmalzried et al 1998), especially in women, where the errors can rise to 34% (Silva et al 2002). Some have an activation threshold that can be adjusted to try to prevent this but it tends to be subject-specific. Thus, pedometers are only really useful for measuring the approximate number of steps taken over prolonged periods, i.e. *activity monitoring*. New accelerometer and gyro sensors offer the possibility of long-term ambulatory monitoring (Coleman et al 1999, Aminian et al 2002, Macko et al 2002, Kirtley 2002), and several products using these sensors are now available: e.g. FitSense *FS-1* (FitSense Technology Inc., Southborough, MA), and Nike *sdm[triax 100]* (Nike, Portland, OR). In both cases, a wristwatch calculates the TSPs after receiving radio signals from a small pod attached to the subject's shoe (Fig. 1.7). They are mainly aimed at runners to track their workout but can be useful clinically, and the data can be recorded on the watch and downloaded later to a computer.

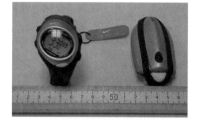

Figure 1.7 Nike *sdm [triax 100]* (Nike, Portland, OR). The wristwatch calculates the wearer's speed from radio signals received from a sensor in the shoe pod.

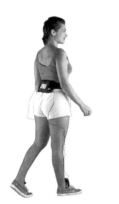

Figure 1.8 *Stride Analyzer* footswitch-based portable gait analysis system (B & L Engineering, Tustin, CA)

Ultrasound can also be used to measure the speed of a walking person, in a similar fashion to police radar guns (Huitema et al 2002). Small fluctuations in the recorded speed can then be used to determine cadence, and compute stride length. Global Positioning Satellites have even been used (Terrier et al 2000) to measure walking speed outdoors.

The temporal parameters of gait (stance, swing and double support times) are more difficult to measure accurately. Footswitches (Hausdorff et al 1995, Blanc et al 1999) on the toe and heel can be used. They make an electrical contact when that part of the foot is loaded, e.g. *Stride Analyzer* (B & L Engineering, Tustin, CA; cost US$9,900; Fig. 1.8) calculates velocity, cadence, stride length, the duration of single and double support for each limb, and the pattern of contact for each foot (Hill et al 1994, Goldie et al 1996). Alternatively, video can be used together with a time code generator (Wall & Crosbie 1996).

One method that has recently become very popular uses a special *instrumented walkway*, e.g. *GaitMat II*™ (E.Q. Inc., Chalfont, PA; cost US$14,500) and *GAITRite*™ (CIR Systems Inc., Clifton, NJ; cost US$14,000; Fig. 1.9). The *GaitMat II* uses an array of 38 rows × 256 switches to record each footfall

Figure 1.9 *GAITRite* pressure sensor array instrumented carpet (CIR Systems Inc., Clifton, NJ).

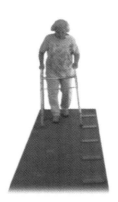

(giving a spatial resolution of 15 mm), with dimensions of 384 × 60 × 3 cm high in three hinged sections. *GAITRite*™ uses a pressure-sensing array arranged in 48 rows of 288 sensors to record the imprint of each footfall with six different levels of pressure (McDonough et al 2001). It is only 3 mm thick, so can be rolled up and transported. The most common mat, 4 m long, weighs 20 kg in its case, but a 7 m version is also available.

NORMATIVE VALUES

It has to be said that despite all the technology that is available and the simplicity of measuring the TSPs with a stopwatch, they are, in fact, rarely measured in routine clinical practice. One possible reason for this is that although several studies have reported normative values, there is unfortunately no good consensus about what the normative *ranges* should be. A person's natural gait is very dependent on the environment, for example, people tend to walk faster on a long walkway (Murray et al 1966, 1969, 1970), and slower on a short one (Oberg et al 1993), and are also influenced by the size of the room. Consequently, outdoor studies (e.g. Finley & Cody 1970, Waters et al 1988, Hausdorff et al 1999) invariably report higher speeds and stride lengths than indoor studies (Grieve & Gear 1966, Oberg et al 1993). This is rather frustrating, and means that normal values should really be obtained for each laboratory or clinic. Bearing this in mind, Table 1.1 is a rough guide, given a typical (ca. 5 m) walkway length.

It's easy to remember 1.5 m/s, 1.5 m and 120 steps/min (i.e. one stride/s) as a quick rule of thumb.

Table 1.1 Approximate normative ranges for the TSPs

	Speed (m/s)	Cadence (steps/min)	Stride length (m)
Men	1.3–1.6	110–115	1.4–1.6
Women	1.2–1.5	115–120	1.3–1.5

EFFECT OF SPEED

Walking speed is related to both cadence and the stride length, so it can be increased by a more rapid cadence, longer stride length, or both. In healthy people (those with no gait disorder) both parameters increase with speed. Cadence increases linearly (Fig. 1.10) but stride length increases logarithmically (Fig. 1.11), changing a lot at low speeds, but tending to level off at higher speeds.

Figure 1.10 Cadence increases linearly with speed.

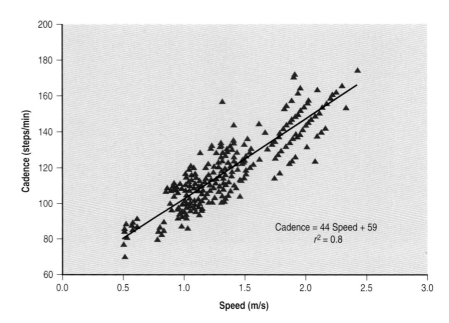

Figure 1.11 Stride length also increases with speed, but the relationship is logarithmic rather than linear.

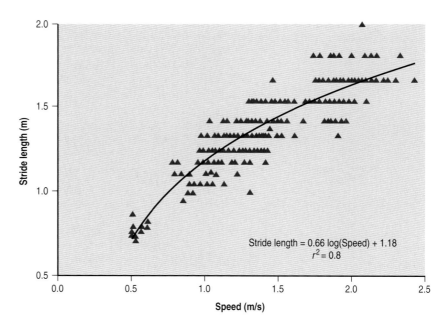

EFFECT OF SPEED ON THE TEMPORAL PHASES OF GAIT

As speed increases the double support time (along with stance duration) decreases. When double support reaches zero, running begins, and with further speed increase, the double support phase becomes negative (i.e. it becomes a *flight* phase). Some useful relationships (Blanc et al 1999) are given in Table 1.2.

Table 1.2 Relationship between speed and the temporal parameters

Variable	Men	Women
Stance duration (%)	71 × stride time (s) – 11.3	71 × stride time – 10.9
Double support (%)	41 × stride time (s) – 20.3	41 × stride time – 20.0

CLINICAL POINTER – BALANCE COMPENSATION

Stance phase is also slightly longer while walking in bare feet compared to when wearing shoes (Eisenhardt et al 1996). Shoes provide a slightly increased base of support, which helps balance. As balance is compromised, both stance and double support increase to provide an increased support time. This is an example of a *compensation strategy*.

? MCQ 1.6

Which gait would you expect to have the longest double support?
(a) Barefoot at 1 m/s
(b) With shoes at 1 m/s
(c) Barefoot at 1.5 m/s
(d) With shoes at 1.5 m/s

EFFECT OF AGE: MATURATION

The average onset of walking in children is about 11 months (mean 329 ± 46 days), and, interestingly, baby-walkers seem to delay this by about 21 days (Garrett et al 2002). Using a normative range of Mean ± 3 SD, this would suggest that a baby should walk before around (329 + 3 × 46) = 467 days (i.e. 16 months). In practice, parents are usually reassured up until the child is 18 months old (Sutherland et al 1980, 1988).

To determine the age at which gait matures (i.e. becomes adult-like) we need to remove the effect of size since children are smaller than adults (Sutherland 1996). This technique is called *normalization*.

Probably the best (but not always used!) method involves converting gait variables into *dimensionless* quantities (Hof 1996, Sutherland 1996, Pierrynowski & Galea 2001, Stansfield et al 2003). For example, normalized stride or step length is obtained by dividing by lower-limb length, l, measured from anterior superior iliac spine (ASIS) to medial malleolus (Fig. 1.12). Walking speed must be divided by $\sqrt{(gl)}$ where g is the acceleration due to gravity (9.81 m/s^2), whereas cadence is divided by $\sqrt{(g/l)}$. When this is done, it appears that the

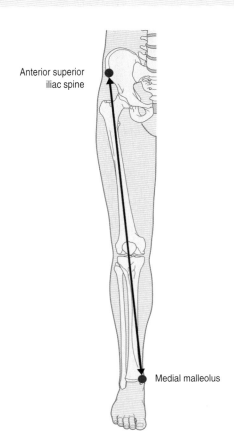

Figure 1.12 Lower-limb length is measured from ASIS to medial malleolus.

Anterior superior
iliac spine

Medial malleolus

temporal–spatial parameters stabilize at around 4–5 years of age (Figs 1.13, 1.14, 1.15).

An alternative approach to normalization involves plotting the TSPs on a *nomogram*, such as those developed by the Shriners groups of hospitals (Todd et al 1989, Johanson et al 1994).

In the clinic, a useful rule of thumb to remember is that a child's natural stride length should be about 90% of their height (Fig. 1.16).

Figure 1.13 After normalization, walking speed is seen to stabilize at around 4 years of age (data from Sutherland 1994).

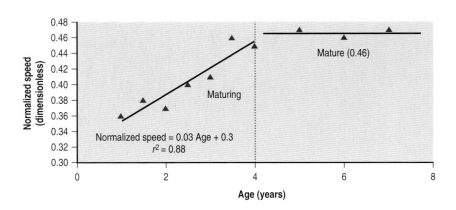

Figure 1.14 Normalized stride length also stabilizes by around 4 years of age (data from Sutherland 1994).

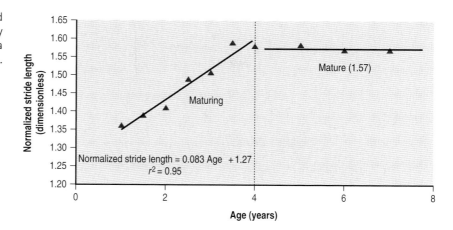

Figure 1.15 Normalized cadence stabilizes by around 5 years of age (data from Sutherland 1994).

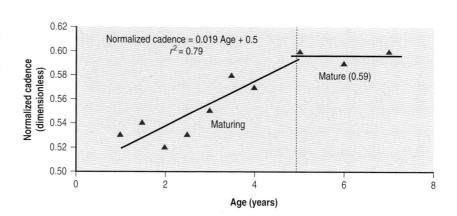

Figure 1.16 An approximate guide to normal stride length in children is 90% of height (data from Hausdorff et al 1999).

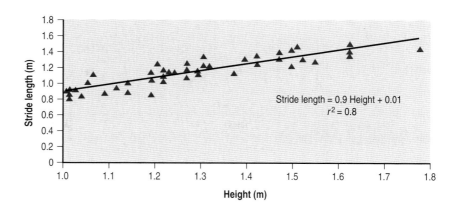

Remember Menelaus's 'rule of thumb':

Total adult height = Height at age 2y × 2

The distal femoral epiphysis contributes 10 mm/y (70% of femur growth), while the proximal tibial epiphysis generates 6 mm/y (60% of tibia growth). Growth ceases at 14–15 years in girls and 16–17 years in boys.

CLINICAL POINTER – DEGENERATION OF GAIT

Natural walking speed remains relatively stable until about age 70 (Winter et al 1990, Leiper & Craik 1991); it then declines about 15% per decade (Fig. 1.17). Healthy subjects can increase their speed by as much as 44% above natural pace (Finley et al 1969). However, maximal speed declines earlier and more steeply: about 20% per decade after the age of 50. Cadence does not change with age (maintaining its relationship to lower-limb length), so stride length must be the source of the decreased speed.

One place where walking speed really matters is the pedestrian crossing. Most crossings are designed for a walking speed of around 1.2 m/s, meaning that about 15% of elderly pedestrians have difficulty getting across before the lights change (Coffin & Morrall 1995).

As people age, balance slowly deteriorates, and this is reflected in the temporal parameters. Stance accounts for 59% of gait cycle at age 20, and 63% at age 70, with double support duration increasing from 18% to 26% (Murray et al 1969). Interestingly, reduced stride length, reduced speed and increased double support time seem to be associated with *fear* of falling, rather than falling itself (Maki 1997).

Figure 1.17 Natural walking speed remains fairly constant, but fast speed declines after age 50 years (data from Oberg et al 1993).

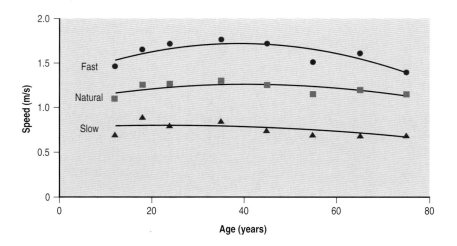

Gait as a biometric?

Biometrics is the science of recognizing people by their biological attributes. Most biometrics applications require the subject's cooperation, e.g. people must put their finger onto a scanner to read their fingerprint. Video surveillance cameras can monitor people without their knowledge, but they require human operators to monitor the images for suspicious events. In an effort to automate the process, attention has therefore turned to gait, and especially the ratio of stride (or step) length to cadence (the so-called *walk ratio*) (Fig. 1.18). This may be a signature that may discriminate between, e.g., humans and non-humans, adults and children, men and women, walking and running, etc., and it may eventually be possible to detect aggressive or malevolent behaviour. Watch out – Big Brother may be analysing your gait!

Figure 1.18 Relationship between individual stride length and cadence. (Reproduced by permission of BenAbdelkader et al 2002.)

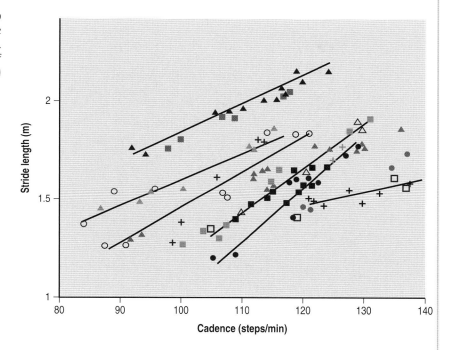

BenAbdelkader C, Cutler R, Davis L 2002 Stride and cadence as a biometric in automatic person identification and verification. Proceedings of the International Conference on Pattern Recognition, 11–15 August, Québec City, Canada

VARIABILITY OF THE TSPs

As with all gait variables, it is important to bear in mind the natural biological variability that is invariably observed when a measurement is repeated several times. Variation can occur within the same subject (*intra-subject*), or in a group of subjects (*inter-subject*). Not surprisingly, the latter is usually higher, because people walk differently. The amount of variation is also usually less when the measurements are taken at the same time (*intra-session*) versus a different time of day or different day (*inter-session* variation). Since there is bound to be some measurement error, the variation recorded will also depend to some extent on the *method* (e.g. instructions given, environment, length of walkway, etc.), *operator* (e.g. whether the same person takes the measurement, and how skilled the person is) and *instrument* (stopwatch or some more sophisticated method) used.

Gait is more variable in the early years, but gradually stabilizes with maturity (see Figs 1.13–1.15). The CV of stride time falls from around 6% in 3- to 4-year-olds, to around 2% in 11- to 14-year-olds (Haussdorff et al 1999). In the elderly, increased variability seems to be associated with risk of falling (Hausdorff et al 1997a,b), with speed variability the single best predictor of falls (Maki 1997).

Is walking fractal?

Gait cycle duration is rarely constant, and until recently these step-to-step fluctuations were just assumed to be random noise superimposed upon a constant walking rhythm. Another possibility is that there might be some underlying complex temporal structure to the variation, i.e. *non-linear*, or *fractal* phenomena. If this were the case, there would be a 'memory effect' – the stride time at any instant would depend on previous stride times. Fractal behaviour, such as has already been observed in long duration heart rate recordings from 24-hour Holter monitoring, may confer important biological advantages related to adaptability.

Long-term measurement of stride time has been done using in-shoe footswitches (Peng et al 1999). A process known as *Detrended Fluctuation Analysis* (DFA) was then used. This is a bit complicated, but basically involves dividing the time series (gait cycle duration plotted against time) into boxes of equal length, *n*. In each box a straight line is fitted to the data (representing the trend in that box), finally resulting in a quantity called *F(n)*. The relationship between *log F(n)* to *log n* is usually found to be a straight line. The slope of this line, α, has been determined to be 0.5 for random noise,

Figure 1.19

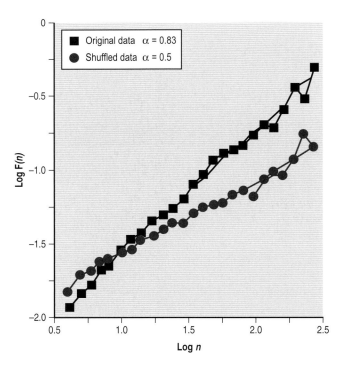

with higher values indicative of long-range correlations (memory) in the data. It turns out that $\alpha = 0.83$ for the gait data, suggesting that there is indeed some pattern to the seemingly random variation in stride time. When the data are randomly shuffled to remove any memory effect, α falls to 0.5 as expected (Fig 1.19).

It is possible that there may be clinical significance in this finding, because values of α were found to be closer to 0.5 (more random) for elderly people compared to young subjects, and in patients with Parkinson's disease and Huntington's chorea (Hausdorff et al 1998).

Peng C-K, Hausdorff J M, Goldberger A L 1999 Fractal mechanisms in neural control: human heartbeat and gait dynamics in health and disease. In: Walleczek J (ed) Non-linear dynamics, self-organization, and biomedicine. Cambridge University Press, Cambridge
Hausdorff J M, Cudkowicz M E, Firtion R et al 1998 Gait variability and basal ganglia disorders: stride-to-stride variations of gait cycle timing in Parkinson's and Huntington's disease. Movement Disorders 13:428–437

TREADMILL GAIT

Many times in rehabilitation, subjects are asked to walk on a treadmill – the advantages being safety (because a harness and/or handrails can be used), less space is required, and walking speed can be directly controlled. Gait on a treadmill is not quite the same as *free* walking, however. In particular, the stride length on a treadmill (or more correctly, *contact or support length*) is shorter and cadence higher for a given walking speed (White et al 1998, Alton et al 1998). Contact length = 0.665 + 0.25 × belt speed, so for a speed of 1.5 m/s, contact length would be only 1.04 m (Kram & Powell 1989). Conversely, cadence increases by 7% in adults and 10% in children compared to overground walking, while stance phase duration decreases by 5% in adults but curiously remains unchanged in children (Stolze et al 1997).

 ### DEBATING POINT

Debate the advantages and disadvantages of making gait measurements on:
– Overground walking
– Treadmill gait

CONTROL OF THE TSPs

Since both stride length and cadence are under voluntary control, they can be manipulated by external cues (Zijlstra et al 1995). Subjects will, for example, synchronize their cadence to the rhythmic sound from a metronome (*frequency modulation*, FM), or adjust their step length to lines drawn on the walkway (*amplitude modulation*, AM). Interestingly, the normal temporal parameters of gait (stance, swing and double support percentages) are maintained (*invariant*) during FM but not AM.

More information comes from experiments with a split-belt treadmill, in which the left and right legs move at different speeds (Zijlstra & Dietz 1995). Although this sounds impossible, subjects are easily able to automatically adapt their walking pattern after only a few seconds even when one belt moves at four times the speed of the other. Stance phase duration is found to increase on the slower belt and decrease on the faster side in order to keep the contact lengths equal on each limb. Presumably, afferent feedback (perhaps from pressure receptors on the sole of the foot, or joint spray endings) via the spinal cord is responsible for this adaptation.

These experiments suggest that a central pattern generator (CPG) provides the basic stepping rhythm, but its rhythm is modified by feedback according to the biomechanical context.

CLINICAL POINTER – POINTER-INTERPRETATION OF THE TSPs IN DISEASE

Walking speed is easily measured and has been shown to correlate well with function. Sometimes walking speed alone can be misleading, since it is a product of cadence and stride length. Most gait problems result in a decreased stride length, and so an increased cadence is a common compensation to maintain speed. In some diseases (e.g. the *festinating gait* of Parkinson's disease), the increase in cadence is very marked (Morris et al 1996, 1999). It is therefore best to measure all three parameters (Table 1.3).

As mentioned previously, stance duration is often *increased* when balance is compromised (*dysequilibrium*) due to vestibular, cerebellar (*ataxia*) or non-specific instability. Conversely, it is *decreased* if the leg or prosthesis on that side is unstable or painful (*antalgic* gait), and the contralateral stance duration will be prolonged to compensate (Table 1.4).

Table 1.3 Interpretation of TSPs in gait disorders

Speed	Stride length	Cadence	Conclusion
N	N	N	Normal gait
N	↓	↑	Compensated gait
↓	↓	↑	Inadequately compensated gait
↓	↓	↓	Severe gait impairment

Table 1.4 Interpretation of temporal measures in gait disorders

Stance duration	Conclusion
↓	Ipsilateral pain or instability
↑	Dysequilibrium or contralateral instability

? MCQ 1.7

What is the most likely diagnosis in a patient with stance duration = 55%?
(a) Ataxia
(b) Antalgic gait
(c) Balance problem
(d) Child

The *step width* (mediolateral distance between the heels in double support) also tends to increase with dysequilibrium in order to increase the *base of support* (Fig. 1.20), although this may only become evident at higher speeds (Krebs et al 2002). Normal step width varies with age, so it's best to normalize it by dividing by pelvic width (measured between the ASIS): normal < 0.5, i.e. less than half the pelvic width.

Interpretation of *step length* sometimes causes confusion. Since the legs are connected together at the pelvis, both legs must travel the same distance (unless the subject is walking in a circle), so the right stride length must equal the left stride length (give or take inter-stride variation). The right and left *step* lengths can be quite different, however, because of the way they are defined (Fig. 1.21).

It should not be assumed that the side with the longer step length is healthier. Sometimes the sound side has a longer step length, but not always, so step length differences are useful only as a measure of *symmetry*. For example, the *step length ratio* (SLR) of the shorter to the longer step length is useful for tracking a patient's progress through their rehabilitation, the ratio rising closer to 1 as the gait improves. Other symmetry indices have been described (Dewar & Judge 1980, Herzog et al 1989, Hesse et al 1999) using variables such as right and left stride times or double support times, but the SLR is probably the most widely used. These indices provide simple overall outcome measures that can even be used as biofeedback to inform the patient of their progress during gait training (Dingwell et al 1996).

Figure 1.20 Step width is increased in disorders of balance in order to increase the base of support

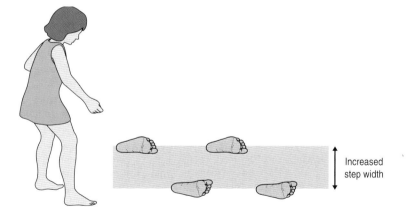

Increased step width

Figure 1.21 In this gait, right *step* length is shorter than the left, but note that the *stride* lengths are still equal.

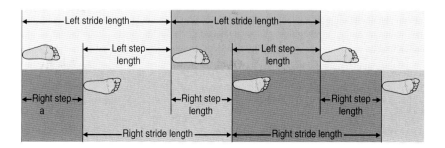

MCQ 1.8

What is the SLR of a patient with right step length of 50 cm and 30 cm on the left?

(a) 0.3
(b) 0.5
(c) 0.6
(d) 1.67

UPPER-LIMB MOTION

The function of the upper-limbs during locomotion has intrigued several researchers over the years (Elftman 1939, Capozzo 1993). At natural walking speed, the upper-limbs swing with the contralateral limb at a frequency equal to the cadence, whilst at slow speeds (at least in some people) they swing in phase with the ipsilateral limb at twice the cadence (Webb & Tuttle 1989, Webb et al 1994). The speed at which arm swing pattern switches from 2:1 in-phase to 1:1 anti-phase is approximately that of the natural pendulum frequency of the upper-limbs (around 0.5 Hz). This is an another example of a dynamic systems phenomenon, which is typically accompanied by catastrophic flags such hysteresis and critical fluctuations that indicate instability around the transition frequency. Amplitude of arm swing increases with walking speed (Donker et al 2001), in order to counteract the angular momentum generated by the lower-limbs (Capozzo 1993, Donker et al 2002).

★ KEY POINTS

★ The gait cycle is divided into stance and swing phases

★ Stance phase consists of single limb support and initial and final double support phases

★ Walking speed can be calculated by multiplying stride length by cadence (expressed in strides/s)

★ Normalization reduces the variability caused by differences in body height

★ The normalized temporal-spatial parameters remain fairly constant from 5 to 70 years of age

★ Gait symmetry may be assessed by the ratio between right and left step lengths or times

References

Alton F, Baldey, Caplan S, Morrissey M C 1998 A kinematic comparison of overground and treadmill walking. Clinical Biomechanics 13:434–440

Aminian K, Najafi B, Büla C et al 2002 Spatio-temporal parameters of gait measured by an ambulatory system using miniature gyroscopes. Journal of Biomechanics 35(5):689–699

Blanc Y, Balmer C, Landis T, Vingerhoets F 1999 Temporal parameters and patterns of the foot roll over during walking: normative data for healthy adults. Gait & Posture 10(2):97–108

Capozzo A 1993 The forces and couples in the human trunk during level walking. Journal of Biomechanics 16:265–277

Coffin A, Morrall J 1995 Walking speeds of elderly pedestrians at crosswalks. Transportation Research Record 1487:63–67

Coleman K, Smith D, Boone D et al 1999 Step activity monitor: long-term, continuous recording of ambulatory function. Journal of Rehabilitation Research and Development 36:8–18

Dewar M E, Judge G 1980 Temporal asymmetry as a gait quality indicator. Medical and Biological Engineering and Computing 18:689–693

Dingwell J B, Davis B L, Frazier D M 1996 Use of an instrumented treadmill for real-time gait symmetry evaluation and feedback in normal and below-knee amputee subjects. Prosthetics and Orthotics International 20:101–110

Donker S, Beek P, Wagenaar R, Mulder T 2001 Coordination between arm and leg movements during locomotion. Journal of Motor Behavior 33:86–103

Donker S, Mulder T, Nienhuis B, Duysens J 2002 Adaptations in arm movements for added mass to wrist or ankle during walking. Experimental Brain Research 146:26–31

Eisenhardt J R, Cook D, Pregler I, Foehl H C 1996 Changes in temporal gait characteristics and pressure distribution for bare feet versus various heel heights. Gait & Posture 4(4):280–286

Elftman H 1939 The function of the arms in walking. Human Biology 11:525–535

Finley F R, Cody K A 1970 Locomotive characteristics of urban pedestrians. Archives of Physical Medicine and Rehabilitation 51:423–426

Finley F R, Cody K A, Finizie R 1969 Locomotive patterns in elderly women. Archives of Physical Medicine and Rehabilitation 50:140–146

Garrett M, McElroy A M, Staines A 2002 Locomotor milestones and babywalkers: cross sectional study. British Medical Journal 324:1494

Goldberger A L, Amaral L A N, Glass L et al 2000 PhysioBank, PhysioToolkit, and PhysioNet: components of a new research resource for complex physiologic signals. Circulation 101(23):215–220 .

Goldie P A, Matyas T A, Evans O W 1996 Deficit and change in gait velocity during rehabilitation after stroke. Archives of Physical Medicine and Rehabilitation 77:1074–1082

Grieve D, Gear R 1966 The relationships between length of stride, step frequency, time of swing, and speed of walking for children and adults. Ergonomics 5(9):379

Hausdorff J M, Ladin Z, Wei J Y 1995 Footswitch system for measurement of the temporal parameters of gait. Journal of Biomechanics 28:347–351

Hausdorff J M, Edelberg H E, Mitchell S, Wei J Y 1997a Increased gait instability in community dwelling elderly fallers. Archives of Physical Medicine and Rehabilitation 78:278–283

Hausdorff J M, Mitchell S L, Firtion R et al 1997b Altered fractal dynamics of gait: reduced stride interval correlations with aging and Huntington's disease. Journal of Applied Physiology 82:262–269

Hausdorff J M, Zemany L, Peng C-K, Goldberger A L 1999 Maturation of gait dynamics: stride-to-stride variability and its temporal organization in children. Journal of Applied Physiology 86:1040–1047

Herzog W, Nigg B M, Read L J 1989 Asymmetries in ground reaction force patterns in normal human gait. Medicine and Science in Sports and Exercise 21(1):110–114

Hesse S, Konrad M K, Uhlenbrock D 1999 Treadmill walking with partial body support versus floor walking in hemiparetic subjects. Archives of Physical Medicine and Rehabilitation 80:421–427

Hill K D, Goldie P A, Baker P A, Greenwood K M 1994 Retest reliability of the temporal and distance characteristics of hemiplegic gait using a footswitch system. Archives of Physical Medicine and Rehabilitation 75:577–583

Hof A L 1996 Scaling gait data to body size. Gait & Posture 4(3):222–223

Huitema R B, Hof A L, Postema K 2002 Ultrasonic motion analysis system – measurement of temporal and spatial gait parameters. Journal of Biomechanics 35(6):837–842

Johanson M E, St Helen R, Lamoreux L W et al 1994 Normal stride length as a function of walking speed. Gait & Posture 2:51

Kaufman K R, Chambers H G, Sutherland D H 1996 variability of temporal distance measurements in pathological gait studies. Gait & Posture 4(2):169–169

Kirtley C 2002 New technology in gait analysis, in physical medicine and rehabilitation. State of the Art Reviews 16(2):361–373

Kirtley C, Whittle M W, Jefferson R J 1985 Influence of walking speed on gait parameters. Journal of Biomedical Engineering 7(4):282–288

Kram R, Powell A J 1989 A treadmill-mounted force platform. Journal of Applied Physiology 67:1692–1698

Krebs D E, Goldvasser D, Lockert J D, Portnoy L G, Gill-Body K M 2002 Is base of support greater in unsteady gait? Physical Therapy 82(2):138–147

Leiper C, Craik R 1991 Relationships between physical activity and temporal-distance charactericstics of walking in elderly women. Physical Therapy 71:791

McDonough A L, Batavia M, Chen F C et al 2001 The validity and reliability of the GAITRite system's measurements: a preliminary evaluation. Archives of Physical Medicine and Rehabilitation 82:419–425

Macko M F, Haeuber E, Shaughnessy M et al 2002 microprocessor-based ambulatory activity monitoring in stroke patients. Medicine and Science in Sports and Exercise 34(3):394–399

Maki B E 1997 Gait changes in older adults: predictors of falls or indicators of fear? Journal of the American Geriatrics Society 45:313–320

Mitchell S B, Sanders J E 2000 An accurate inexpensive system for the assessment of walking speed. Journal of Prosthetics and Orthotics 12(4):117–119

Morris M E, Iansek I, Matyas T A, Summers J J 1996 Stride length regulation in Parkinson's disease: normalization strategies and underlying mechanisms. Brain 119:551–568

Morris M E, McGinley J, Huxhan F et al. 1999 Constraints on the kinetic, kinematic and spatiotemporal parameters of gait in Parkinson's disease. Human Movement Science 18:461–468

Murray M P, Kory R C, Clarkson B H, Sepic S B 1966 Comparison of free and fast speed walking patterns of normal men. American Journal of Physical Medicine 45:8–24

Murray M P, Kory R C, Clarkson B H 1969 Walking pattern in healthy old men. Journal of Gerontology 24:169–178

Murray M P, Kory R C, Sepic S B 1970 Walking patterns of normal women. Archives of Physical Medicine and Rehabilitation 51:637–650

Oberg T, Karsznia A, Oberg K 1993 Basic gait parameters: reference data for normal subjects 10–79 years of age. Journal of Rehabilitation Research and Development 30:210–233

Pierrynowski M R, Galea V 2001 Enhancing the ability of gait analyses to differentiate between groups: scaling data to body size. Gait & Posture 13:193–201

Rose-Jacobs R 1983 Development of gait at slow, free, and fast speeds in 3- and 5-year-old children. Physical Therapy 63:1251–1259

Schmalzried T P, Szuszczewicz E S, Northfield M R et al 1998 Quantitative assessment of walking activity after total hip or knee replacement. Journal of Bone and Joint Surgery 80A:54–59

Sekiya N, Nagasaki H 1998 Reproducibility of the walking patterns of normal young adults: test-retest reliability of the walk ratio (step-length/step-rate), Gait & Posture 7(3):225–227

Sequeira M M, Rickenbach M, Wietlisbach V et al 1995 Physical activity assessment using a pedometer and its comparison with a questionnaire in a large population survey. American Journal of Epidemiology 142:989–999

Silva M, Shepherd E F, Jackson W O et al 2002 Average patient walking activity approaches 2 million cycles per year: pedometers under-record walking activity. Journal of Arthroplasty 17(6):693–697

Stansfield B W, Hillman S J, Hazlewood M E et al 2003 Normalisation of gait data in children. Gait & Posture 17(1):81–87

Stolze H, Kuhtz-Buschbeck J P, Mondwurf C et al 1997 Gait analysis during treadmill and overground locomotion in children and adults. Electroencephalography and Clinical Neurophysiology 105(6):490–497

Sutherland D 1994 In Rose J, Gamble J G (eds.) Human walking, 2nd edn. Williams & Wilkins, Baltimore

Sutherland D 1996 Dimensionless gait measurements and gait maturity. Gait & Posture 4(3):209–211

Sutherland D H, Olshen R A, Cooper L, Woo S 1980 The development of mature gait. Journal of Bone and Joint Surgery 62A:336–353

Sutherland D H, Olshen R A, Biden E N, Wyatt M P 1988 The development of mature walking. J B Lippincott, Philadelphia

Terrier P, Ladetto Q, Merminod B, Schutz Y 2000 High-precision satellite positioning system as a new tool to study the biomechanics of human locomotion. Journal of Biomechanics 33(12):1717–1722

Todd F N, Lamoreux L W, Skinner S R et al 1989 Variations in the gait of normal children. Journal of Bone and Joint Surgery 71A:196–204

Wall J C, Crosbie J 1996 Accuracy and reliability of temporal gait measurement. Gait & Posture 4(4):293–296

Waters R L, Lumsford B R, Perry J, Byrd R 1988 Energy–speed relationship of walking: standard tables. Journal of Orthopedic Research 5:215–222

Webb D, Tuttle R H 1989 The effects of stride frequency on the motion of the upper limbs in human walking. American Journal of Physiology and Anthropology 78:321–322

Webb D, Tuttle R H, Baksh M 1994 Pendular activity of human upper-limbs during slow and normal walking. American Journal of Physiology and Anthropology 93:477–489

White S, Yack H J, Tucker C A, Lin H Y 1998 Comparison of vertical ground reaction forces during overground and treadmill walking. Medicine and Science in Sports and Exercise 30(10):1537–1542

Winter D A, Patla A E, Frank J S, Walt S E 1990
Biomechanical walking changes in the fit and
healthy elderly. Physical Therapy 70:340–347

Zijlstra W, Dietz V 1995 Adaptability of the human
stride cycle during split-belt walking Gait & Posture
3(4):250–257

Zijlstra W, Rutgers A W F, Hof A L, Van Weerden T W
1995 Voluntary and involuntary adaptation of
walking to temporal and spatial constraints. Gait &
Posture 3(1):13–18

Chapter **2**

Measurement of gait kinematics

Movement never lies.

Martha Graham

OBJECTIVES

- Awareness of the advantages and disadvantages of methods available for measuring joint kinematics
- Understanding of the techniques used in analysing gait using digital video
- Understanding of the theory and practical considerations involved in filtering kinematic data
- Know the typical patterns of joint motion during normal gait
- Appreciation of the errors and limitations of two-dimensional analysis

MEASUREMENT OF KINEMATICS

The term *kinematics* simply means a description of the gait in terms of the angles, positions (displacements), velocities and accelerations of the body segments and joints. Several techniques are available for the measurement of gait kinematics.

Electrogoniometers (sometimes called *elgons*) are probably the simplest method, being just an electronic version of an ordinary clinical goniometer. The most basic consists of a *potentiometer* (like the volume control on a radio) mounted on two brackets which are strapped to the body segments either side of the joint, e.g. the *Gait Analysis System* by MIE Medical Research Ltd, Leeds, UK (Fig. 2.1). Although such systems

Figure 2.1 Gait analysis system by MIE Medical Research Ltd (Leeds, UK), in which motion is recorded by potentiometers aligned with the joint axes.

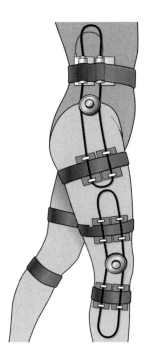

are relatively cheap and give immediate (real-time) results, their fundamental limitation lies in the need for accurate alignment of the potentiometer spindle with the joint axis of rotation (Chao 1980). This is not always constant and may change with the joint angle. The knee joint is a good example of this (Fig. 2.2) – its axis of rotation moves as it flexes due to the femur gliding over the tibia (Blankevoort et al 1988).

Moreover, the straps may move during gait and can be an encumbrance to the subject, psychologically if not mechanically, and attaching them can be quite tedious. Although it is possible to obtain three-dimensional (3D, i.e. sagittal, frontal and transverse plane) data with these devices (Chao 1980), they are mainly used for 2D (sagittal plane) measurements.

Figure 2.2 The centre of rotation of the knee moves in a semicircular pathway (evolute) over the femoral condyle due to a combination of gliding and rolling of the femur on the tibia.

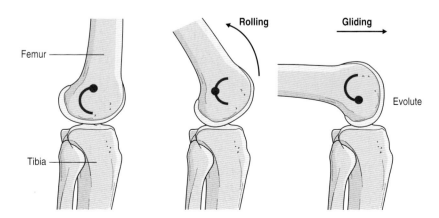

Cinema

If the word kinematics sounds like cinema, that's because both words come from the same Greek root, *kinema*, for movement. Cinema actually started as an offshoot of a method devised for measuring the kinematics of racehorses. In 1872, Leland Stanford, then Governor of California, wondered whether a trotting horse ever had all four feet off the ground. He offered $10,000 to anyone who could photograph his famous horse, *Occident,* trotting at full speed (about 30 m/s). At the time, photographers used collodion wet-plate film that needed at least 20 seconds exposure. An English photographer, Eadweard Muybridge, took on the challenge, and after several experiments at Stanford's Palo Alto ranch, succeeded in getting the shutter speed down to 1/500th of a second. Later, he arranged for the horse's motion to break threads that released the shutters on a battery of 12 cameras in rapid succession.

Even with the aid of the bright Californian sunshine, the picture was shadowy and indistinct, but Stanford was satisfied that he could indeed discern that all four legs were off the ground. It was the first moving picture. Later, at the University of Pennsylvania, Muybridge perfected the process further, and took an astonishing 20,000 pictures of animals, men, women and children (Fig. 2.3) during various activities, including gait. The pictures were displayed at the 1893 Columbian Exhibition in Chicago, using a device called a *zoopraxiscope* to project them onto a screen.

Figure 2.3   Walking boy by Eadweard Muybridge (from the collections of the University of Pennsylvania Archives).

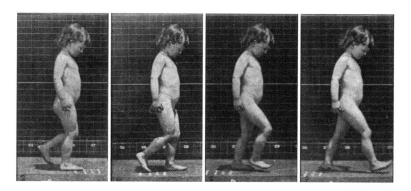

Muybridge didn't make much money out of his invention (he was eventually tried for the murder of his wife's lover) but two French brothers, Louis and Auguste Lumière, did. Their short film, *Sortie d'Usine* ('Leaving the Factory'), shot in what is now known as the *Rue du Premier Film*, Lyon, on March 19, 1895, was the first to use the *cinematograph* process, which was eventually shortened to *cinema.* Sixteen years later, the Nestor Film Company took over the old Blondeau Tavern on Sunset Boulevard and Hollywood was born.

Eadweard Muybridge 1887 The Human Figure in Motion, Dover Publications, Inc., republished 1989

Biometrics Ltd (formerly Penny and Giles, Gwent, UK) makes an improved flexible electrogoniometer, which consists of two small end blocks connected to a 12–18 mm strain gauged metal strip (Fig. 2.4). The

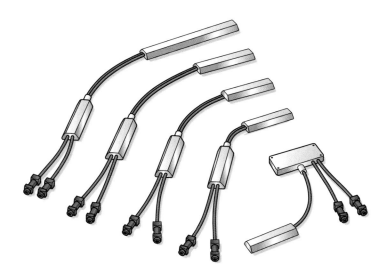

Figure 2.4 Flexible electrogoniometers from Biometrics Ltd.

end blocks are simply attached to the skin adjacent to each side of the joint using double-sided tape, so there is no need for alignment with the joint centre. Single and twin axis versions are available in various sizes, and they also make torsiometers for measuring rotation. Another device (*Shape-tape* by Measurand, Canada) makes use of an optical fibre that affects the transmission of light when it bends.

These are certainly much better than the potentiometer-based systems, but they still can still be quite encumbering to the subject because of the necessary cabling. They are useful for measuring the motion of one or two joints. Note that all electrogoniometer systems are also fundamentally limited in that while they can record *relative* motion between adjacent body segments (joint angles), they cannot measure the *absolute* motion of body segments in space. Examples of these are motions of the pelvic and trunk, e.g. pelvic tilt and trunk flexion.

? MCQ 2.1

Which of the following is a body *segment*?
(a) Foot
(b) Ankle
(c) Knee
(d) Hip

In order to measure absolute motion of body segments, measurements must be taken with respect to a fixed *global reference system*. There are basically four ways to do this:

- Optical. *Vicon Motion Systems* (Oxford, UK), *Motion Analysis Corp.* (Santa Rosa, CA, USA), *Peak Performance* (Denver, CO, USA), *CODA mpx30* (Charnwood Dynamics Ltd, Loughborough, UK), *Optotrak* (Northern Digital Inc., Waterloo, ON, Canada), B|T|S (Milan, Italy), *SIMI Reality Motion Systems* GmbH (Unterschleissheim, Germany), *Ariel Dynamics, Inc.* (Trabuco Canyon, CA, USA), *eMotion* (Padova,

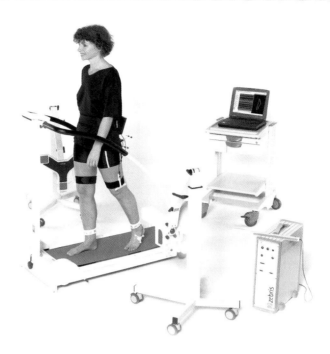

Figure 2.5 *Zebris* ultrasonic motion analysis system, which utilizes the delay in sound transmission through air to triangulate the position of ultrasound emitting markers.

Italy), *PhoeniX Technologies* (Burnaby, BC, Canada), *Spica Technology Corp.* (Hawaii, USA), *zFlo* (Quincy, MA, USA).
- Electromagnetic. *FasTrak* (Polhemus, USA), *Flock of Birds and MotionStar Wireless* (Ascension Technology Corp., VT, USA)
- Ultrasonic. *Zebris* (zebris Medizintechnik GmbH, Tuebingen, Germany) (Fig. 2.5).
- Inertial. The latest, and still somewhat experimental technique, using a combination of miniature MEMS (micro-electro-mechanical systems) sensors (Kirtley 2002; *xSense*, Enschede, Netherlands).

Of these, optical methods are presently the most popular for clinical gait analysis. Although originally cine film was used (Sutherland & Hagy 1972), these days the most popular measurement systems are based on video-based *photogrammetry*. Nearly all the main products commercially now available for gait analysis are based on this method, so it is important to understand the main principles used. To do this, it's worth carrying out a simple 2D (sagittal plane) analysis of gait using one camera.

DEBATING POINT

Debate the advantages and disadvantages of the following for recording gait kinematics:
- Electrogoniometers
- Ultrasound and electromagnetic tracking
- Optical (video-based) measurement
- Inertial systems

Video

Television pictures are made up of thousands of tiny dots, or *pixels*. In the video camera, the image is scanned from left to right, one row at a time at a *frame rate* of 25 fps (frames per second, or Hz) in the European PAL and SECAM systems or 30 fps in the American NTSC system. To speed the process up a bit, the camera skips every other row and then goes back and fills in the gaps (a process called *interlacing*). This generates two *fields*, which the eye sees as one frame (picture) (Fig. 2.6). It is possible in software to separate the two interlaced fields and thereby achieve double the rate to 50 or 60 fps, respectively. To achieve faster frame rates for analysing running and other sports, resolution must usually be sacrificed (e.g. JVC DVL-9x00 or Basler A601 DVL-9x00 cameras, which allow 100 fps).

To record digital video, some sort of *frame grabber* is required to convert the analogue TV picture into a digital computer file, and this is usually a card inserted into the back of a desktop PC or the PCMCIA slot of a laptop computer. AVI is usually used as the container file format. Note that the .WMV (Windows Media Video) format uses Microsoft's own MPEG-4 codec, which is not compatible with others.

Since there are 720×576 pixels in Europe and 720×480 in the US in each full screen picture, this makes for a lot of information (*data-rate* or *bandwidth*) in Mbits/s or Mb/s (1 megabyte, Mb = 8 Mbits) and some sort of compression, using a CODEC (compression-decompression algorithm) must be performed to reduce the resulting file size. This may be implemented in hardware (*MPEG 4*) or software (e.g. *Cinepak, Intel Indeo* or *DV*) and inevitably involves a trade-off between quality and file size.

Digital video (DV) camcorders record directly to digital format. The data can then be quickly downloaded to the PC through a *FireWire* (IEEE 1394) port (up to 80 Mb/s), and it is possible to collect data from up to three cameras simultaneously. Not all PCs are equipped with FireWire at present, however.

Many digital still cameras are capable of recording short clips of video to a memory card, but only a few are capable of recording at 30 fps (the interlaced fields are not separated). The temporal accuracy of these cameras can be unreliable, however, which limits their use for biomechanics. One quick way to check this is to record a short clip of a stopwatch reading in 1/100ths of a second. The time between each picture should be constant.

To be useful for gait analysis work, a camera must have a shutter speed that can be manually set to 1/500 s (or faster) to prevent blurring. This is sometimes called 'sports' mode. It should also be possible to set the focus manually. If markers are used, it helps to be able to adjust the diaphragm (or *stop*) to enhance contrast with the background.

Figure 2.6

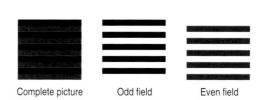

Complete picture   Odd field   Even field

FILTERING

It is impossible to be perfectly accurate in digitizing the position of the markers. These small inaccuracies in each coordinate lead to what is called *digitization noise* in the results. Luckily this noise tends to be high frequency whereas the signal (the marker trajectories) is relatively low frequency. So the noise can be reduced by low-pass filtering, letting the low frequencies in the signal through and blocking the high-frequency noise (Fig. 2.7).

Figure 2.7 Frequency spectrum of the marker trajectory data.

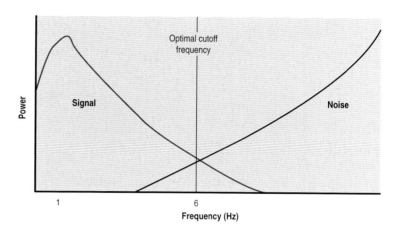

The most common type of filter used in gait analysis is a critically-damped 2nd order Butterworth low-pass filter (Winter et al 1974). It's not really necessary to know the details of how this works, but it should be understood that the choice of cutoff frequency that separates the wanted signal and the unwanted noise is *empirical*. This means that the decision depends on the sort of data being filtered. If it is too low, the data will be over-smoothed, while if it is too high too much of the noise will remain. It has been found by experience that the optimal cutoff is about six times the stride frequency of the gait. So, for a normal gait at 120 steps per minute, i.e. stride frequency of 1 Hz, the cutoff should be about 6 Hz.

? MCQ 2.2

What would be the optimal cutoff frequency for a gait with a cadence of 160 steps per minute?
(a) 1 Hz
(b) 6 Hz
(c) 8 Hz
(d) 12 Hz

CALCULATION OF SEGMENT ANGLES

The next job is to convert the marker trajectories into segment angles (Fig. 2.8). This is done by trigonometry, specifically the tangent function (opposite over adjacent):

$$\tan \theta = (y_d - y_p)/(x_d - x_p)$$

Notice that for consistency the angle is always measured counterclockwise from the right horizontal. In practice, a related tangent function, *atan2*, is needed because of the way the tangent function behaves when the angle is greater than 90°.

CALCULATION OF JOINT ANGLES

Each joint (ankle, knee, hip) angle is calculated as shown in Figure 2.9. The angle must then be transformed to the clinical convention, based on the anatomical position. For the ankle, this means subtracting 90°.

? MCQ 2.3

What is the ankle angle if the foot is at 30° and the shank at 120°?
(a) 0°
(b) 60°
(c) 90°
(d) 150°

Figure 2.8 Segment angles are calculated by trigonometry.

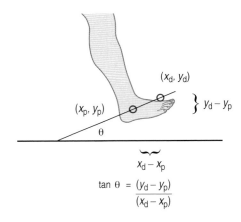

$$\tan \theta = \frac{(y_d - y_p)}{(x_d - x_p)}$$

Figure 2.9 Joint angles are calculated from the difference between adjacent segment angles.

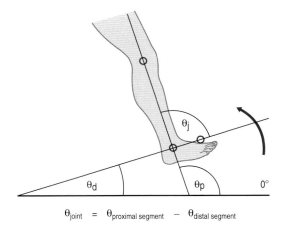

$$\theta_{joint} = \theta_{proximal\ segment} - \theta_{distal\ segment}$$

Figure 2.10   2D gait kinematics during normal gait.

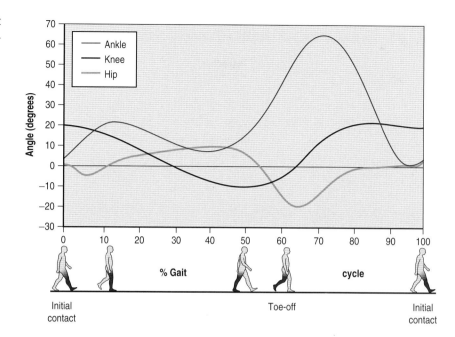

NORMAL GAIT KINEMATICS

The joint kinematics of normal gait are shown in Figure 2.10. Note the key findings:

- The hip angle curve is approximately sinusoidal, going from flexion at initial contact to extension at contralateral initial contact (50% cycle) and back to flexion for the next ipsilateral initial contact.
- The knee angle shows two peaks: stance phase and swing phase flexion, with the latter being much larger than the former.
- The ankle angle is neutral (0°) at initial contact, after which it plantarflexes slightly, before dorsiflexing through stance, until around contralateral initial contact, when it suddenly plantarflexes. In swing phase it returns to neutral. Traditionally, ankle joint kinematics are divided into three rockers (Perry 1992):
  - 1st: rapid plantarflexion immediately following contact
  - 2nd: gradual dorsiflexion from early to mid stance phase
  - 3rd: sudden plantarflexion around toe-off.

? MCQ 2.4

What would happen to the knee angle if the data were to be filtered at 3 Hz instead of 6 Hz?

(a) There would be more noise in the recording
(b) The peaks will be increased in amplitude
(c) The peaks will be decreased in amplitude
(d) No change

VARIABILITY OF 2D KINEMATICS

Not surprisingly, the variability in the recorded joint angles is lower for a given individual (*intra*-subject) compared to that of a group of people (*inter*-subject), as shown in Table 2.1 (Winter 1983, 1984, 1991). Notice, too, that the variability expressed as average SD is highest at the hip and knee, and lowest at the ankle, yet the %CV is lowest at the knee. This demonstrates one weakness of the use of CV as a measure of variation – it can be misleadingly large when the mean of the measurement (e.g. hip or ankle angle) is close to zero.

LIMITATIONS OF 2D ANALYSIS

Although much valuable pioneering work on gait was performed using these techniques, 2D analysis is currently rarely used for clinical or research purposes, and 3D techniques are now accepted as standard. There are two major reasons for this: parallax error and perspective error.

PARALLAX ERROR

Parallax error occurs when objects move away from the optical axis of the camera (Fig. 2.11). Of course, it is impossible to completely eliminate parallax error but it should be minimized by aligning the optical axis of the camera with the central part of the motion, and zooming the lens in as much as possible to record only the required motion.

PERSPECTIVE ERROR

Perspective error is the apparent change in length of an object when it moves out of the calibrated plane (Fig. 2.12).

Notice that the error increases as the out-of-plane distance, d, increases, but decreases as the distance to the camera is increased. To keep perspective error to a minimum, therefore, the camera should be kept as far from the subject as possible, zooming in to compensate for the image size. It should also be mounted exactly perpendicular to the calibrated plane.

In 2D analysis, it is assumed that all the motion takes place in the calibrated plane (e.g. the sagittal plane, or more precisely the plane of progression in which the subject is walking). Some disorders (such as deformities and spasticity) make it difficult for the patient to walk in a sagittal plane, further contributing to these out-of-plane errors. It is possible to estimate and correct for perspective errors by monitoring the

Table 2.1 Variability in joint angles, expressed as average standard deviation (degrees) and coefficient of variation (%) for the three major joint angles during normal gait (Winter 1983)

Joint angle	Intra-subject (one person)	Inter-subject (group of people)
Hip	± 3° (21%)	± 6° (52%)
Knee	± 2° (8%)	± 5° (23%)
Ankle	± 1° (16%)	± 4° (72%)

Figure 2.11 Parallax error increases toward the periphery of the camera image. In this case, the camera axis is aligned with the centre of the thigh and so, while motion of the hip and knee is recorded reasonably well, errors (dashed lines) are worse for the foot and shoulder trajectories (adapted from Sih et al 2001).

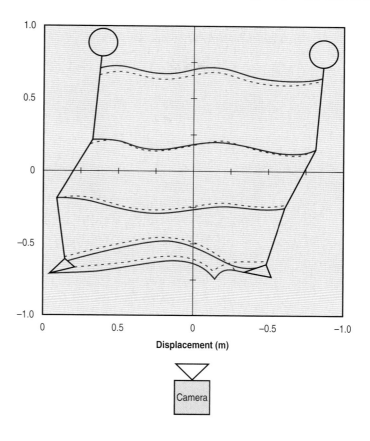

Displacement (m)

Figure 2.12 Perspective error caused by out-of-plane movement. The segment length, l, is reduced by an amount e when it moves out of the calibrated plane by a distance d. The error can be reduced by increasing the camera distance, c.

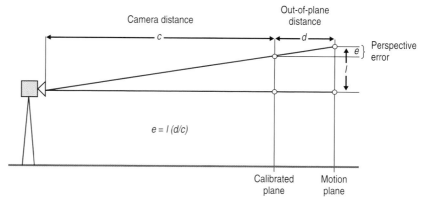

$$e = l \,(d/c)$$

segment length, since any increase or decrease suggests out-of-plane motion (Li et al 1990), although this is difficult to implement in practice.

Measurement of frontal plane motion is even more problematic (Cornwall & McPoil 1994, Mannon et al 1997) because the body moves toward or away from the calibrated plane (Fig. 2.13). This perspective error can be minimized by limiting the measurement to the period immediately prior to and following heel-strike (Cornwall & McPoil 1993, Kappel-Bargas et al 1998), when the foot is within the calibrated plane.

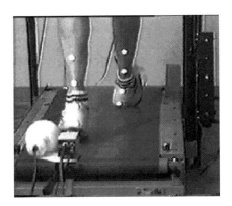

Figure 2.13 Measuring frontal plane motion (rearfoot eversion/inversion) by 2D kinematics (even on a treadmill) is prone to error because of perspective error caused by a large amount of out-of-plane motion. This can be minimized by limiting the measurement to the period immediately prior to and following heel-strike.

Although transverse motion, recorded by an overhead camera, is not so affected, it is even more difficult in practice because the upper-body obscures lower-limb motion (Sawert et al 1995).

Due to these limitations, 3D systems have become increasingly more popular. Unfortunately, the equipment necessary is very expensive (in the region of $100,000) and is therefore restricted to universities and specialist centres. Nevertheless, even for the clinician without access to such facilities, the insights from 3D analyses are so illuminating that it is worth understanding the techniques involved.

KEY POINTS

★ Kinematic measurements include linear and angular displacement, velocity and acceleration

★ Electrogoniometers, electromagnetic, ultrasonic and optical tracking systems can be used

★ In optical systems, skin marker locations are digitized from images recorded by a video camera

★ Filtering is required to reduce digitization and other noise in the marker trajectories

★ Parallax and perspective errors limit the use of 2D measurements

References

Blankevoort L, Huiske R, de Lange A 1988 The envelope of passive knee joint motion. Journal of Biomechanics 21(9):705–720

Chao E Y S 1980 Justification of triaxial goniometer for the measurement of joint rotation. Journal of Biomechanics 13:989–1006

Cornwall M W, McPoil T G 1993 Reducing 2-dimensional rearfoot motion variability during walking. Journal of the American Podiatry Association 83:394–397

Cornwall M W, McPoil T G 1994 Comparison of 2-dimensional and 3-dimensional rearfoot motion during walking. Clinical Biomechanics 10:36–40

Kappel-Bargas A, Woolf R D, Cornwall M W, McPoil T G 1998 The influence of the windlass mechanism on rearfoot motion during normal walking. Clinical Biomechanics 13:190–194

Kirtley C 2002 New technology in gait analysis, in physical medicine and rehabilitation. State of the Art Reviews 16(2):361–373

Kirtley C, Smith R A 2001 Application of multimedia to the study of human movement. Multimedia Tools and Applications 14(3):259–268

Li J A, Bryant J T, Stevenson J M 1990 Single camera photogrammetric technique for restricted 3D motion analysis. Journal of Biomedical Engineering 12:69–74

Mannon K, Anderson T, Cheetham P et al 1997 A comparison of two motion analysis systems for the measurement of two-dimensional rearfoot motion during walking. Foot and Ankle International 18:427–431

Perry J 1992 Gait analysis, normal and pathological function. Slack, Thorofare, NJ

Sawert M K, Cornwall M W, McPoil T G 1995 The validation of two-dimensional measurement of transverse tibial rotation during walking using three-dimensional movement analysis. The Lower Extremity 2:285–291

Sih B L, Hubbard M, Williams K R 2001 Correcting out-of-plane errors in two-dimensional imaging using nonimage-related information. Journal of Biomechanics 34:257–260

Sutherland D H, Hagy J L 1972 Measurement of gait movements from motion picture film. Journal of Bone and Joint Surgery 54A(4):787–797

Winter D A 1983 Biomechnical motor patterns in normal walking. Journal of Motor Behavior 15(4):302–330

Winter D A 1984 Kinematic and kinetic patterns in human gait: variability and compensating effects. Human Movement Science 3:51–76

Winter D A 1991 The biomechanics and motor control of human gait: normal, elderly and pathological. University of Waterloo Press, Ontario, Canada

Winter D A, Sidwall H G, Hobson D A 1974 measurement and reduction of noise in kinematics of locomotion. Journal of Biomechanics 7:157–159

Chapter **3**

Three-dimensional gait analysis

In life, as in art, the beautiful moves in curves.

Edward George Bulwer-Lytton

CHAPTER CONTENTS

OBJECTIVES

- Awareness of the principles used in reconstructing 3D motion from camera images
- Understand how mathematical models are used to derive lower-limb joint angles
- Appreciation of the limitations of such models and the consequences of marker placement errors
- Know the general patterns of 3D joint motion during normal gait
- Awareness of the special problems and typical approaches used in tracking and modelling foot motion

---

The principles involved in performing a 3D gait analysis are similar to the simple 2D one-camera method, with some important differences. Although many clinicians may never set foot in a gait laboratory, let alone use the sophisticated technology available nowadays, some familiarity with the techniques involved is essential for a thorough understanding of gait and interpretation of gait analysis findings.

TRACKING AND RECONSTRUCTION

In a similar way to how the eyes work together to provide 3D binocular vision, the images from two or more 2D camera images are tracked and

Figure 3.1 Arrangement of cameras in a typical 3D gait analysis. The cameras are positioned so that at least two see each marker at any given time. Powerful infra-red light sources around each camera reflect from the retro-reflective markers result in a corresponding bright spot in each image, and these spots are then combined (reconstructed) to generate the 3D trajectories.

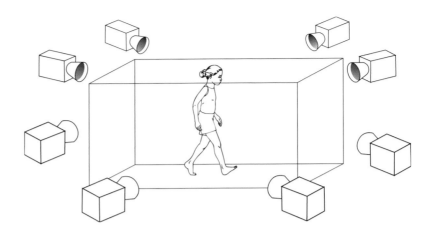

these points are used to *reconstruct* their original 3D trajectories. The mathematics involved are very sophisticated and closely-guarded secrets of the manufacturers but fundamentally involve *calibration* of the volume in which the subject will move (Miller et al 1980). A rod with two markers at a known distance from one another is first waved around in sight of the cameras. This generates a large number of simultaneous equations, which are solved to determine the precise relationship of each camera to the *calibrated volume*, as it is called (Fig. 3.1).

Once this is done, and assuming that the cameras are not moved, any point within this space can then be tracked in 3D so long as it can be seen by at least two cameras. Accuracy of tracking markers is typically around ± 0.1% of the capture volume. Since the length of the capture volume in most adult laboratories is around 5 m, this is equivalent to about ± 5 mm (Ehara et al 1995, 1997). Increases in camera resolution (especially the number of scan lines) and refinements of the calibration and tracking algorithms can be expected to improve this in future. In practice, however, the major limitation on accuracy is the model used for deriving joint motion from skin-mounted markers (Kadaba et al 1990, Growney et al 1997, Holden et al 1997), as well as relative motion between the markers and the underlying bone (soft-tissue motion artefact).

One snag of 2D analysis is that as the arm swings it tends to obscure the hip (greater trochanter) marker. Keeping the arms folded prevents this happening, but it may interfere with the natural gait, particularly in people with walking disorders. In 3D gait analysis, several cameras (typically six or more) are used so that at least two of them can see a marker at any one time. The most advanced motion capture facility in the world at the present time has a total of 72 cameras. It is operated by *Sony Imageworks* for recording the complex action sequences used in computer games.

MODELS

The objective of gait analysis is to track the motion of the body segments (Whittle 1996). Whereas in 2D only two markers are necessary to define the location of each segment, in 3D three are needed. As in 2D, markers placed on the joints can be used to define the two adjacent segments, with the advantage of reducing the number of markers needed (Kadaba et al 1989, Ramakrishnan & Kadaba 1991, Davis et al 1991). This strategy became popular because in the early days of 3D gait analysis (Sutherland 2002), the technology had difficulty tracking more than a few markers, and although the tracking ability of modern systems is much improved, these 'minimal' marker sets continue to be used in most laboratories. The most popular is variously called the *Modified Helen Hayes* (MHH), *Vaughan, Newington, Kadaba, Davis, Gage,* or *Vicon Clinical Manager* (VCM) model (Fig. 3.2).

To see how it works, start at the pelvis. This is defined by markers attached over the right and left anterior superior iliac spine (ASIS) and the spinous process of the second sacral vertebra (S2). These *bony landmarks* were chosen because they are relatively easy to locate reliably (at least in non-obese people): the ASIS is prominent at the anterior end of the iliac crest, while skin dimples indicate the level of S2 (Fig. 3.3). Note that if any

Figure 3.2   The Modified Helen Hayes model.

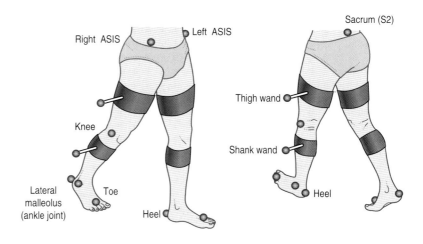

Figure 3.3   Markers on the left and right ASIS and S2 form a triangle which defines the pelvis in three dimensions.

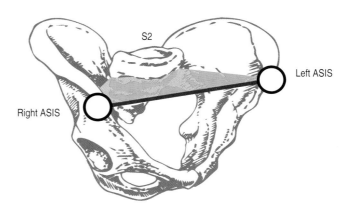

of these markers is misplaced, the recorded pelvic angle (with respect to the room or global coordinate system) will be incorrect (Foti et al 2001). For example, mistakenly attaching the sacral marker to S1 rather than S2 will introduce an anterior pelvic tilt artefact into the recorded angles.

The thigh is more difficult to define because there are very few easily identified bony landmarks. Moreover, the hip joint is deep, hidden under layers of muscle and tendon. These problems are still a challenge to modern gait analysis and many strategies have been designed to solve them. In the MHH model, regression equations define the location of the hip joint centre (HJC), based on the location of the two ASIS markers, S2 marker and the height of the subject (Bell et al 1990, Davis et al 1991, Vaughan et al 1992). These equations were developed from measurements of normal pelvic x-rays, making the MHH dependent on the accuracy of anthropometry: there is an implicit assumption that the subject's pelvis has the same proportions as the x-rays from which the equations were derived. Indeed, the error in HJC estimation is often as high as ± 1 or even ± 2 cm (Seidel et al 1995, Stagni et al 2000, Feiser et al 2000). This is an important limitation of such *anthropometric* models.

Defining the HJC is very useful, though, because it also defines the location of the femoral head (assuming that it doesn't move out of the acetabulum – probably a reasonable assumption for most hip joints). So, two more points are needed to complete the triangle defining the thigh segment. The lateral femoral condyle is one bony landmark that is quite easily identified, and moreover, this can double as the knee joint centre (KJC) because the axis of rotation of the knee passes through here. Finding it can be a little tricky, and is generally done by asking the subject to alternately flex and extend the knee until a point is found with minimal movement. The model then uses the measured knee width between medial and lateral femoral condyles to calculate the position of the KJC.

There are not many options left for the third thigh marker. The medial femoral condyle would be ideal, except that it would likely be knocked off by the contralateral knee as it swings through. At first glance, the greater trochanter seems ideal, but it has a tendency to move under the skin as the thigh rotates. A further consideration is that the three markers should not be *colinear*. This means that they should not lie in a straight line, otherwise rotation would not be recorded. This requirement means that the third marker should preferably be offset some distance from the other two. The solution used by the MHH set is to attach the third marker on a short stick, or *wand*, which is then attached to the thigh by a Velcro strap (Fig. 3.4). This is hardly ideal, it must be said, because such a wand will tend to wobble as the subject walks, but it is assumed that this vibration can be removed by low-pass filtering (Karlsson & Tranberg 1999).

There is a further complication to the attachment of the thigh wand, in that it has to also define the frontal plane of the femur. This sounds straightforward, but in practice can be difficult to achieve (Baker et al 1999). One technique involves the use of a mirror to line up the wand with the knee marker and the HJC, assuming the location of the latter is to be indicated in the sagittal plane by the greater trochanter (Fig. 3.5).

Figure 3.4 The thigh wand serves two functions. It defines the frontal plane of the thigh, and allows rotations to be measured.

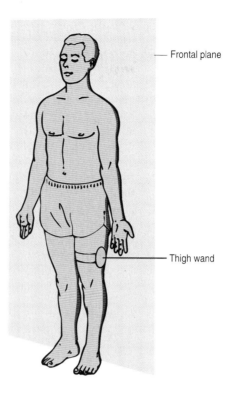

Frontal plane

Thigh wand

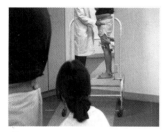

Figure 3.5 Ensuring that the thigh wand is lined up with the frontal plane of the thigh with the aid of a mirror. The assistant is indicating the greater trochanter with a finger while the wand is aligned with this and the knee marker.

The rest of the markers are fairly straightforward to attach. The lateral malleolus defines the ankle joint centre (AJC), and together with the knee marker and another wand (this time strapped to the calf) forms a triangle defining the shank. Finally, a marker between the second and third metatarsal heads and the calcaneus (os calcis) heel defines the foot. These should be placed at the same height to ensure that the ankle angle is correctly measured (Fig. 3.6).

By now it should be apparent that there are an uncomfortably large number of assumptions involved in the MHH model. Moreover, it relies on subjective decisions (on the part of the gait analyser) in the placement of many of the markers (Growney et al 1997, Kirtley 2002). One study found a variation of well over 10° in the angles recorded by different laboratories (Gorton et al 2000), with training leading to only modest improvements in accuracy (Gorton et al 2001). Hip angles seem especially sensitive to marker attachment (Fig. 3.7, Table 3.1).

? MCQ 3.1

What would be the effect of attaching the sacral marker to S3 instead of S2?
(a) Anterior pelvic tilt
(b) Posterior pelvic tilt
(c) Increased hip flexion
(d) Upward obliquity

For these reasons, some laboratories prefer alternative models. Of these, the most common is the *Cleveland Clinic* (CC) set (Fig. 3.8), which

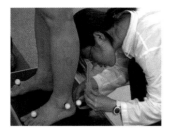

Figure 3.6 Attaching the foot markers.

uses the same three pelvis markers, but dispenses with the thigh and shank wands in favour of a *marker cluster* or triad (*fiducial* tracking). This is simply a set of three orthogonal markers (each at 90° to each other) that are strapped around the respective segment. Although such clusters are attached to soft tissue rather than over bony landmarks, and so are inclined to move slightly with underlying muscle contraction, they are less sensitive to placement errors and appear to track the underlying bone more faithfully (Manal et al 2000).

To obviate the reliance on anthropometry, some researchers have advocated the use of functional HJC determination algorithms (Leardini et al 1999a, Piazza et al 2001). Briefly, these involve asking the subject to move the hip through a range of flexion/extension and abduction/adduction, in order to generate a set of simultaneous equations that are solved for the HJC. This is not without its problems, however, since it is rare for the mathematics to result in a single solution – instead, a cloud of possible values is generated and some averaging technique must be used to choose

Figure 3.7 Some effects of misplaced markers on 3D kinematics and kinetics (Kirtley 2002).

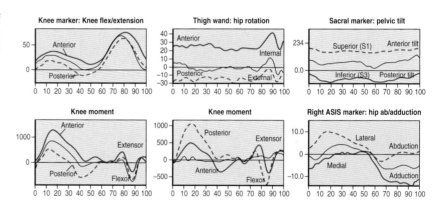

Table 3.1 Summary of the effects of misplaced markers (Kirtley 2002)

Error	Effect
ASIS marker too high	Ipsilateral upward obliquity
	Contralateral downward obliquity
	Pelvic tilt more posterior
	Ipsilateral hip adduction
	Contralateral hip adduction
	Reduced hip flexion (bilaterally)
Sacral marker too high	Pelvic tilt more anterior
	Increased hip flexion (bilaterally)
Thigh wand too anterior	Ipsilateral hip internal rotation
	Reduced ipsilateral knee flexion
	Knee varus (adduction) artefact
Knee marker too anterior	Increased hip and knee flexion and ankle dorsiflexion
Heel marker too high	Increased ankle plantarflexion

Figure 3.8 The Cleveland Clinic marker set, which is based around marker clusters on the thigh and shank segments.

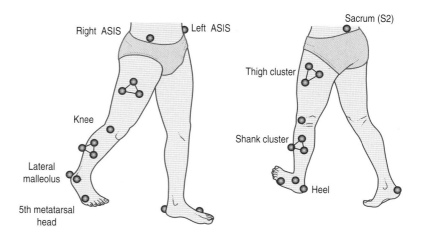

which one is the closest to reality. It can also be difficult for patients with spasticity or arthritis to produce the required range of motion at the hip. A useful compromise is to try a functional determination but default to the anthropometric solution if the result is unsatisfactory (e.g. standard deviation too great).

So-called *six-degree-of-freedom* (6DoF) models acknowledge the difficulties of determining joint centres of rotation by simply tracking the adjacent segments. This approach is facilitated by software such as *Move3D* (National Institutes of Health, Bethesda, MD, USA) and its successor, *Visual3D* (C-Motion, Rockville, MD, USA). In this approach, the bones are tracked separately with no assumptions being made about joint constraints, often resulting in joints that 'dislocate'. Although this is clearly not happening in the real world, the proponents of such models point out that such artefacts are also present, but hidden by the joint constraints of other models. By visualizing the disarticulation, errors in tracking the bones are revealed for all to see.

Despite all its weaknesses and potential inaccuracies, the MHH model continues to be used for most routine 3D clinical gait analysis. It has the advantage of being quite quick to apply (after an initial training period), which is particularly important when the patient is a child, and with experience many of its difficulties and idiosyncrasies can be overcome.

DEBATING POINT

Research and debate the advantages and disadvantages of the following for clinical gait analysis:
- Anthropometric models such as the MHH
- Fiducial models such as the CC set
- Six-degree-of-freedom models such as the NIH approach.

THE ANATOMICAL POSITION

The convention for displaying graphs of kinematics of gait is based on the anatomical position standing with feet forward. In this posture all joints are defined to be in their neutral position (0°). The convention in Table 3.2 is then followed.

The pelvis is a body segment rather than a joint, and its terminology is a bit messy – sagittal plane motion about a mediolateral axis passing through both hip joints is called tilt, while frontal plane motion is variously called *obliquity*, *list* or *lateral tilt*. To specify the direction, the pelvis is divided into a right and left *hemipelvis*. Of course, whatever happens to one hemipelvis, the opposite happens on the contralateral side. So, an upward obliquity on the right is the same as a downward obliquity on the left, and an internal rotation on the right is the same as an external rotation on the left.

NORMAL 3D KINEMATICS

Figure 3.9 shows typical results from a 3D kinematic study. The pattern of sagittal plane angles can be seen to be very similar to those measured by 2D methods. In addition, pelvic and hip motion in the three planes is revealed, along with the angulation of the foot with the line of progression (foot progression angle).

EFFECT OF SPEED

The main effect of increasing walking speed on joint kinematics is found at the knee and ankle. The stance phase knee flexion increases with speed, while the rapid ankle plantarflexion around toe-off (3rd rocker) occurs earlier and is deeper (Fig. 3.10).

INTEGRATIVE KINEMATIC MEASURES

A comprehensive 3D kinematic analysis generates so much data that it can sometimes be bewildering. The clinician often wants to know how

Table 3.2   The convention for displaying graphs of kinematics of gait

Plane	Sagittal	Frontal	Transverse
Axis	Mediolateral	Anteroposterior	Vertical
Positive angles	Flexion	Adduction	Internal rotation
Negative angles	Extension	Abduction	External rotation
Positive pelvis angles	Anterior tilt	Upward obliquity	Internal rotation
Negative pelvis angles	Posterior tilt	Downward obliquity	External rotation
Positive ankle angle	Dorsiflexion	Inversion	Internal rotation
Negative ankle angle	Plantarflexion	Eversion	External rotation

Figure 3.9 3D lower-limb kinematics recorded using the Cleveland Clinic model. Normative range is shown as mean ± 1 SD.

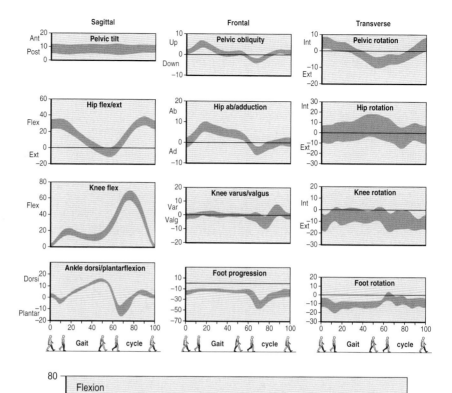

Figure 3.10 Effect of walking speed on knee and ankle kinematics. As speed increases, the stance phase knee flexion increases. At the ankle, there is less dorsiflexion in late stance, 3rd rocker plantarflexion occurs earlier, and the degree of plantarflexion is slightly increased (data from Stansfield et al 2001, with permission).

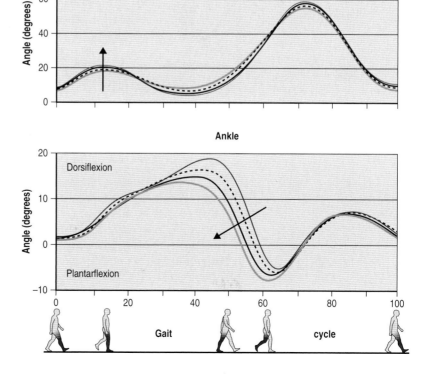

different from normal the patient's gait is, and whether it is improving or worsening. The normalcy index (Schutte et al 2000) is a single number summarizing all the curves by the statistical procedure of principle components analysis. Interestingly, gaits with closely similar joint kinematics can appear much different to the naked eye (Troje 2002), indicating a pattern recognition function that remains to be exploited in conventional gait analysis.

The foot and ankle merit special attention for the following reasons:

FOOT KINEMATICS

- The foot is the interface between body and floor
- Motion of the joints of the foot and ankle are complex and difficult to quantify
- The foot and ankle perform particularly important functions in the gait cycle
- Disorders of the foot and ankle are very common.

Currently, nearly all gait laboratories model the foot as a single rigid body. This is clearly too simplistic, but until now there really was little alternative. There are three reasons for this:

1. The foot is effectively a bag containing 26 separate bones. If markers were placed on all of them, they would merge together in the camera images. It is possible to use small markers (diameter 10 mm or even 5 mm), but even modern 3D motion analysis systems still have trouble tracking several of these close together. The talus is impossible to track because it is completely surrounded by other bones.
2. Even if all these markers could be tracked, it is doubtful that they would faithfully reflect the underlying bony motion. The skin of the foot moves greatly over the bones (skin–bone interface artefact), and the magnitude of the resulting errors can be quite large (Holden et al 1997, Reinschmidt et al 1997). Skin markers tend to overestimate both linear (translation) and angular motion.
3. The joints of the foot do not act as simple hinge joints, but have complex articular surfaces (Inmann et al 1981).

A useful compromise between these extremes of modelling is to treat the foot as three functional segments: rear-, mid- and forefoot (Scott & Winter 1991, 1993, Wu et al 2002). Several models have been described which utilize around a dozen markers, and tracking can be achieved by zooming the cameras in on the foot region (Fig. 3.11). Unfortunately, this is usually at the expense of excluding swing phase motion and the rest of the lower-limbs (Dul & Johnson 1985, Siegler et al 1988, Scott & Winter 1991, 1993, Leardini et al 1999b, Cornwall & McPoil 1999). A new generation of digital cameras (with higher resolution in terms of the number of pixels in the image), as well as miniature electromagnetic tracking systems (Fig. 3.12), are now making possible more sophisticated foot models (Nawoczenskiet al 1998, Carson et al 2001, MacWilliams et al 2003, Theologis et al 2003).

Figure 3.11 3D model for tracking foot kinematics (redrawn from MacWilliams et al 2003, with permission).

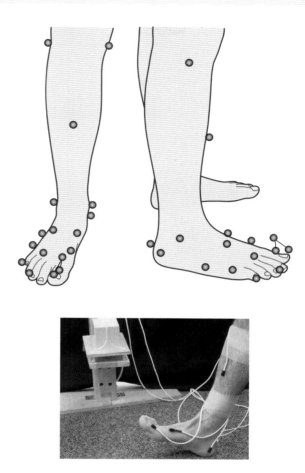

Figure 3.12 Flock of Birds electromagnetic tracking system. The cube in the background is a source for an electromagnetic field, which is used to derive 3D position and angle data at each sensor ('bird'). An advantage of this approach is that only one bird need be attached to each foot segment, whereas optical systems require a minimum of three reflective markers (photo courtesy of Dr D A Nawoczenski).

TERMINOLOGY

The terminology used for foot kinematics can be quite confusing because the foot anatomy is so complicated (consisting of 26 bones, not including sesamoids) and several terms are often used for the same joint or motion. Table 3.3 is an attempt to summarize and define the terms commonly in use. Although the axes of rotation of the major foot joints differ quite widely between subjects, Figure 3.13 indicates the approximate directions.

DEFINITION OF THE NEUTRAL POSITION

Due to its axis, the subtalar joint can compensate for deformities at the other joints (Root et al 1977). For example, a varus or valgus deformity may only become visible with the foot positioned in subtalar joint neutral (STJN). The question then arises: how to define STJN? Unfortunately, clinical methods for determining STJN position are unreliable (Elveru et al 1988, Lattanza et al 1998). One solution would be to simply bisect the measured range of motion between eversion and inversion (Astrom

Table 3.3   Summary of the various terminologies used for foot kinematics*

Term	Definition	Synonyms
Ankle joint	Tibiotalar + fibulotalar + tibiofibular joints	Talocrural joint
Subtalar joint	Talocalcaneal + talonavicular joints	
Ankle joint complex	Ankle + subtalar joints	Often, confusingly, also termed 'ankle joint'
Midtarsal joint	Talonavicular + calcaneocuboid joints	Transverse tarsal joint, Chopart's joint
Tarsometatarsal joint	Between cuneiforms/cuboid and metatarsals (1st, 2nd and 3rd metatarsocuneiform + 4th and 5th metatarsotarsocuboid joints)	Lisfranc's joint
Metatarsophalangeal joint	Joints between the each of the five metatarsals and proximal phalanx	Midfoot break, metatarsophalangeal break
Extension	Sagittal plane motion (toes up)	Dorsiflexion
Flexion	Sagittal plane motion (toes down)	Plantarflexion
Abduction	Transverse plane motion (forefoot rotates externally)	
Adduction	Transverse plane motion (forefoot rotates internally)	
Eversion	Frontal plane motion at the subtalar joint (sole faces laterally)	Hindfoot eversion, pronation, valgus
Inversion	Frontal plane motion at the subtalar joint (sole faces medially)	Hindfoot inversion, supination, varus
Valgus	Everted hind or forefoot	
Varus	Inverted hind or forefoot	
Pronation	Eversion + dorsiflexion + abduction	Eversion, valgus
Supination	Inversion + plantarflexion + adduction	Inversion, varus
Forefoot supination	Frontal plane motion at the metatarsophalangeal joint (dorsiflexion of medial toes more than lateral)	Midfoot break, forefoot varus

*It should be noted that there is currently some confusion in the terminology for foot motion, with eversion, pronation and valgus (and inversion, supination and varus) being sometimes used interchangeably. Strictly speaking, eversion/inversion refers to subtalar motion alone, while pronation/supination refers to triplanar (sagittal, frontal and transverse) motion at the ankle complex and transverse tarsal joints. The terms varus and valgus tend to be used for structural deformities of the hind or forefoot.

& Arvidson 1995). Since the hindfoot inverts more than everts, a ratio of one-third to two-thirds subtalar joint eversion to inversion has also been proposed (Root el al 1977), but this of course ignores individual variation. Another solution is to use the angle between the calcaneus and the floor: the resting calcaneal stance position (RCSP), rearfoot or calcaneal angle (calcaneus to tibia). Unfortunately, clinical assessment of calcaneal angle does not seem to correlate very well with radiographic measurements (Taylor et al 2001).

Figure 3.13 Approximate directions of the axes of rotation of the major foot joints.

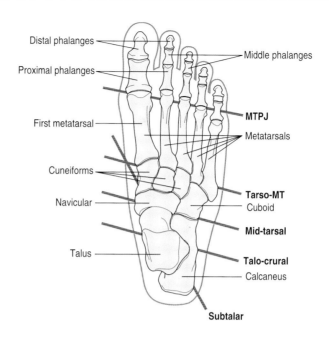

Distal phalanges
Middle phalanges
Proximal phalanges
MTPJ
First metatarsal
Metatarsals
Cuneiforms
Tarso-MT
Navicular
Cuboid
Mid-tarsal
Talus
Talo-crural
Calcaneus
Subtalar

NORMAL FOOT KINEMATICS

Results from studies of foot kinematics so far performed tend to show the largest motion taking place at the hindfoot (talocrural and subtalar joints) and forefoot (metatarsophalangeal joints), with relatively less motion occurring at the midtarsal joint (Fig. 3.14). Hindfoot inversion takes place around 50% cycle (Kepple et al 1990, Lafortune et al 1994, McPoil & Cornwall 1994, 1996a,b, Pierrynowski & Smith 1996, Mannon et al 1997).

The key events are as follows:

- Subtalar eversion at initial contact
- Midtarsal dorsiflexion during mid-stance
- Talonavicular locking
- Metatarsophalangeal dorsiflexion in late stance, which tenses the plantar fascia
- Subtalar inversion in late stance to further lock the foot
- Plantarflexion for push-off.

ANKLE COMPLEX MOTION

An excellent early study of ankle kinematics was performed using a 3D electrogoniometer (Wright et al 1964).

The combination of the talocrural and subtalar joints forms a universal joint, which automatically adapts to rotation about any axis by sharing the movement between the two joints. The talocrural axis passes approximately through the malleoli, across the transverse dimension of the foot, such that it rotates primarily in the sagittal plane. The axis of rotation of the subtalar joint varies somewhat from person to person, but is roughly aligned with the longitudinal axis of the foot, such that it rotates approximately in the frontal plane. Since the majority of ankle motion in walking occurs in the sagittal plane, subtalar motion is minimal when the foot is aligned with the plane of progression. However, with toeing-out, the subtalar axis rotates laterally and its action becomes progressively more sagittal, resulting in an increased range of motion (Fig. 3.15).

Figure 3.14   (A) 3D foot sagittal plane motion, (B) 3D foot frontal plane motion, (C) 3D foot transverse plane motion (redrawn from MacWilliams et al 2003, with permission).

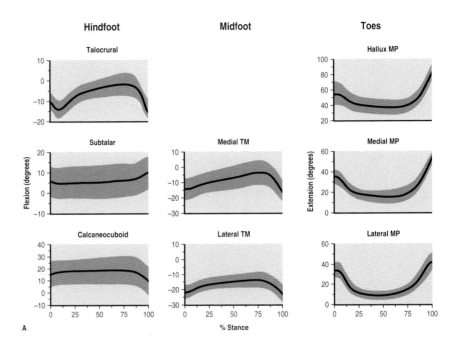

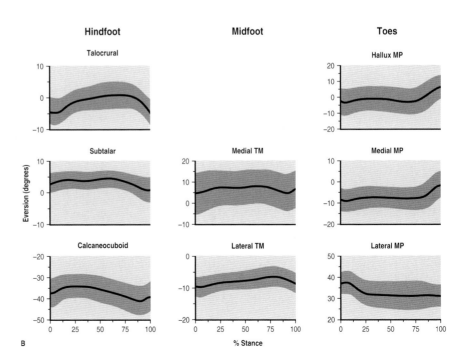

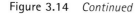

Figure 3.14   *Continued*

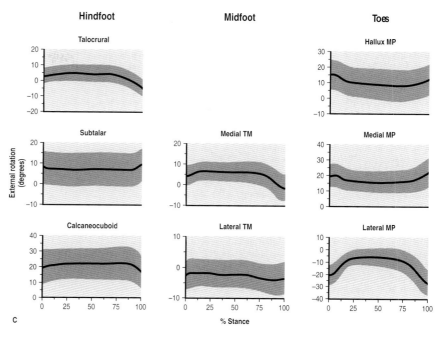

c

Figure 3.15   Foot progression angle affects subtalar joint motion, with toeing-out increasing its range of motion (data from Wright et al 1964).

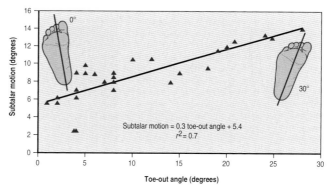

Thus, out-toeing provides a compensatory mechanism for limitation of ankle (talocrural) motion, allowing the motion to occur at the subtalar joint instead.

AXIAL COUPLING AND THE TORQUE CONVERTER EFFECT

Due to the inclination in the subtalar axis, internal rotation of the tibia is coupled to eversion of the foot (Nigg et al 1993, Nester et al 2000). Moreover, during closed-chain activities, when the foot is fixed on the floor, this mechanism becomes a kinetic coupling: axial moment at the distal tibia is converted into frontal plane foot moments (or vice versa). Moment (torque) is transmitted via the anterior talofibular and superior deltoid ligaments (Huson et al 1986). This axial coupling between tibia and foot seems to remain intact following a subtalar arthrodesis, suggesting that the mechanism arises from more than just the subtalar joint

(Hintermann & Nigg 1995). It has been postulated that this torque converter effect may be a risk factor for knee injury in people with excessive eversion, by increasing internal rotation stresses on the joint (Kilmartin & Wallace 1994).

LOCKING OF THE MIDTARSAL JOINT

The midtarsal joint has two axes of rotation. When the subtalar joint is everted these axes are approximately parallel, allowing a large range of motion. When the subtalar joint is inverted the two axes are oblique to each other, which effectively 'locks' the midtarsal joint (Huson 2000).

Walking simulators

The difficulties of measuring foot motion in vivo have led some researchers to turn to sophisticated in vitro preparations, in which a cadaver foot is mounted on a pneumatic piston (Fig. 3.16). This delivers a vertical load to the specimen foot through a metal rod in the tibia to simulate the ground reaction force. Forces are applied through the tendons (e.g. *tibialis posterior/anterior, flexor hallucis longus, extensor/flexor digitorum longus, peroneus brevis/longus* and *tendoachilles,* in a sequence resembling in vivo muscle activation. By inserting K-wires into the bones, individual motion of these small bones (e.g. cuboid, cuneiforms, metatarsals) can be directly measured.

Figure 3.16

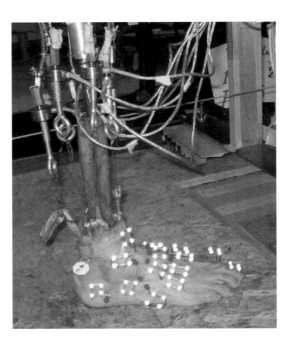

Kim K-J, Kitaoka H B, Luo Z-P et al 2001 In vitro simulation of the stance phase in human gait. Journal of Musculoskeletal Research 5(2):113–121

KEY POINTS

★ 3D gait analysis requires the use of a model mapping skin markers to the underlying bone

★ The two most popular models are the modified Helen Hayes and Cleveland Clinic

★ Accuracy of a 3D gait analysis is crucially dependent on correct marker placement

★ The foot is usually modelled as a single segment or divided into three sub-segments

References

Astrom M, Arvidson T 1995 Alignment and joint motion in the normal foot. Journal of Orthopaedic and Sports Physical Therapy 22(5):216–222

Baker R, Finney L, Orr J 1999 A new method for determining hip rotation profile. Human Movement Science 18:655–667

Bell A L, Petersen D R, Brand R A 1990 A comparison of the accuracy of several hip centre location prediction methods. Journal of Biomechanics 23:617–621

Carson M, Harrington M, Thomson N, Theologis T 2001 A four segment in vivo foot model for Clinical Gait Analysis. Journal of Biomechanics 34:1299–1307

Cornwall M W, McPoil T G 1999 Three-dimensional movement of the foot during the stance phase of walking. Journal of the American Podiatry Association 89:56–66

Davis R, Ounpuu S, Tyburski D, Gage J 1991 A gait analysis data collection and reduction technique. Human Movement Science 10:575–587

Dul J, Johnson G E 1985 A kinematic model of the human ankle. Journal of Biomedical Engineering 7:137–143

Ehara Y, Fujimoto H, Miyazaki S et al 1995 Technical note. Comparison of the performance of 3D camera systems, Gait & Posture 3(3):166–169

Ehara Y, Fujimoto H, Miyazaki S et al 1997 Comparison of the performance of 3D camera systems II. Gait & Posture 5(3):251–255

Elveru R A, Rothstein J M, Lamb R L, Riddle D L 1988 Methods for taking subtalar joint measurements. A clinical report. Physical Therapy 68:678–682

Fieser L, Quigley E, Wyatt M, Sutherland D, Chambers H G 2000 comparison of hip joint centers determined from surface anatomy and CT scans. Gait & Posture 11:119–120

Foti T, Davis R B, Davids J R, Farrell M E 2001 Assessment of methods to describe the angular position of the pelvis during gait in children with hemiplegia. Gait & Posture 13:270

Gorton G, Hebert D, Goode B 2000 Assessment of the kinematic variability between 12 Shriner's motion analysis laboratories. Gait & Posture 13(3):247

Gorton G, Hebert D, Goode B 2001 Assessment of the kinematic variability between 12 Shriner's motion analysis laboratories. Part 2: Short term follow-up. Gait & Posture 16(S1):S65–66

Growney E, Meglan D, Johnson M et al 1997 Repeated measures of adult normal walking using a video tracking system. Gait & Posture 6(2):147–162

Hintermann B, Nigg B M 1995 Influence of arthrodesis on kinematics of the axially loaded ankle complex during dorsiflexion/plantarflexion. Foot and Ankle 16:633

Holden J P, Orsini J A, Siegel K L et al 1997 Surface movement errors in kinematic and kinetic measurements of gait. Gait & Posture 5:217–227

Huson A 2000 Biomechanics of the tarsal mechanism. A key to the function of the normal human foot. Journal of the American Podiatric Medical Association 90(1):12–21

Huson A, van Langelaan E J, Spoor C W 1986 Tibiotalar delay and tarsal gearing. Journal of Anatomy 149:244–245

Inmann V T, Ralston H J, Todd F 1981 Human walking. Williams and Wilkins, Baltimore MD.

Kadaba M, Ramakrishnan H, Wootten M et al 1989 Repeatability of kinematic, kinetic, and electromyographic data in normal adult gait. Journal of Orthopaedic Research 7(6):849–860

Kadaba M, Ramakrishnan H, Wootten M 1990 Measurement of lower extremity kinematics during level walking. Journal of Orthopaedic Research 8(3):383–391

Karlsson D, Tranberg R 1999 On skin movement artifact-resonant frequencies of skin markers attached to the leg. Human Movement Science 18:627–635

Kepple T M, Stanhope S J, Lohmann-Siegel K N, Roman N L 1990 A video-based technique for measuring ankle-subtalar motion during stance. Journal of Biomedical Engineering 12(4):273–280

Kilmartin T E, Wallace W A 1994 The scientific basis for the use of biomechanical foot orthoses in the treatment of lower limb sports injuries – a review of the literature. British Journal of Sports Medicine 28(3):180–184

Kirtley C 2002 Sensitivity of the modified Helen Hayes model to marker placement errors. Seventh International Symposium on the 3-D Analysis of Human Movement, Newcastle, UK, July 10–12

Lafortune M A, Cavanagh P R, Sommer H J, Laenak A 1994 Foot inversion-eversion and knee kinematics during walking. Journal of Orthopaedic Research 12:412–420

Lattanza L, Gray G W, Kanther R M 1998 Closed versus open kinematic chain measurements of subtalar joint eversion: implications for clinical practice. Journal of Orthopaedic and Sports Physical Therapy 9(9):310–314

Leardini A, Cappozzo A, Catani F et al 1999a Validation of a functional method for the estimation of hip joint centre location. Journal of Biomechanics 32:99–103

Leardini A, Benedetti M G, Catani F et al 1999b An anatomically based protocol for the description of foot segment kinematics during gait. Clinical Biomechanics 14(8):528–536

MacWilliams B, Cowley M, Nicholson D 2003 Foot kinematics and kinetics during adolescent gait. Gait & Posture 17:214–224

Manal K, McClay I, Stanhope S et al 2000 Comparison of surface mounted markers and attachment methods in estimating tibial rotations during walking: an in vivo study. Gait & Posture 11(1):38–45

Mannon K, Anderson T, Cheetham P et al 1997 A comparison of two motion analysis systems for the measurement of two-dimensional rearfoot motion during walking. Foot and Ankle 18:427–431

McPoil T, Cornwall M W 1994 Relationship between neutral subtalar joint position and pattern of rearfoot motion during gait. Foot and Ankle 15:141–145

McPoil T G, Cornwall M W 1996a Relationship between the static rearfoot angle in one-leg standing and the pattern of rearfoot motion during walking. Journal of Orthopaedic and Sports Physical Therapy 23:370–375

McPoil T G, Cornwall M W 1996b The relationship between static lower extremity measurements and the pattern of rearfoot motion during walking. Journal of Orthopaedic and Sports Physical Therapy 24:309–314

Miller N R, Shapiro R, McLaughlin T M 1980 A technique for obtaining spatial kinematic parameters of segments of biomechanical systems from cinematographic data. Journal of Biomechanics 13:535–547

Nawoczenski D A, Saltzman C L, Cook T M 1998 The effect of foot structure on the three-dimensional kinematic coupling behavior of the leg and rear foot. Physical Therapy 78:404–416

Nester C J, Hutchins S, Bowker P 2000 Shank rotation: a measure of rearfoot motion during normal walking. Foot and Ankle 21:578–783

Nigg B M, Cole G, Nachbauer W 1993 Effects of arch height of the foot on angular motion of the lower extremities in running. Journal of Biomechanics 26:909–916

Piazza S J, Okita N, Cavanagh P R 2001 Accuracy of the functional method of hip joint center location: effects of limited motion and varied implementation. Journal of Biomechanics 34(7):967–973

Pierrynowski M R, Smith S B 1996 Rear foot inversion/eversion during gait relative to the subtalar joint neutral position. Foot and Ankle International 17(7):406–412

Ramakrishnan H K, Kadaba M P 1991 On the estimation of joint kinematics during gait. Journal of Biomechanics 24(10):969–977

Reinschmidt C, van den Bogert A J, Lundberg A et al 1997 Tibiofemoral and tibiocalcaneal motion during walking: external vs. skeletal markers. Gait & Posture 6:98–109

Root M L, Orien E P, Weed J H 1977 Clinical biomechanics: normal and abnormal function of the foot, vol. 2. Clinical Biomechanics Corporation, Los Angeles

Schutte L M, Narayanan U, Stout J L et al 2000 An index for quantifying deviations from normal gait. Gait & Posture 11(1):25–31

Scott S H, Winter D A 1991 Talocrural and talocalcaneal joint kinematics and kinetics during the stance phase of walking. Journal of Biomechanics 24(8):743–752

Scott S H, Winter D A 1993 Biomechanical model of the human foot: kinematics and kinetics during the stance phase of walking. Journal of Biomechanics 26(9):1091–1104

Seidel G K, Marchinda D M, Dijkers M, Soutas-Little R W 1995 Hip joint center location from palpable bony landmarks – a cadaver study. Journal of Biomechanics 28(8):995–998

Siegler S, Chen J, Schneck C D 1988 The three-dimensional kinematics and flexibility chanaracteristics of the human ankle and subtalar joints. Part I: kinematics. Journal of Biomechanical Engineering 110:364–373

Stagni S, Leardini A, Cappozzo A et al 2000 Effects of hip joint centre mislocation on gait analysis results. Journal of Biomechanics 33(11):1479–1487

Stansfield B W, Hillman S J, Hazlewood M E et al 2001 Sagittal joint kinematics, moments, and powers are predominantly characterized by speed of progression, not age. J Paediatric Orthopaedics 21:403–411

Sutherland D 2002 The evolution of clinical gait analysis – Part II Kinematics. Gait & Posture 16:159–179

Taylor M K F, Bojescul J A, Howard R S et al 2001 Measurement of isolated subtalar range of motion: A cadaver study. Foot and Ankle International 22(5):426–432

Theologis T N, Harrington M E, Thompson N, Benson M K 2003 Dynamic foot movement in children treated for congenital talipes equinovarus. Journal of Bone and Joint Surgery 85B:572–577

Troje N F 2002 Decomposing biological motion: A framework for analysis and synthesis of human gait patterns. Journal of Vision 2:371–387

Vaughan C L, Davis B L, O'Connor J 1992 Dynamics of human gait. Human Kinetics Press, Champaign, Illinois

Whittle MW 1996 Clinical gait analysis: a review. Human Movement Science 15:369–387

Wright D G, Desai S M, Henderson W H 1964 Action of the subtalar and ankle-joint complex during the stance phase of walking. Journal of Bone and Joint Surgery 46A(2):361–382

Wu G, Siegler S, Allard P et al 2002 ISB recommendation on definitions of joint coordinate system of various joints for the reporting of human joint motion-part I: ankle, hip, and spine. Journal of Biomechanics 35(4):543–548

Chapter **4**

Biomechanics of standing

He that stands upon a slippery place makes nice of no vile hold to stay him up.

Shakespeare

OBJECTIVES

- Understand how the ground reaction force arises
- Know how the external joint moment is calculated from the ground reaction force
- Understand how the external moment is balanced by an internal muscle moment
- Know how to infer muscle action from the location of the ground reaction force
- Understand normal ankle and knee action during quiet standing

It is helpful to analyse standing before looking further at walking, since standing illustrates many of biomechanics fundamentals that are needed to understand gait.

THE GROUND REACTION FORCE

When a person is standing completely still (so-called *quiet* standing – Fig. 4.1), the ground produces a reaction force equal and opposite to their body weight – a consequence of Newton's Third Law.

This ground reaction force (GRF) is really an average of all the forces or pressure under the feet. Pressure is not borne evenly by all parts of the sole, but is concentrated in two main regions: the heel and the ball

Figure 4.1 During quiet standing, body weight acting downwards gives rise to an equal and opposite *reaction*, called the ground reaction force (GRF).

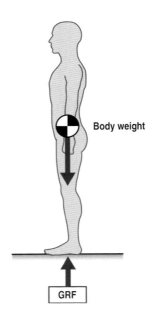

Body weight

GRF

(metatarsophalangeal joints). The location of the centre of pressure (CoP) marks the line of action of the GRF, and in normal quiet standing is about 5 cm anterior to the ankle joint (under the navicular bone). Note that there is very little *actual* pressure in this region (the instep) – the CoP is a purely mathematical concept. It is, however, an extremely useful one.

Evolution of bipedal stance

Standing up is what makes us human. So when did it evolve and why?

This turns out to be a surprisingly difficult question to answer. In 1978, Mary Leakey made the sensational discovery of ancient footprints extending more than 20 m, fossilized in cement-like volcanic ash on the arid Laetoli plain in Tanzania. The footprints were remarkable evidence of an adult couple strolling with their child across Africa around 3.7 million years ago. They probably belonged to the human ancestor (protohominid) *Australopithecus afarensis*, whose famous skeleton, *Lucy*, had been discovered four years previously. Lucy lived in the Pliocene, when climate change in the Rift valley caused tropical forests to be replaced by patches of savannah (open grassland).

The pattern of indentation in the footsteps is a rough guide to the amount of pressure transmitted by each region of the sole. A Laetoli footprint is shown here (Fig. 4.2, left) compared to a modern human print (Fig. 4.2, right), with darker areas reflecting greater weight bearing. Although the toes were longer than ours, the big toe was in alignment with the others, showing that the mechanism of weight transfer through the foot during walking was remarkably similar to ours.

It is thought that bipedal stance and locomotion aided these Australopithecines in moving from one clump of trees to another because they could see over the long grass and so spot any predators. Later, other advantages were evident: freeing the hands allowed them to be used for

Figure 4.2

making and using tools, and for carrying food and babies. Another theory holds that the brain became overheated as it enlarged in size, and standing helped keep it cool. We'll probably never know for certain, but those ancient evocative footprints at Laetoli will forever keep us wondering!

Abitbol M M 1995 Speculation on posture, locomotion, energy consumption, and blood flow in early hominids. Gait & Posture 3(1):29–37

ANKLE MOMENT

Whenever a force is applied some distance away from a joint or fulcrum, it will tend to rotate the joint in the direction of the force. This effect is called the *moment of force*, or simply the *joint moment*. In normal standing, with the CoP 5 cm anterior to the ankle joint, the foot will tend to dorsiflex (Fig. 4.3).

Figure 4.3   The ground reaction force typically acts about 5 cm anterior to the ankle joint, which causes an external dorsiflexor moment.

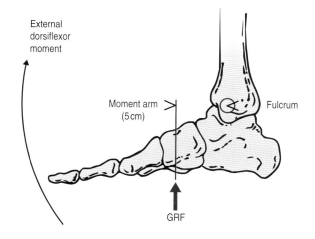

External dorsiflexor moment

Moment arm (5 cm)

Fulcrum

GRF

Standing in space

The GRF is caused by gravity – so what happens in the zero-*g* conditions of space flight?

Astronauts have long reported problems with increased sway while standing when they return from space flight. Inflight experiments aboard the space shuttle and *Mir* space station, in which bungee cords were used to simulate gravity, have revealed disordered responses to perturbations. Interestingly, these abnormalities improved when foot pressure was artificially applied to the feet, and special boots may be used in future to help prevent the problems with postural control on return to earth. These may also prove helpful for patients who need to undergo prolonged periods of bed rest.

Layne C S, Mulavara A P, McDonald P V et al 2001 The effect of long duration spaceflight on postural control during self-generated perturbations. Journal of Applied Physiology 90(3):997–1006

Figure 4.4 The external dorsiflexor moment is balanced by an internal plantarflexor moment generated by the plantarflexors (*gastrocnemius* + *soleus*) through the Achilles tendon.

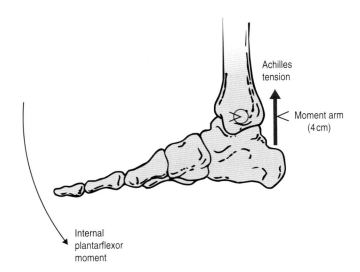

Since there is no movement in quiet standing, there must be an equal and opposite opposing moment (Newton's Third Law again). This moment is produced by tension (force) in the Achilles tendon (Fig. 4.4), which inserts onto the calcaneus bone on the opposite (posterior) aspect of the ankle joint. In effect, the two forces (ground reaction and Achilles tendon tension) act as an inverted see-saw (Fig. 4.5). The *external* moment at the ankle due to the GRV can be calculated quite simply:

$$\text{Ankle Moment} = \text{GRF} \times \text{Moment Arm of GRF}$$
$$= mgd$$

where m = body mass, g = acceleration due to gravity (9.81 m/s^2 – let's round it off to 10 to keep things simple) and d is the moment arm of the GRF (5 cm in this case). If the weight is borne symmetrically on the two feet, this total moment will need to be divided by two. So, we have:

$$\text{Ankle Moment} = (mgd)/2$$
So, if body mass = 80 kg, the moment at the ankle
$$= 80 \times 10 \times 0.05/2 = 20 \text{ N m}$$

? MCQ 4.1

What would be the ankle moment if the GRF passes through the ankle joint?
(a) 20 N m
(b) −20 N m
(c) 0 N m
(d) 1 N m

TENDON AND MUSCLE FORCES

This external moment at the ankle must be exactly balanced by the internal moment produced by the Achilles tendon force (Fig. 4.6).

From dissecting cadavers, it is known that the moment arm of the Achilles tendon (when the foot is *plantigrade*, i.e. ankle at 0°) is about 4 cm (you can estimate it yourself by measuring the distance between your

Figure 4.5 The external (ground reaction) and internal (Achilles tendon) forces act like an inverted see-saw at the ankle joint and need to be balanced during standing.

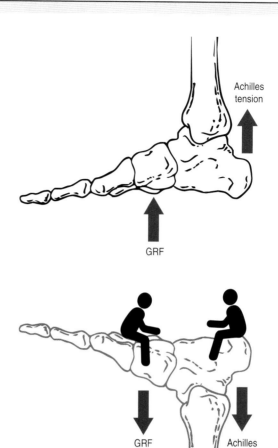

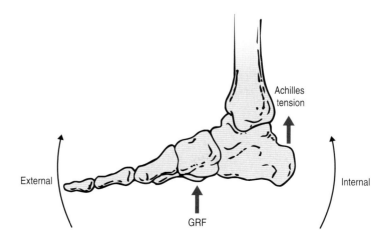

Figure 4.6 Balanced equilibrium between external and internal moments at the ankle.

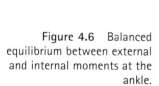

lateral malleolus and Achilles tendon). We can now estimate the force (tension) in the Achilles tendon:

Since, Ankle Moment = Tendon Force × Tendon Moment Arm
Tendon Force = Ankle Moment/Tendon Moment Arm
= 20/0.04, or 500 N

Although this force is transmitted via the Achilles tendon, it is, of course, mostly generated by muscle, since tendon is a passive structure. The muscles that insert onto it are the *soleus* and *gastrocnemius* (often called collectively the plantarflexors, or *triceps surae*). So, we now know that these muscles (in each leg) are contracting during normal quiet standing to provide a total force of 1000 N. This is quite a lot of force – equivalent to a weight of 100 kg, i.e. 20 kg more than body mass, so it's a surprising finding.

? MCQ 4.2

What is the tension in *each* Achilles tendon in a person of mass 60 kg standing symmetrically?
(a) 150 N
(b) 300 N
(c) 375 N
(d) 750 N

Tendon moment arms

The tendon moment arm does not have a fixed value – it changes slightly according to the angle of the joint (Fig. 4.7; from Maganaris et al 1998). In

Figure 4.7 (Reproduced by permission from Maganaris C N, Baltzopoulos V, Sargeant A J 1998 Changes in Achilles tendon moment arm from rest to maximum isometric plantarflexion: In vivo observations in man. Journal of Physiology 510:977–985, Blackwell Publishing).

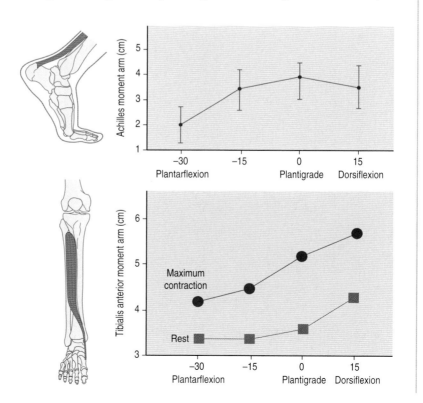

standing, the foot is plantigrade (flat on the ground) so the ankle is in neutral (0°), and the Achilles tendon lies approximately 4 cm posterior to the ankle joint axis. At other angles, the calcaneus rotates and moves the tendon insertion closer to the ankle joint axis. The *tibialis anterior* tendon moment arm is even more variable, because of the way it wraps under the retinaculum in front of the ankle. Its moment arm depends on the strength of the contraction as well as the ankle angle.

Maganaris C N, Baltzopoulos V, Sargeant A J 1998 Changes in Achilles tendon moment arm from rest to maximum isometric plantarflexion: In vivo observations in man. Journal of Physiology 510:977–985

Maganaris C N 2000 In vivo measurement-based estimations of the moment arm in the human tibialis anterior muscle-tendon unit. Journal of Biomechanics 33:375–379

CONTROL OF STANDING

The GRF isn't always 5 cm anterior to the ankle joint. If, for example, an external force (perturbation) – a gust of wind or a nudge from someone – pushes the person forwards, their body weight, and hence GRF, will also move forwards. The plantarflexors must balance the GRF to prevent collapse, so when it moves further forwards they must contract more strongly to generate a larger ankle moment. For example, say the GRF moves to 7 cm anterior to the ankle (Fig. 4.8).

The external moment is now:

$$\text{Ankle Moment} = \text{GRF Moment Arm of GRF}$$
$$= (mgd)/2$$
$$= 80 \times 10 \times 0.07/2$$
$$= 28 \text{ N m}$$

The new tendon force can now be calculated:

$$\text{Tendon Force} = \text{Ankle Moment/Tendon Moment Arm}$$
$$= 28/0.04, \text{ or } 700 \text{ N}$$

Figure 4.8   When the GRF acts further in front of the ankle, the external moment is increased, requiring a complementary increase in internal moment generated by increased tension in the Achilles tendon.

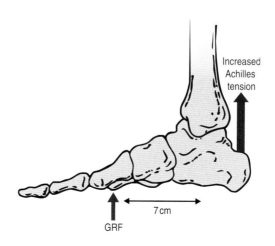

Increased Achilles tension

7 cm

GRF

? MCQ 4.3

What would be the new tendon force in the person of mass 60 kg?
(a) 150 N
(b) 350 N
(c) 375 N
(d) 525 N

The opposite can happen, too, of course. If a gust of wind blows the person backwards, the GRF may even move posteriorly – until it is

Figure 4.9 When the GRF passes behind the ankle joint, the external moment becomes plantarflexor, and must be resisted by an internal dorsiflexor moment, e.g. from *tibialis anterior* tension.

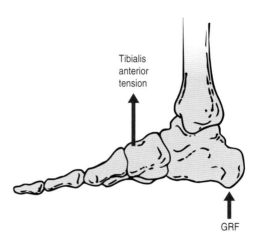

underneath the heel (Fig. 4.9). Now the GRF tends to *plantarflex* the ankle, and a restraining *dorsiflexor* moment is needed from muscles such as the *tibialis anterior* (TA).

Assuming that the TA tendon inserts 5 cm anterior to the ankle, if the GRF is 3 cm posterior to the ankle joint, the tendon force in an 80 kg person must now be:

$$\text{Tendon Force} = \text{Ankle Moment/Tendon Moment Arm}$$
$$= 80 \times 10 \times 0.03/(2 \times 0.05), \text{ or } 240 \text{ N}$$

? MCQ 4.4

What would be the TA tendon force for an 80 kg person if the GRF were 1 cm behind the ankle joint?
(a) 50 N
(b) 80 N
(c) 150 N
(d) 500 N

PROXIMAL JOINT MOMENTS

The same principle applies to the knee and hip joints. The internal joint moment at each joint must be equal and opposite to the moment exerted by the GRF. However, in quiet standing, the GRF usually passes pretty close to these joints, so the joint moments required are very small, and very little muscle action is needed.

Figure 4.10 During a squat, the GRF passes behind the knee. The moment arm is the perpendicular distance from the joint to line of the force – in this case 10 cm.

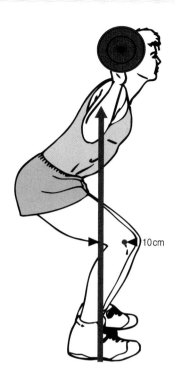

In a squatting posture (Fig. 4.10), the GRF now passes behind (posterior to) the knee joint, so the moment is now given by:

$$\text{Knee Moment} = \text{Force} \times \text{Moment Arm of GRF at knee}$$
$$= (mgd)/2$$

For example, assuming symmetrical standing, with a body mass of 80 kg (800 N) and the GRF passing 10 cm posterior to the knee, then

$$\text{Joint Moment} = 800 \times 0.1/2 = 40 \, \text{Nm}$$

Clearly, the knee will tend to collapse (flex) in this posture – in other words, this *external* moment is flexor. So, just as at the ankle, a muscle must generate an *internal* moment to maintain equilibrium. Since the external moment is flexor, the internal muscle moment must be extensor. In other words, the quadriceps muscle is contracting.

Rule of thumb: the active muscle is always the one on the opposite side of the joint to the GRF.

 MCQ 4.5

Which statement is true when the GRF is anterior to the hip joint?
(a) External moment is extensor
(b) Internal moment is flexor
(c) Active muscle is *iliopsoas*
(d) Active muscle is *gluteus maximus*

What happens if the GRF passes in front of the knee joint? By the rule of thumb, the flexors of the knee (hamstrings) must be active. However, the knee is a little special, in that in most people it cannot extend beyond

Figure 4.11 The posterior capsule ligaments prevent hyperextension.

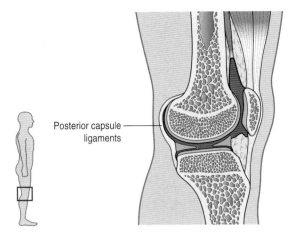

Posterior capsule ligaments

0°. The strong posterior capsule ligaments (Fig. 4.11) become taut at this angle and so prevent any hyperextension.

Thus, in the standing position, whenever the GRF passes anteriorly, the knee is *passively* stable and no muscle action is necessary. In this way, the knee and ankle work together – by maintaining the GRF forward of the ankle and slightly forward of the knee, the constant (*tonic*) contraction of the plantarflexors simplifies the control of standing considerably. Only occasional (*phasic*) contractions of the quadriceps muscle are needed when the GRF passes posterior to the knee axis in order to bring it back to the stable position.

KEY POINTS

★ In quiet standing the ground reaction force is equal and opposite to body weight

★ The centre of pressure falls about 5 cm anterior to the ankle joint

★ An external moment acts on the ankle equal to the force multiplied by the CoP

★ A balancing internal moment is generated by muscle tension on the opposite side of the joint

★ The internal moment is equal to the muscle tension multiplied by its lever arm at the joint

★ At the knee, the posterior capsule ligaments prevent hyperextension

Chapter **5**

The ground reaction in normal gait

OBJECTIVES

- Understand the relationship between force and acceleration
- Be familiar with vector representation of forces
- Understand how forces are resolved into their components
- Be familiar with the operation of a force platform
- Know the typical path of the centre of pressure in gait
- Know the effect of speed on the ground reaction
- Understand the origin of shock and how it is absorbed by the body

In quiet standing, the ground reaction is constant, being equal and opposite to body weight. During normal gait, however, it changes with the gait cycle, resembling the shape of a letter 'M' (Fig. 5.1). Notice what happens in each of the time periods A to E:

A. During initial double support, the force quickly rises as weight is transferred from the contralateral limb.

Figure 5.1   The vertical ground reaction force during normal gait varies above and below resting body weight. The left scale shows the force in newtons (N), while the right scale shows the normalized force obtained by dividing it by body weight (*mg*) and expressed as a percentage (data from Winter 1991).

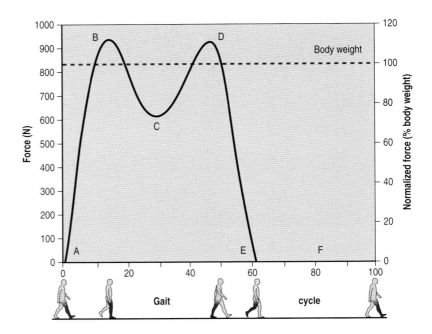

B. The force rises above resting body weight in early stance.
C. The force falls below resting body weight during mid-stance.
D. The force rises above resting body weight once again in late stance.
E. During terminal double support, the force quickly falls as weight is transferred to the contralateral limb.
F. Swing phase: the foot is off the ground so there is no ground reaction force.

Any rise or fall of the force above or below body weight must mean that there is some extra acceleration. A good way to get a feel for this is to take a trip on an elevator. If you can, take a set of bathroom scales to measure your weight, otherwise just concentrate on feeling what happens at each stage (Fig. 5.2). Note the following:

A. The subject's resting weight. Although bathroom scales are calibrated in kg (mass), they really measure force. To calculate the load in newtons the reading needs to be multiplied by *g* (about 10 m/s²). So, for example, a person of mass 70 kg has a weight (ground reaction) of *mg* = 700 N but the scales *read* 70 kg.
B. Press the button to go up. Weight increases, because it is now added to by an amount $F = ma$, where *a* is the acceleration upwards (the slope of the speed graph is upwards, i.e. positive). If, for example, $a = 2$ m/s², the new weight will be $700 + 70 \times 2 = 840$ N (the scales will read 84 kg). The actual value will depend on the acceleration of the elevator.
C. Once the elevator reaches its constant speed, acceleration falls back to zero, and body weight falls back to its resting value (700 N).

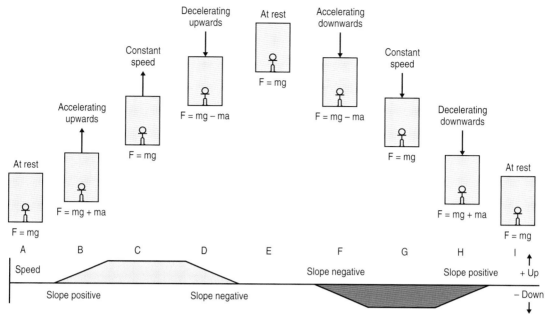

Figure 5.2   Changes in body weight during an elevator ride.

D. As the elevator approaches the requested floor, it slows down (decelerates). This is another way of saying that the acceleration, *a*, is now negative (the slope of the speed graph is now negative). Body weight is therefore *decreased* by an amount −*ma*, i.e. 700 − 70 × 2 = 660 N (and the scales will show 66 kg).

E. Once the elevator comes to rest again, body weight returns to its resting value.

F. Now press the button to descend. There is now a downward acceleration, i.e. *a* is negative. So body weight falls by −*ma* (to 660 N).

G. As the elevator speed plateaus, weight once again returns to normal.

H. On approaching the lower floor, the elevator is decelerating downwards. This is equivalent to accelerating upwards, so body weight increases once again by an amount +*ma* (to 840 N).

By now, it should be clear that the ground reaction varies above and below resting body weight according to vertical acceleration. Moreover, note that the reaction force is not affected by constant speed up or down (as happens when the elevator travels between floors).

? MCQ 5.1

What would the scales read if a person of mass 70 kg stands on them inside an elevator accelerating upwards at 2 m/s²? (assume *g* = 10 m/s²)

(a) 84 kg
(b) 70 kg
(c) 66 kg
(d) 35 kg

The spring in your step

The person who walks with short and slow steps is a person who starts his business sluggishly and does not pursue a goal.

Aristotle

Time wounds all heels.

Groucho Marx

The amount of fluctuation in the ground reaction force may be related, amongst other things, to mood. Depressed people seem to have a less pronounced M-shape to their force profiles, perhaps lending support to the adage that happiness is associated with a 'spring in the step' (Sloman et al 1987). Among the factors that were inversely correlated with the amplitude of the GRF fluctuation were mood ($r = -0.32$), sleep disturbance ($r = -0.46$) and indecisiveness ($r = -0.38$). Although the findings are likely due to the depressed subjects walking more slowly (Lemke et al 2000), they do reveal an interesting relationship between motion and emotion.

Ironically, the person who possibly takes the prize for the least 'springy' gait in history is Groucho Marx (Fig. 5.3), the American comedian. His characteristic gait kept vertical accelerations to a minimum, resulting in a 'tabletop' pattern of ground reaction force, with hardly any fluctuation above or below resting body weight. Charlie Chaplin's (Fig. 5.4) gait, on the other hand, seems calculated to generate the most extreme fluctuations in all three components of force.

Sloman L, Pierrynowski M, Berridge M et al 1987 Mood, depressive illness and gait patterns. Canadian Journal of Psychiatry 32:190–193

Lemke M R, Wendorff T, Mieth B et al 2000 Spatiotemporal gait patterns during ground locomotion in major depression compared with healthy controls. Journal of Psychiatric Research 34:277–283

McMahon T A, Valiant G, Frederick E C 1987 Groucho running. Journal of Applied Physiology 62(6):2326–2337

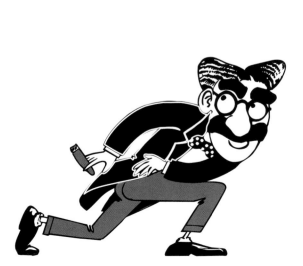

Figure 5.3   Groucho Marx.

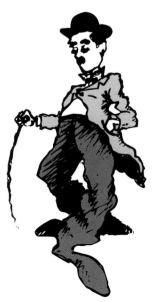

Figure 5.4   Charlie Chaplin.

SHEAR FORCES

In quiet standing, the ground reaction is vertical, since it opposes body weight. When movement occurs, as in walking, other forces act too. These forces are horizontal, rather than vertical, and are called *shear* forces. They are produced due to friction between the foot and the ground. Just as body weight acting downwards generates an equal and opposite upward ground reaction, a shear force that acts anteriorly on the ground causes an equal and opposite *posterior* reaction (Fig. 5.5).

FORCE PLATFORMS

The individual load and the shear components of the GRV can be measured using a *force platform* (sometimes also called a force *plate*) (Fig. 5.6). This is a precision instrument using either strain gauges (e.g. those made by Advanced Medical Technologies, Watertown, MA, USA and Bertec Corp., Columbus, OH, USA) or piezo-electric quartz crystals (e.g. Kistler Instruments, Winterthur, Switzerland) to convert force into electric signals.

Figure 5.5 Shear force caused by friction between the foot and ground.

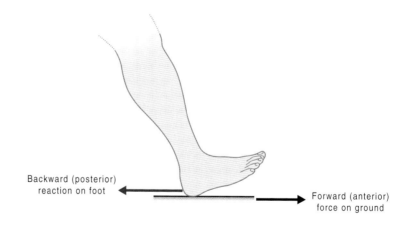

Figure 5.6 Force platform measuring three components of force.

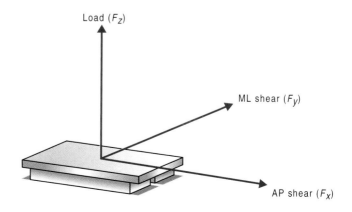

Note that it is possible to describe the forces in two ways: the force *on the platform* (action-orientated) or the *reaction on the body* (reaction-orientated). Although these are equal, they are in opposite directions so will have opposite signs. The latter (reaction on the body) is the convention most often used. In the example, a positive AP shear would indicate a ground reaction directed to the right of the page. The platform can also be mounted longitudinally or transversely, so in most laboratories the *x*-axis component represents AP, and in others the ML shear. To avoid confusion, it is therefore best to label shear forces by F_{AP} and F_{ML} rather than F_x and F_y.

Clean and dirty strikes

One potential problem with assessing someone's gait with a force platform is that a *clean* foot-strike is needed. This means that the foot must land within the boundaries of the platform (Fig. 5.7), otherwise not all the GRF will be recorded. Moreover, if both feet land on the platform during double support (a *double strike*) the force recorded will be a meaningless mixture of the GRF of both sides.

When two or more platforms are used, the best configuration is probably to place them directly adjacent (Fig. 5.8A), allowing a small gap (2–3 mm) between to ensure valid shear measurements. Some laboratories have opted for a staggered arrangement (Fig. 5.8B or C) in order to try to capture two successive foot-strikes. However, this is often too ambitious and may encourage the subject to adapt their step length to strike both platforms.

A short step length (as found in children and many pathological gaits) often leads to a double strike. The chance of this happening can be reduced by using

Figure 5.7

Figure 5.8

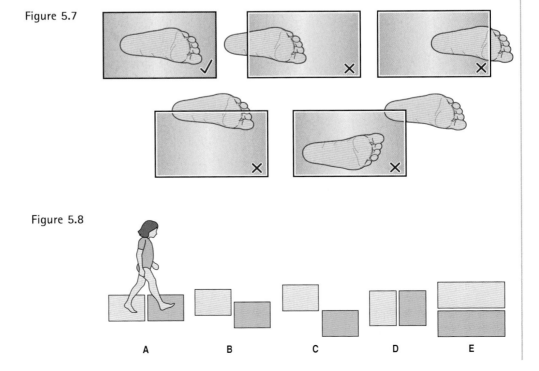

A   B   C   D   E

smaller platforms (Oggero et al 1997) or rotating standard ones (Fig. 5.8D). Some laboratories have two long platforms in parallel (Fig. 5.8E), but this may interfere with the subject's natural gait because they are asked to walk down the centre-line, with each foot (hopefully) striking its respective platform.

People are often very cooperative when their gait is being analysed, and may adjust their stride in order to make a clean strike on the platform (Paul 1996). Several techniques have been devised to discourage this behaviour, although they are rarely completely successful. For example, practice trials are useful to establish a starting point from which a clean strike is more likely, assuming, of course, that stride length is consistent. Nevertheless, subjects will inevitably tend, consciously or subconsciously, to aim for the platform, so some laboratories disguise the platform by covering the walkway with a carpet (Augsburger et al 1996). Unfortunately, this usually means that a lot of trials have to be discarded until a clean strike is obtained, and the subject can become tired, especially if he or she has a walking disorder. The effect of targeting is, in practice, probably quite minimal (Grabiner et al 1996 a,b, Wearing et al 2003).

Augsburger S, Oeffinger D, Edester B et al 1996 The effects of carpet on a motion analysis laboratory floor and forceplates. Gait & Posture 4(2):190–191

Grabiner M D, Davis B L, Lundin T M, Feuerbach J W 1996a. Visual guidance to forceplates does not increase ground reaction force variability. Journal of Biomechanics 28:115–117

Grabiner M D, Davis B L, Lundin T M, Feuerbach J W 1996b. Author's response. Journal of Biomechanics 29(6):833

Oggero E, Pagnacco G, Morr D R, Simon S R, Berme N 1997 Probability of valid gait data acquisition using currently available force plates. Biomedical Sciences Instrumentation 34:392–397

Paul J P 1996 Letter to the editor (about the study by Grabiner et al 1996b). Journal of Biomechanics 29(6):833

Wearing S C, Smeathers J E, Urry S R 2003 Frequency-domain analysis detects previously unidentified changes in ground reaction force with visually guided foot placement. Journal of Applied Biomechanics 19(1):71–78

SHEAR COMPONENTS IN NORMAL GAIT

A typical recording of all three ground reaction components during normal gait is shown in Figure 5.9. It can be seen that the shear components are much smaller than the load (vertical reaction). Notice too, that while the load is always positive (because gravity only acts downwards), the shear components can switch direction. For example, the AP (or *fore–aft*) shear is directed posteriorly (braking) in the first 50% of stance (i.e. 35% cycle) but anteriorly (propulsive) in late stance. ML shear is almost always directed medially in response to lateral motion of the body. Its size is proportional to stride width (Carlsöö et al 1974).

NORMATIVE VALUES

Normative ranges for the mean (in % body weight) and standard deviation at each peak of the three force components, along with the time (in % gait cycle) at which the peak occurs, are given in Table 5.1 (Giakas & Baltzopoulos 1997).

Figure 5.9 The three components of the ground reaction force during normal gait.

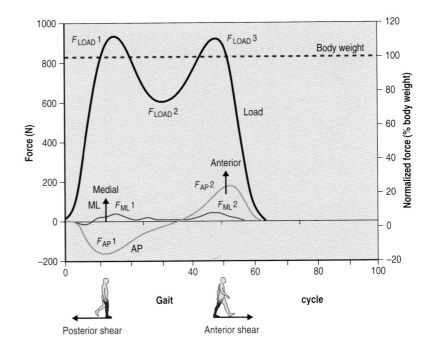

Table 5.1 Normative ranges for the force peaks of each component of the GRF (from Giakas & Baltzopoulos 1997)

Force (% BW)	Mean ± 1 SD	Time (% cycle)	Mean ± 1 SD
$F_{LOAD}1$	117 ± 9	$T_{LOAD}1$	23 ± 2
$F_{LOAD}2$	75 ± 6	$T_{LOAD}2$	48 ± 3
$F_{LOAD}3$	109 ± 5	$T_{LOAD}3$	76 ± 2
$F_{AP}1$	−19 ± 3	$T_{AP}1$	17 ± 2
$F_{AP}2$	22 ± 3	$T_{AP}2$	86 ± 2
$F_{ML}1$	5 ± 1	$T_{ML}1$	5 ± 0.5
$F_{ML}2$	4 ± 1	$T_{ML}2$	44 ± 15

VECTORS

Looking at more than one graph at the same time can be a bit confusing. Luckily, there is a nice way to combine them back together again into a single force, called the *ground reaction vector* (GRV). Its size (magnitude) can be calculated by the Pythagoras theorem (the square of the hypotenuse of a right-angled triangle equals the sum of the squares of the other two sides), whilst its direction (θ) is given by the tangent of the load divided by the shear (Fig. 5.10).

Alternatively, the total GRV can be *resolved* into its components by trigonometry. Sometimes it's more helpful to think of the total GRV while at other times it is more useful to think of it in terms of its components, so it's worth getting a feel for how this conversion works.

Figure 5.10 The GRV is the geometric sum of the load and shear components.

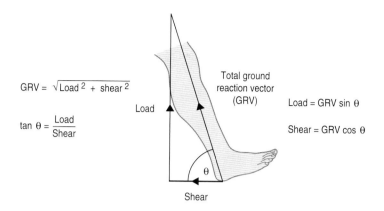

$$GRV = \sqrt{\text{Load}^2 + \text{shear}^2}$$

$$\tan \theta = \frac{\text{Load}}{\text{Shear}}$$

Load

Total ground
reaction vector
(GRV)

Load = GRV sin θ

Shear = GRV cos θ

θ

Shear

? MCQ 5.2

What is the total GRV if the load is 400 N and the shear 300 N?
(a) 100 N
(b) 200 N
(c) 500 N
(d) 700 N

CENTRE OF PRESSURE

During normal gait, the Centre of Pressure (CoP) moves from the lateral border of the heel at initial contact, along the foot to the big toe (hallux) at toe-off (Fig. 5.11). Remember that the CoP is the mean of all the pressure applied to the sole of the foot (centre of foot pressure). So, if the foot pronates the pathway of the CoP will tend to move medially, whereas on supination it will tend to move toward the lateral border.

Figure 5.11 Pathway of the Centre of Pressure (CoP) in normal gait. Starting at the lateral border of the heel at initial contact, it moves along the centre of the foot, until at the metatarsophalangeal joints it turns medial to finish under the hallux at toe-off. When the foot pronates, the CoP moves medially, while in supination it moves laterally.

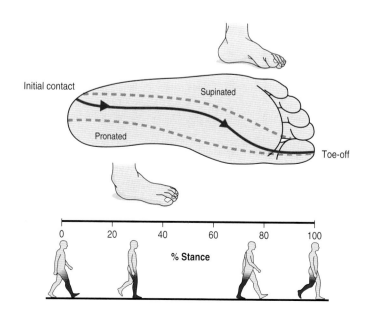

BUTTERFLY DIAGRAM

The changes in size and orientation of the GRV through the gait cycle can be summarized by constructing a 'butterfly' or Pedotti (Boccardi et al 1977, Pedotti 1977) diagram (Fig. 5.12). The diagram also shows that the forward speed of the CoP (indicated by the spacing at the base of each vector) is not constant: it tends to slow down, or linger, over the instep and the metatarsophalangeal joints (MTPJs).

EFFECT OF SPEED

The main effect of speed on the vertical GRF (Fig. 5.13) seems to be to increase the braking peak and to decrease further the force during

Figure 5.12   Butterfly or Pedotti diagram. Each arrow represents the GRV at each point in the gait cycle, the base of each vector being the CoP at that point in time. Notice that the progress of the vector is not constant – it slows down over the instep and metatarsophalangeal areas.

Figure 5.13   Effect of speed on the load (vertical GRF) during normal walking. Note that the time axis is limited to the stance phase in this figure (all GRFs are, of course, zero in swing) (redrawn from Stansfield et al 2001, with permission).

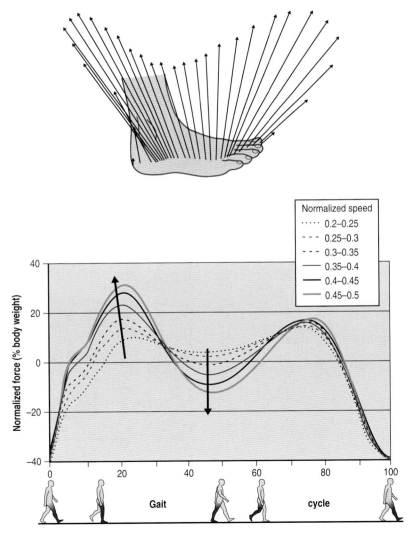

mid-stance. The final (propulsive) peak is almost unaffected by walking speed. Both the braking and propulsive peaks of the AP shear increase with walking speed (Fig. 5.14).

Not surprisingly, AP shear is closely related to stride length (Martin & Marsh 1992), with

braking AP shear (in % body weight) = 31 − normalized SL × 8.36

and

propulsive AP shear = 30 × normalized SL − 6.4 ($r^2 = 0.99$)

TOTAL BODY GRF

A single force platform records the GRF on one limb, but it should be noted that during double support the total force on the body is the sum of the GRF on each foot. This can only be seen if two or more force platforms are used to capture successive footfalls (Fig. 5.15). In contrast to the usual smooth pattern of the GRF recorded from a single limb, the total GRF is seen to be quite irregular during these periods.

ACCURACY OF FORCE PLATFORM MEASUREMENTS

In general, force platforms are extremely accurate instruments. However, they need to be mounted correctly to obtain valid results (Gill & O'Connor 1997, Fairburn et al 2000). This is done by firmly attaching the platform to concrete (usually in a specially constructed trench beneath

Figure 5.14   Effect of speed on the anteroposterior (AP) shear force during normal walking (redrawn from Stansfield et al 2001, with permission).

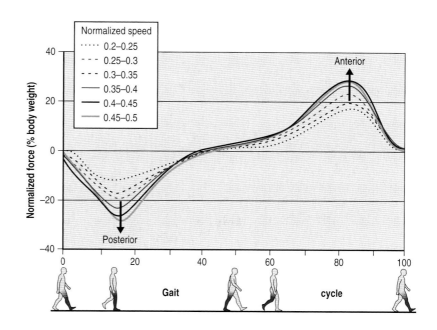

Figure 5.15 During double support phase, the total GRF on the body is the sum of the GRF from each side (dashed lines), as revealed in this recording from a person walking across three force platforms. Notice that the individual force curves are quite smooth while the total force is somewhat irregular during double support.

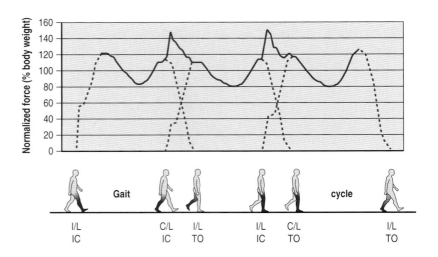

the gait laboratory floor) (Fig. 5.16). If this is not done the natural frequency of the platform may fall, causing a phenomenon called *ringing*. This is caused by resonance of the platform, and will result in an artefact in the force recorded. It is possible to buy specially designed portable force platforms, but these inevitably suffer from a lower natural frequency.

TREADMILL FORCE PLATFORMS

A few companies have recently introduced treadmills with built-in force platforms. Kistler Gaitway (Kistler Gmbh, Winterthur, Switzerland) has one piezo-electric platform under the belt that is capable of measuring vertical load, while AMTI (Newton, MA, USA) is also sensitive to shear forces. The ADAL3D dynamometric treadmill has split belts, each equipped with separate transducers, and is able to continuously measure the three forces and moments under each limb.

Figure 5.16 Mounting a force platform on concrete in a trench under the walkway.

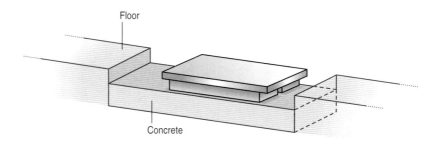

CLINICAL POINTER – INTERPRETATION OF THE GRF IN DISEASE

Although the GRF is a very *sensitive* measure of walking pathology, its *specificity* is low, since it is a whole body measure that integrates the motion (acceleration) of all body segments.

- The integral (area under the curve) of the force, called the *impulse*, is useful for quality control purposes. It is generally desired that subjects are tested at equilibrium, i.e. walking at a constant speed, neither speeding up nor slowing down. This can be verified by checking that the AP impulse over a complete gait cycle is zero (Seliktar et al 1979). It has to be said that this is rarely done in practice because it would require many trials to be discarded and repeated.
- Butterfly diagrams enjoyed a brief period of popularity some years ago (Khodadadeh 1988) but seem to be rarely used these days.
- Surprisingly, the GRF profile of the left and right sides are not necessarily symmetrical, even in healthy individuals (Herzog et al 1989), making its use for detecting unilateral pathology questionable.
- Force platforms can be used to determine the whole body centre of mass (see chapter 9).
- By far the most important use for force platforms is, in combination with the gait kinematics, to determine muscle activity by calculating the joint moments.

KEY POINTS

★ Forces are proportional to acceleration: $F = ma$

★ The ground reaction force is composed of a vertical load, anteroposterior shear and mediolateral shear

★ These three components can be combined to form a ground reaction vector

★ During normal gait, the vertical load component rises and falls about body weight

★ The anteroposterior shear force is directed backwards then forwards during stance phase

★ The centre of pressure is the mean of all foot pressure, and moves from heel to hallux

References

Boccardi S, Chiesa G, Pedotti A 1977 New procedure for evaluation of normal and abnormal gait. American Journal of Physical Medicine 56:163–182

Carlsöö S, Dahllöf A G, Holm J 1974 Kinetic analysis of the gait in patients with hemiparesis and in patients with intermittent claudication. Scandinavian Journal of Rehabilitation Medicine 6(4):166–179

Fairburn P S, Palmer R, Whybrow J et al 2000 A prototype system for testing force platform dynamic performance. Gait & Posture 12(1):25–33

Giakas G, Baltzopoulos V 1997 Time and frequency domain analysis of ground reaction forces during walking: an investigation of variability and symmetry. Gait & Posture 5: 189–197

Gill H S, O'Connor J J 1997 A new testing rig for force platform calibration and accuracy tests, Gait & Posture 5(3):228–232

Herzog W, Nigg B M, Read L J, Olsen E 1989 Asymmetries in ground reaction force patterns in normal human gait. Medicine and Science in Sports and Exercise 21(1):110–114

Khodadadeh S 1988 Vector (butterfly) diagrams for osteoarthritic gait. Journal of Medical Engineering and Technology 12(1):15–19

Martin P E, Marsh A P 1992 Step length and frequency effects on ground reaction forces during walking. Journal of Biomechanics 25(10):1237–1239

Pedotti A 1977 Simple equipment used in clinical practice for evaluation of locomotion. IEEE Transactions in Biomedical Engineering BME 24:5

Seliktar R, Yekutiel M, Bar A 1979 Gait consistency test based on the impulse-momentum theorem. Prosthetics and Orthotics International 3:91–98

Stansfield B W, Hazlewood M E, Hillman S J et al 2001 Normalised speed, not age, characterizes ground reaction force patterns in 5–12 year old children walking at self selected speeds, Journal of Paediatric Orthopaedics 21(3):395–402

Winter D A 1991 The biomechanics and motor control of human gait: normal, elderly and pathological. University of Waterloo Press, Ontario, Canada

Chapter 6

Plantar pressure measurement

He had a foot forming almost a straight line with the leg, which, however, did not prevent it from being turned in, so that it was an equinus together with something of a varus, or else a slight varus with a strong tendency to equinus. But with this equinus, wide in foot like a horse's hoof, with rugose skin, dry tendons, and large toes, on which the black nails looked as if made of iron, the clubfoot ran about like a deer from morn till night.

Gustave Flaubert *(Madame Bovary)*

OBJECTIVES

- Know how pressure is distributed over the sole of the normal foot
- Appreciation of the benefits and limitations of presently available measurement equipment
- Know the commonly used measures used for interpretation of plantar pressure measurements
- Understand the principles involved in the use of plantar pressure measurement in diabetic care
- Know the typical patterns of plantar pressure in common foot disorders

The sole of the foot is uniquely responsible for transmitting forces from the ground to the body, and so the distribution of pressure over its surface is naturally of great interest. From earliest times, people have noticed that the deepest parts of footprints correspond to the highest pressures, and a pioneering researcher (Beely 1882) requested his patients to step on a linen bag filled with quick-setting plaster of Paris. He concluded that in standing the heel and the heads of the 2nd and 3rd metatarsals (MTHs) bore the greatest pressures. In the early 20th century Seitz observed changes in blood flow through the capillaries of the sole as an indication of pressure and Basler reported that the skin becomes completely ischaemic under a pressure of about 10 kPa.

The first dynamic pressure studies during walking were performed using a rubber mat (Elftman 1934, Morton 1952), and popularized for clinical use by Harris and Beath (Barrett 1976, Evanski & Waugh 1980, Silvino et al 1980). Later, optical techniques (*pedobarography*) were developed, exploiting the ability of pressure on a plastic film to polarize or reflect light, which was observed by a video camera below a glass platform (Arcan & Brull 1976, Betts et al 1980, Franks et al 1983). In recent years, matrix arrays of force or pressure transducers (*electrodynography*) have become popular (Soames & Atha 1981).

METHODS OF MEASURING PLANTAR PRESSURES

There are basically five means of operation used by currently available pressure sensors:

- Optical – the oldest method (*pedobarography*), which relies on the ability of pressure to cause interference patterns on light reflected from plastic film (Betts et al 1980)
- Capacitive – which relies on the change of electrical capacitance when two plates are pressed together (Hennig & Rosenbaum 1991, Cavanagh & Ulbrecht 1994)
- Piezo-resistive – in which the resistance of a special conductive ink is changed on application of pressure (Lord et al 1992, Young 1993, Ashruf 2002)
- Piezo-electric – in which pressure on a ceramic (quartz or polyvinylidene fluoride, PvDF) crystal generates an electrical voltage (Hennig et al 1982, Manouel et al 1992, Lanshammer et al 1993, Akhlaghi & Pepper 1996).
- Laser (Hughes et al 2000).

Piezo-electric sensors are potentially the most accurate. Unfortunately, nobody has yet succeeded in making a flat plate commercial sensor. In the *Parotec* system (Paromed Medizintechnik GmbH, Germany) piezo-electric pressure sensors are mounted within small fluid *hydrocells* (Chesnin et al 2000). This has some advantages and some disadvantages. One advantage is that the sensor responds to shear (friction) as well as vertical loading (though they cannot be distinguished; the pressure measured is a summation of all components). A disadvantage is that the insole is a little thicker than other systems. The array size is also currently limited to just 32 sensors, which cover only 23% of the sole area. A non-commercial system, *Gaitscan*, uses small square sandwiches of PvDF film between copper plates and is capable of independent measurement of shear and vertical load (Akhlaghi & Pepper 1996).

In addition to the type of sensor, there are two design options available:

- Flat-plate systems, which are mounted or placed on the floor in a similar manner to force platforms (Cavanagh & Hennig 1982), measure the pressure between the (usually bare) foot and the floor (Fig. 6.1).
- Insole systems, which are worn inside the shoe, record the pressures between the foot and shoe sole (Fig. 6.2). These have the added advantages of being able to record multiple steps, and whilst wearing a functional foot orthosis (Cavanagh 1992, Akhlagi & Pepper 1996).

Figure 6.1 Flat plate type of plantar pressure measurement system (reproduced by permission of *HRMat*, Tekscan Inc., South Boston, MA, USA).

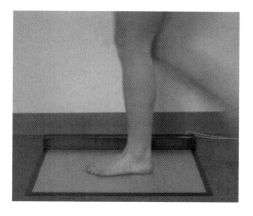

Figure 6.2 Insole plantar pressure measurement (reproduced by permission of *F-Scan*, Tekscan Inc., South Boston, MA, USA).

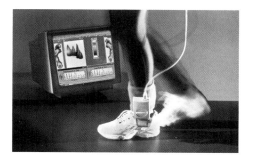

Hobbling gods

Why do the women of Elis summon Dionysus in their hymns to come among them with his bull-foot?

Plutarch (*Greek Questions*)

Psychiatrist: Your son has an Oedipus complex.

Yiddish Mother: Oedipus, Shmoedipus, so long as he loves his mother!

Lamed gods are common in many cultures, and the heel seems to be have been especially holy. Jacob (Ja-aceb meaning 'heel-god' in Hebrew) became king after his wrestling match with an angel left him with a dislocated hip (Genesis 30: 25 & 33: 4). The resulting leg length discrepancy would have caused him to walk on the forefoot of the affected side, with his sacred heel lifted off the ground. The weakness of Achilles ('swift of foot') was, of course, the heel that was held when he was being immortalized by his mother dipping him into the River Styx.

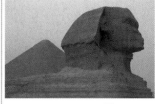

Figure 6.3

Hephæstus (or Vulcan) was born from Hera's thigh with his clubfeet facing backwards. She threw him off Mount Olympus for being so ugly (Iliad 14.395). In his underwater smithy, he crafted golden leg-braces and high-heeled shoes, as well as building two golden robots to help him move around.

When the Theban king Laios asked the Delphic oracle whether he would have a son, the oracle replied that he would, but that this son was destined to kill his father. So Laius drove a spike through the baby's ankles, bound them together with a leather thong, and gave the baby to a herdsman to expose on Mt Cithaeron. The peasant named him Oedipus: Oidus means swollen and pous means foot. Oido also means 'I know', and Oedipus later answered the riddle of the Sphinx (Fig. 6.3): Which animal has one voice, but two, three or four feet, being slowest on three? Perhaps inspired by his own disability, he answered correctly: Man (who walks on four feet as a baby, and aided by a stick as an old man), becoming the new ruler and taking the hand of his widowed mother, Jocasta (Odyssey 11.271–280). Freud later used the term Oedipus complex to describe a man in love with his mother.

Talus (whose name is given to the ankle bone) was a giant on the island of Crete. His weak spot was a vein above one ankle, through which his *ichor* (life-blood of an immortal) flowed. He died when Medea's pin pierced his heel. On reading Ovid's account in 1640, the Oxford parson Francis Potter proposed the idea of blood transfusion, going on to conduct transfusion experiments between animals and humans!

Like Talus, Orion was a giant from Crete. After boasting that he would exterminate all the animals on Earth, he was punished by the Earth Goddess, Gaia, who sent Scorpio, a giant scorpion, to sting Orion on his heel, which is marked by Rigel (Arabic for foot), the brightest star in the Orion constellation (Fig. 6.4). The constellation Eridanus is the blood flowing from his wound.

Figure 6.4

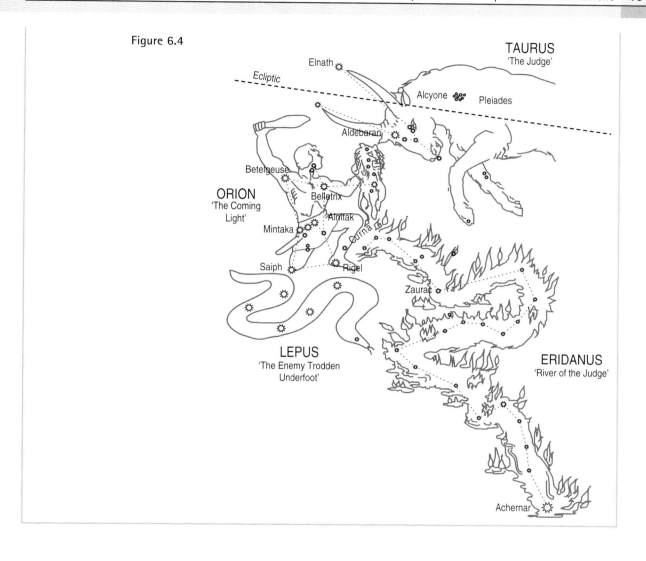

UNITS OF PRESSURE

Pressure is defined as the force per unit area, i.e.:

Pressure = Force/Area

It follows that pressure can be reduced either by reducing the force applied (not usually practical) or, more usefully, increasing the area over which forces acts.

The SI unit of pressure is the pascal (Pa), the pressure exerted by a force of 1 N over an area of 1 m^2 (1 N/m^2). Since this is an extremely low pressure, the kilopascal (kPa), the pressure exerted by a force of 0.1 N over an area of 1 cm^2 (0.1 N/cm^2), is more often used:

$$\text{Pressure} = 0.1/(10^{-2})^2$$
$$= 0.1 \times 10^4 = 10^3 = 1000 \text{ Pa or 1 kPa}$$

Since weight = mg (where g is the acceleration due to gravity = 9.81 m/s²), this is equivalent to a weight of about 0.01 kg, similar to that of a coin acting over an area approximately equal to a fingertip. A continuously applied pressure of 15–20 kPa is sufficient to stop arterial blood flow and pain occurs when plantar pressure exceeds 255 kPa (Bauman et al 1963, Silvino et al 1980).

Rather confusingly, several other units are in common use for pressure. For example, blood pressure is measured in mmHg, the height of a column of mercury in millimetres. Pressure in a fluid column is calculated by:

$$\text{Pressure} = \rho g h$$

where ρ is the density of the fluid, g = 9.81 m/s² and h is the height of the column in metres. The relative density of mercury is 13.6, meaning that it is 13.6 times denser than water, which has a density of 1000 kg/m³. So, the pressure in Pa due to a mercury column of 1 mm (0.001 m) = 13.6 × 1000 × 9.81 × 0.001 = 133 Pa or 0.13 kPa.

Table 6.1 summarizes the various conversion factors between each of these units, along with some others that can be useful for getting a feel for what pressures mean in practice.

? | **MCQ 6.1**

Express mean arterial pressure (100 mmHg) in kPa (use g = 9.81 m/s²).
(a) 13
(b) 7.5
(c) 130
(d) 750

LIMITATIONS OF PRESSURE SENSORS

It is important to be aware of several limitations from which pressure sensors, unlike force transducers such as force platforms, tend to suffer (Ahoni et al 1998). Manufacturers are sometimes reluctant to quote the specifications of their sensors or report calibration curves. A calibration curve can be obtained by cycling the sensor through a range of known

Table 6.1 Multiplication factors for conversion between the various units used for reporting plantar pressure (mbar = millibar; mmHg = millimetres of mercury; mmH₂0 = millimetres of water; atm = atmospheres)

Unit	kPa	N/cm²	mbar	kg/cm²	psi	mmHg	mmH₂0	atm
kPa	1	0.1	10	0.01	0.14	7.5	102	0.01
N/cm²	10	1	100	0.1	1.45	75	1020	0.1
mbar	0.1	0.01	1	0.001	0.015	0.75	10	0.001
kg/cm²	98.1	9.81	981	1	14.2	735	10,000	0.97
psi	6.9	0.69	69	0.07	1	52	703	0.068
mmHg	0.13	0.013	1.3	0.00134	0.02	1	13.6	0.0013
mmH₂0	0.01	0.001	0.1	0.0001	0.0014	0.074	1	0.0001
atm	101	10.1	1,013	1.03	14.7	760	10,332	1

pressures in a materials testing system (Fig. 6.5). The following parameters are generally used to characterize the performance of the sensor:

- Calibrated or Dynamic Range: the range of pressure values that the sensor is designed to measure. This range is defined by the manufacturer, and performance is not guaranteed outside this range. In general, a range of 0–1000 kPa is needed for gait assessment (Duckworth et al 1982).

- Maximum pressure rating: high levels of pressure may irreversibly damage the sensor.

- Accuracy: the maximum difference between the actual (known) pressure (as measured by some *gold standard* technique) and that measured by the sensor, expressed as a percentage of the calibrated range of the sensor.

- Linearity: the maximum discrepancy between sensor readings from a straight line (linear regression).

- Hysteresis: the difference between the measured pressure during loading compared to that measured during unloading. Hysteresis is a particular problem of in-shoe sensors, which by their nature must conform to the shape of the foot and shoe (Woodburn & Helliwell 1996). Such flexibility is inevitably accompanied by a tendency for the elastomer material in the sensor to exhibit *viscoelastic* properties with a *memory* or *time-dependent* effect (Buis & Convery 1996). Readings obtained from the sensor thus reflect, to some degree, its past history. This is a major reason why most in-shoe sensors must be replaced after a certain number of examinations.

- Creep or Drift: a related problem to hysteresis is a tendency for sensor readings to gradually change over time when a constant load is applied. Most foot pressure systems use the body mass of the subject

Figure 6.5 Generalized calibration curve of a typical transducer used in plantar pressure measurement.

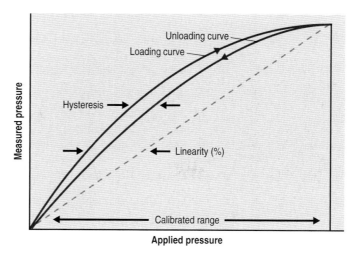

to re-calibrate the sensors and so correct for drift. A related problem of piezo-electric systems, charge leakage, makes them less suitable for static tests.

- Dynamic response: the ability of the sensor to respond to rapid changes in loading (such as occur at initial contact). This is a function of the natural frequency of the sensor, which should be as high as possible to avoid resonance (Antonsson & Mann 1985). There may also be a phase shift, in which the output of the sensor lags behind the changes in applied load. In general, metal or ceramic sensors are stiffer and so have a higher natural frequency than polymer (plastic or rubber) sensors.

- Curvature artefacts: some sensors are designed to be thin in order to conform to the contour of the sole. Whilst this has advantages in terms of validity because the effect of the sensor on the pressure measured is minimal, the bending of the sensors can generate spurious data (artefacts). This can be avoided to some extent by applying a metal backing to the sensors, but of course this makes them more rigid (Zhu et al 1995).

- Crosstalk: this means that load applied to one sensor affects the readings from those adjacent to it. It may be mechanical, due to deformation of the sensor array (a common problem in optical pedobarography), or electrical (especially in capacitative systems), due to the characteristics of the amplifier and other electronic hardware used to transfer the data to the computer.

- Off-axis stresses: a matrix of sensors is designed to respond to loads at the centre of each sensor. In reality, the pressure is distributed over the sensor such that some falls at its edge, which may result in inaccuracies. In general, the smaller the sensor the less susceptible it is to off-axis stresses.

- Temperature: temperature can have a marked effect on some (especially piezo-electric) sensors and may be monitored simultaneously (e.g. Parotec) in order to correct the readings.

- Size: it has been suggested that the optimal sensor diameter for recording plantar pressures during gait should be less than 6 mm, with larger sensors likely to underestimate peak plantar pressures (PPPs), especially under the toes (Davis et al 1996).

Several flat-plate and insole systems utilize force sensitive resistor (piezo-resistive) technology. *F-Scan* (Tekscan Inc., South Boston, MA, USA) has an array of 960 individual FSR elements per foot (4 sensors per cm²). The insole system can be trimmed to fit shoe size, is extremely thin (less than 0.2 mm) and conforms to the foot shape (Hsiao et al 2002). This is usually advantageous, though can sometimes give rise to inaccuracies due to bending of the insole. Each sensor is sampled at 165 Hz (which entails some 316,800 individual sensor readings per second). The insoles can be reused for up to 10 examinations. An untethered version (*F-Scan Mobile*) records the data to memory in a small ankle cuff and waist band.

This version scans both feet up to 500 Hz and can record up to 20,000 samples.

Capacitative systems operate on the change of capacitance when two electrical plates are squeezed together. The *EMED* system (Novel GmbH, Munich, Germany) has a resolution of 1–4 sensors/cm^2. Sampling rate is 25 or 50 Hz, pressure range 1–99 N/cm^2, accuracy ± 7%, hysteresis <3%, and crosstalk −40 dB. By comparison, the insole *Pedar* system has up to 1024 sensors, sampled at up to 20,000 sensors/second, and pedar-mobile allows up to 60 minutes of data storage on a small changeable PCMCIA card. A recent advance offers Bluetooth wireless telemetry system with a range of 50–100 m.

CALIBRATION

Given the limitations of pressure sensors, frequent and routine calibration is important. There are two approaches (Urry 1999):

- Static calibration (step loading) in which the output is recorded when known loads (e.g. body weight or air/fluid-filled bladder) are applied, provides a means by which to assess accuracy and linearity.
- Dynamic calibration with a cycle of loading and unloading or sudden impulsive loading reveals the frequency response of the system.

COLLECTION PROTOCOLS

In the midgait approach, data are collected during steady-state after the subject has walked a few steps. A mean of three steps raises reliability coefficients above 0.7 (Mueller & Strube 1996). In the two-step method, data are collected from the subject's second step (Bryant et al 1999). Clearly, the former is preferable whenever possible, but often patients are unable to take the required number of steps. The two-step method appears to be almost as reliable as the midgait method (Bryant et al 1999). It has two subtypes: the *gait initiation protocol* (in which data are collected from the trailing foot) and *gait termination protocol* (in which data are collected from the leading foot). Whilst having minimal effect on forefoot pressures, the former seems to alter the relative timing of the pressure pattern, whereas the latter preserves the timing but may result in reduced forefoot pressures (Wearing et al 1999).

METHODS FOR DISPLAYING PLANTAR PRESSURES

Several methods have been developed for the display of plantar pressures. Isobars can be drawn (similar to a weather map) to connect points of equal pressure, building up a contour map of pressure (Fig. 6.6). A colour scale provides an indication of the peak pressure at each sensor.

Three-dimensional mountain plots, in which height corresponds to pressure, are another way of displaying this information (Fig. 6.7).

CAUSES OF INCREASED PEAK PRESSURE

In general, pressures are determined by foot structure and function. Heel pressure is affected by heel-strike velocity, longitudinal arch structure, thickness of the heel pad and age. Midfoot pressure is dominated by arch structure, while metatarsal head pressure is mainly determined by talocrural joint motion and gastrocnemius activity, and hallux pressure by first metatarsophalangeal joint motion (Morag & Cavanagh 1999, Mueller et al 2002).

EFFECT OF PRESSURE ON TISSUE

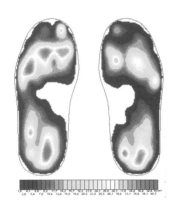

Figure 6.6   Contour display, in which areas are coloured according to the peak pressure (reproduced by permission of T & T medilogic Medizintechnik GmbH, Schönefeld, Germany).

There are five basic tissue responses to increasing pressure (Mueller & Maluf 2002):

- atrophy
- maintenance
- hypertrophy (callus formation)
- injury (ulcer formation)
- death (necrosis).

Moreover, injury can occur for three reasons (Mueller 1999):

- extremely high pressures resulting from trauma (i.e. stepping on a tack)
- low pressures for a very long duration (i.e. ischaemic wounds from wearing shoes that are too tight)
- repetitive pressures of moderate magnitude repeated thousands of times (i.e. such as might come from walking).

It follows that there is no single threshold value of pressure that can be considered a safe limit, since it depends on how long and how frequently the pressure is applied, as well as the direction of the loading (Mueller 1999). Moreover, the presence of bony deformities and impaired oxygenation undoubtedly make the skin more susceptible to ulcer formation (Bauman et al 1963, McNeely et al 1995).

Nevertheless, many researchers have sought to come up with a 'rule of thumb' cutoff, above which injury is more likely. Such an arbitrary threshold will necessarily have limited *sensitivity* (meaning that it will fail to detect some of those at risk for an ulcer – false negatives) and *specificity* (it will wrongly label some healthy people as being at risk – false positives). For example, a value of 700 kPa (70 N/cm^2 or 102 psi) has been found to result in a sensitivity of 70%, missing 30% of those at risk, and a specificity of 65%, wrongly diagnosing 35% of healthy people (Armstrong et al 1998). While lower thresholds, such as 300 kPa, are likely to have higher sensitivity they will also have inevitably a lower specificity, resulting in more unnecessary interventions and expense.

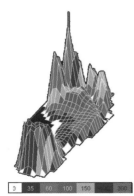

Figure 6.7   3D 'mountain' plot of peak pressure (reproduced by permission of Novel GmbH, Munich, Germany).

Pressure studies are often used to evaluate the efficacy of interventions designed to reduce peak pressures. In addition to total contact orthoses and extra-depth shoes, which aim to spread the pressure over the largest possible area, metatarsal pads can be attached to the orthosis immediately proximal to the MTPJ region to unload the prominent metatarsal heads. Rocker-bottom soles on the shoe can also help minimize metatarsophalangeal joint dorsiflexion and maximize foot contact area during late stance phase (Hayda et al 1994). Unloading the MTPJ region tends to increase pressure over the heel, but fortunately the heel fat pad protects this region and ulcers are uncommon under the heel.

The presence of shear stress dramatically reduces the pressure threshold at which an ulcer forms (Dinsdale 1974, Davis 1993, Murray et al 1996). Unfortunately, there are currently no systems on the market capable of measuring shear, although the *Parotec* system records a combination of load and shear. Research using specially built instrumentation (Lord et al 1992, Perry et al 2002) has shown that the greatest shear stresses (up to around 50 kPa, or 20% of typical vertical pressures) occur under the medial metatarsal heads and the lowest under the toes. Peak load and shear usually occur at the same site, but not necessarily (Perry et al 2002).

Surprisingly, plantar pressures do not seem to correlate with measures of perceived comfort (Jordon & Bartlett 1995), and this is presently a source of some frustration to footwear manufacturers.

PRESSURE–TIME INTEGRALS

Since the amount of tissue damage is related not only to the magnitude of pressure but also to the duration of exposure, an integral of the pressure (*pressure–time integral*) over the gait cycle would seem more likely to be related to ulceration risk. Many commercial systems now report PTIs, but as yet, there do not appear to have been any studies confirming that they are better predictors of pathology than peak pressures.

A *coronal index* can be calculated by comparing the pressure–time integral under the medial to the lateral column of the foot (Chang et al 2002). It seems to be well correlated with clinical assessment, providing better information than radiographic measurements in differentiating clinical categories (severe varus, varus, neutral, valgus, and severe valgus). It has the added advantage of summarizing the pressure distribution with a single number.

MASKS

Masks may be applied in order to calculate the total pressure (either peak or pressure–time integral) recorded by the sensors in a given area (Barnett 1998): e.g. heel, midfoot, metatarsophalangeal joints (MTPJs) and toes (Figs 6.8 and 6.9). This provides a means by which to standardize reporting and summarize the large amount of raw sensor data.

SYNCHRONIZATION WITH VIDEO AND OTHER BIOMECHANICAL MEASURES

Some commercial systems now enable the plantar pressure distribution to be displayed simultaneously with a video image.

Figure 6.8 Pressure masks, which show the total pressure over a given region of the sole (reproduced by permission of Novel GmbH, Munich, Germany).

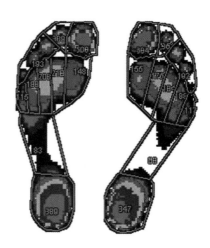

Figure 6.9 Regional analysis of pressure by the use of pressure maps (reproduced by permission of Novel GmbH, Munich, Germany).

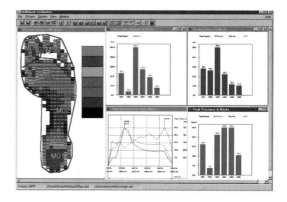

NORMAL PLANTAR PRESSURES

It is usual to begin a plantar pressure analysis with a static assessment during quiet standing (Bryant et al 2000) (Fig. 6.10). The normal sequence of plantar pressure during walking is shown in Figure 6.11. It can be seen that there is smooth transfer of pressure from heel (a), to lateral midfoot (c), to the metatarsophalangeal area (g), to the toes (h) and finally the hallux (i).

EFFECT OF SPEED

Peak plantar pressures are generally increased with walking speed (Fig. 6.12), especially under the heel, 1st metatarsal, lateral forefoot and hallux. However, pressure falls under lateral midfoot, and there is a tendency for loading to shift medially (Rosenbaum et al 1994, Zhu et al 1995, Perttunen & Komi 2001).

Figure 6.10   Static foot pressures, showing an approximately symmetrical division of pressure between the heel and metatarsophalangeal regions of each foot (reproduced by permission of Zebris Medical GmbH, Isny, Germany).

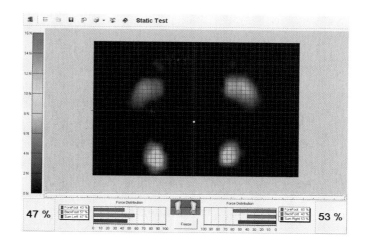

Figure 6.11   Isobar plantar pressure sequence from a healthy subject (reproduced by permission of Novel GmbH, Munich, Germany).

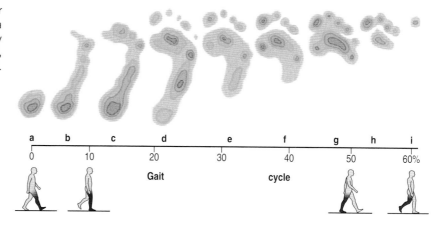

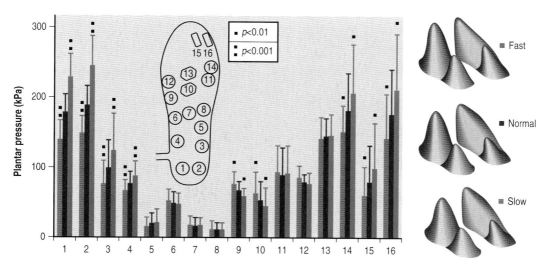

Figure 6.12   Effect of walking speed on plantar pressures, as recorded with a Parotec piezo-electric system (reproduced by permission of Perttunen J, Komi P V 2001 Journal of Human Movement Studies 40:291–305).

MATURATION OF PLANTAR PRESSURES

In order to normalize for body weight and plantar surface area, to facilitate comparisons between individuals of different sizes and ages, a relative vertical impulse (RVI) can be calculated by integrating the signal from a given mask over mask area (A) and gait cycle time (t), and dividing this by the total impulse:

$$RVI_x = I_x / \Sigma I_i, \text{ where } I_i = A_i \int P_i(t) \, dt \text{ for } i = 1 \text{ to the number of masks}$$

RVI is usually expressed in %, i.e. % total foot impulse.

At the onset of walking, much of the foot (the talus, calcaneus and some of the phalanges) is still cartilaginous. The ankle is in valgus, and the longitudinal arch does not form until around 3 years of age (Nakai et al 2000). As a consequence, the load is spread evenly over the sole, and RVIs are lower than in adults, except the midfoot, where the absence of an arch causes raised pressure.

There are three basic patterns in the first year of walking (Fig. 6.13):

- Initial heel-strike, in which there is a peak under the heel at initial contact.

Figure 6.13 Patterns of pressure distribution in three main types of infant gait (Copyright © 2003 by the American Orthopaedic Foot and Ankle Society (AOFAS), originally published in Foot and Ankle International, May 2003, Volume 24, Number 5, pages 449–451 and reproduced here with permission).

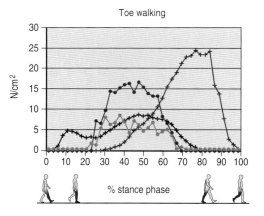

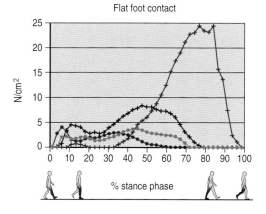

Figure 6.13   *Continued*

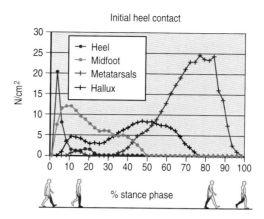

- Plantar contact, in which pressures are simultaneously elevated under heel, midfoot and metatarsals.
- Toe-walking, in which there is pressure under the metatarsals or hallux at initial contact.

As gait matures, pressure decreases under the hallux, 1st metatarsal head, midfoot and heel and rises under the 3rd to 5th metatarsal heads (Fig. 6.14). Toe-walking is rare after 2 years, although plantar contact still occurs. Eventually, a heel–toe gait develops, with a roll-over characterized by a delayed rise in pressure under the metatarsals and hallux, and more pronounced pressure peak under the heel at contact (Hallemans et al 2003). Midfoot RVIs remain elevated above adult values.

Figure 6.14   Comparison of pressure distribution in children compared to adults (Copyright © 2003 by the American Orthopaedic Foot and Ankle Society (AOFAS), originally published in Foot and Ankle International, May 2003, Volume 24, Number 5, pages 449–451 and reproduced here with permission).

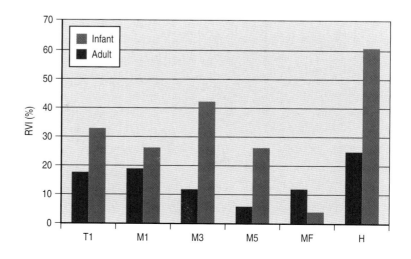

Shoes

According to the gospel of our shoemakers, the big toe ought to be in the place of the third one [Fig. 6.15].

Bernard Rudofsky

In 1938 dozens of sandals were unearthed from beneath ash from the Mt. Mazama volcano in central Oregon. They were carbon-dated to 10,000 years – the oldest shoes yet discovered. They had a flat sole, held on by twisted strings. In 1991, a couple mountaineering in the Ötztal Valley near the border with Austria in the Italian Alps, discovered the well-preserved 5,000 year-old corpse of Ötzi, a Neolithic Iceman. His shoes had oval leather soles and linden bark netting with turned-up edges held in place with a leather thong (Fig. 6.16). Hay was stuffed inside (like socks) as protection against the cold, along with deerskin uppers closed with laces.

In the UK, shoe sizes increase in increments of one-third of an inch, with 13 the largest size. The reason for this is that the barleycorn was the main unit of measurement in Olde England. In 1324, Edward II decreed that 3 barley-

Figure 6.15

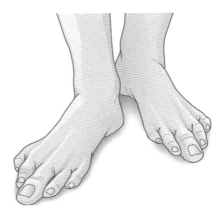

Figure 6.16

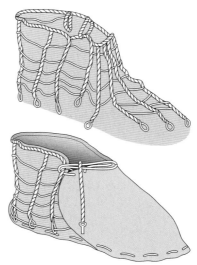

corns, placed end to end, equalled one English inch. Edward's own foot became the standard foot, with a length of 36 barleycorns. The largest size was 39 barleycorns, or size 13, and the rest in steps of one barleycorn (third of an inch). Despite many attempts to standardize measurements (Europe uses the French system based on the *Paris Points*, which is two-thirds of a centimetre), the barleycorn, for all its metrological shortcomings, continues to be used in both the UK and US. Incidentally, right and left shoes only came in with the advent of mass production after the American Civil War (1861–1865), in which 'shoddy' shoes played an important part in the defeat of the Confederate army. For most people, the larger foot is on the opposite side to the dominant hand.

Lateral shoe sizes are even more illogical, with some manufacturers measuring width, while others use girth. Sometimes the unit is ¼ inch, sometimes ³/₁₆ inch, and sometimes something else. The scale does not count upward in a logical, incremental way, but uses letters: AAAA (narrowest), AAA, AA, A, B, C, D, E, EE, EEE, EEEE (no BB or CCC). The National Institute of Advanced Industrial Science and Technology Digital Human Research Center in Japan has recently embarked on an ambitious project to build a comprehensive database of foot shapes and sizes.

Rudofsky B 1971 The unfashionable human body. Doubleday, Garden City, New York
Dowie J 1861 The foot and its covering. Hardwicke, London
Baum I, Spencer A M 1980 Limb dominance: its relationship to foot length. Journal of the American Podiatry Association 70(10):505–507

KEY POINTS

★ In normal standing, plantar loading is shared between the heel and metatarsophalangeal area

★ During normal gait, pressure rises first over the heel, and passes along the lateral border of the foot to the hallux

★ Areas with high plantar pressures are prone to ulceration in diabetic neuropathy

★ In infants, relative impulses are decreased compared to adults due to increased contact area

References

Ahoni J H, Boyko E J, Forsberg R 1998 Reliability of F-Scan in-shoe measurements of plantar pressure. Foot and Ankle 9/10:668–673

Akhlaghi F, Pepper M 1996 In-shoe biaxial shear force measurement: The Kent shear system. Medical and Biological Engineering and Computing 34:315–317

Antonsson E K, Mann R W 1985 The frequency content of gait. Journal of Biomechanics 18:39–47

Arcan M, Brull A 1976 A fundamental characteristic of the human body and foot, the foot-ground pressure pattern. Journal of Biomechanics 9:453–457

Armstrong D G, Peters E J, Athanasiou K A, Lavery L A 1998 Is there a critical level of plantar foot pressure to identify patients at risk for neuropathic foot ulceration? Journal of Foot and Ankle Surgery 37(4):303–307

Ashruf C M A 2002 Thin flexible pressure sensors. Sensor Review 22(4):322–327

Barnett S 1998 International protocol guidelines for plantar pressure measurement. Diabetic Foot 1(4):137–140

Barrett J P 1976 Plantar pressure measurements: rational shoe-wear in patients with rheumatoid arthritis. Journal of the American Medical Association 235:1138–1139

Bauman J H, Girling J P, Brand P W 1963 Plantar pressures and trophic ulceration: an evaluation of footwear. Journal of Bone and Joint Surgery 45(B):652–673

Beely F 1882 Zur Mechanik des Stehens. Longenbeck's Archiv Für Klinische Chirugie 27:457–471

Betts R P, Franks C I, Duckworth J, Burke J 1980 Static and dynamic foot pressure measurement in clinical orthopaedics. Medical and Biological Engineering and Computing 21:566–572

Bryant A, Singer K, Tinley P 1999 Comparison of the reliability of plantar pressure measurements using the two-step and midgait methods of data collection. Foot and Ankle International 20(10):646–650

Bryant A R, Tinley P, Singer K P 2000 Normal values of plantar pressure measurements determined using the EMED-SF system. Journal of the American Podiatry Medical Association 90(6):295–299

Buis A, Convery P 1996 Calibration problems encountered while monitoring stump/socket pressures with force sensing resistors: techniques adopted to minimize inaccuracies. Prosthetics and Orthotics International 21:179–182

Cavanagh P R 1992 In-shoe plantar pressure measurement: a review. The Foot 2:185–194

Cavanagh P R, Hennig E M 1982 A new device for the measurement of pressure distribution on a rigid surface. Medicine and Science in Sports and Exercise 14(2):153

Cavanagh P R, Ulbrecht J S 1994 Clinical plantar pressure measurement in diabetes: rationale and methodology. The Foot 4:123–135

Chang C H, Miller F, Schuyler J 2002 Dynamic pedobarograph in evaluation of varus and valgus foot deformities. Journal of Pediatric Orthopedics 22(6):813–818

Chesnin K J, Selby-Silverstein L, Besser M P 2000 Comparison of an in-shoe pressure measurement device to a force plate: concurrent validity of center of pressure measurements. Gait & Posture 12(2):128–133

Davis B L 1993 Foot ulceration: hypotheses concerning shear and vertical forces acting on adjacent regions of skin. Medical Hypotheses 40:44–47

Davis B L, Cothren R M, Quesada P et al 1996 Frequency content of normal and diabetic plantar pressure profiles: implications for the selection of transducer sizes. Journal of Biomechanics 29(7):979–983

Dinsdale S M 1974 Decubitus ulcers: role of pressure and friction in causation. Archives of Physical Medicine and Rehabilitation 55:147–152

Duckworth T, Betts R P, Franks C I, Burke J 1982 The measurement of pressures under the foot. Foot and Ankle 3:130–141

Elftman H 1934 A cinematic study of the distribution of pressure in the human foot. Anatomical Record 59:481–487

Evanski P M, Waugh T R 1980 The Harris and Beath Footprinting Mat: diagnostic validity and clinical use. Clinical Orthopedics and Related Research 151:265–269

Franks C I, Betts R P, Ducksworth T 1983 Microprocessor-based image processing system for dynamic foot pressure studies. Medical and Biological Engineering and Computing 21:566–572

Hayda R, Tremaine M D, Tremaine K et al 1994 Effect of metatarsal pads and their positioning: a quantitative assessment. Foot and Ankle International 15(10):561–566

Hallemans A, D'Aout K, De Clercq D, Aerts P 2003 Pressure distribution patterns under the feet of new walkers: the first two months of independent walking. Foot and Ankle 24(5):444–453

Hennig E M, Rosenbaum P 1991 Pressure distribution patterns under the feet of children in comparison with adults. Foot and Ankle 11(5):306–311

Hennig E M, Cavanagh P R, Albert H T, MacMillan N H 1982 A piezoelectric method of measuring the vertical contact stress beneath the human foot. Journal of Biomedical Engineering 4:213–222

Hsiao H, Jinhua G, Weatherly M 2002 Accuracy and precision of two in-shoe pressure measurement systems. Ergonomics 45(8):537-555

Hughes R, Rowlands H, McKeekin S 2000 A comparison of two studies of the pressure distribution under the feet of normal subjects using different equipment. Foot and Ankle 14:514–519

Jordon C, Bartlett R 1995 Pressure distribution and perceived comfort in casual footwear. Gait & Posture 3:215–220

Lanshammer H, Turan I, Lindgren U 1993 Assessment of foot disorders using biomechanical analysis of foot loads during locomotion. Clinical Biomechechanics 8:135–141

Lord M, Hosein R, Williams R B 1992 Method for in-shoe shear stress measurement. Journal of Biomedical Engineering 14:181–186

McNeely M J, Boyko E J, Ahroni J H et al 1995 The independent contributions of diabetic neuropathy and vasculopathy in foot ulceration. How great are the risks? Diabetes Care 18(2):216–219

Manouel M, Pearlman H S, Belakhlef A, Brown T 1992 A miniature piezoelectric polymer transducer for in vitro measurement of the dynamic contact stress distribution. Journal of Biomechanics 25:627–635

Morag E, Cavanagh P R 1999 Structural and functional predictors of regional peak pressures under the foot during walking. Journal of Biomechanics 32:359–370

Morton D J 1952 Human locomotion and body form. A study of gravity and man. Williams and Wilkins, Baltimore

Mueller M J 1999 Application of plantar pressure assessment in footwear and insert design. Journal of Orthopaedic and Sports Physical Therapy 29:747–755

Mueller M J, Maluf K S 2002 tissue adaptation to physical stress: a proposed 'physical stress' theory to guide physical therapy practice, education, and rehabilitation research. Physical Therapy 82:383–403

Mueller M J, Strube M J 1996 Generalizability of in-shoe peak pressure measurement using the F-Scan system. Clinical Biomechanics 11(3):159–164

Murray H J, Young M J, Hollis S, Boulton A J M 1996 The association between callus formation, high pressures and neuropathy in diabetic foot ulceration. Diabetic Medicine 13:979–982

Nakai T, Takakura Y, Sugimoto K et al 2000 Morphological changes of the ankle in children as assessed by radiography and arthrography. Journal of Orthopedic Science 5(2):134–138

Perry J E, Hall J O, Davis B L 2002 Simultaneous measurement of plantar pressure and shear forces in diabetic individuals. Gait & Posture 15:101–107

Perttunen J, Komi P V 2001 Effects of walking speed on foot loading patterns. Journal of Human Movement Studies 40:291–305

Rosenbaum D, Hautmann S, Gold M, Claes L 1994 Effects of walking speed on plantar pressure patterns and hindfoot angular motion. Gait & Posture 2:191–197

Silvino N, Evanski P M, Waugh T R 1980 The Harris and beath footprinting mat: diagnostic validity and clinical use. Clinical Orthopedics 151:265–269

Soames R W, Atha J 1981 The role of the antigravity musculature during quiet standing in man. European Journal of Applied Physiology Occupational Physiology 47:159–167

Urry S 1999 Plantar pressure-measurement sensors. Measuring Science Technology R16–32

Wearing S C, Urry S, Smeathers J E, Battistutta D 1999 A comparison of gait initiation and termination methods for obtaining plantar foot pressures. Gait & Posture 10(3):255–263

Woodburn J, Helliwell P S 1996 Observations on the F-scan in-shoe pressure measuring system. Clinical Biomechanics 11:301–304

Young C R 1993 The F-scan system of foot pressure analysis. Clinics in Podiatric Medicine and Surgery 10(3):455–461

Zhu H, Wertsch J J, Harris G F, Alba H M 1995 Walking cadence effect on plantar pressures. Archives of Physical Medicine and Rehabilitation 76:1000–1005

Chapter 7

Joint moment

I am never content until I have constructed a mechanical model of the subject I am studying. If I succeed in making one, I understand. Otherwise, I do not.

Lord Kelvin

OBJECTIVES

- Understand how the ground reaction vector can be used to infer muscle action
- Know the typical pattern of the ground reaction vector during normal gait
- Awareness of the principles used in performing an inverse dynamics analysis of the lower-limb
- Appreciation of the limitations and sources of error in joint moment estimates
- Be able to interpret joint moment curves in physiological terms
- Appreciation of the effect of tendon lever arms in the generation of bone-on-bone forces

VIDEO-VECTOR SYSTEMS

One of the main objectives of gait analysis is to determine muscle activity. Forces are, of course, invisible, but the ground reaction vector (GRV)

Figure 7.1   Video vector synchronization system.

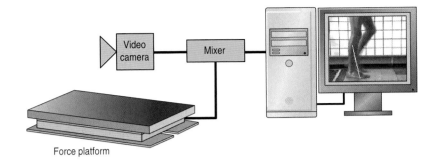

Force platform

can be artificially visualized by superimposing a line on a TV picture (Tait & Rose 1979, Stallard 1987). If this is recorded, the location of the GRV with respect to the joints during gait can be studied (Fig. 7.1). Commercial systems, such as Pro-Vec Plus (MIE Ltd, Leeds, UK) and Digivec (B|T|S Milan, Italy) allow the clinician to view the location of the vector in real time, or record a video for later study.

ESTIMATING MUSCLE ACTIVITY WITH THE GRV

Recall that during quiet standing the location of the GRV with respect to each joint gave an indication of the muscle activity at that joint. This technique can also be used, with some limitations, during gait.

At heel contact (Fig. 7.2A), the GRV is behind the ankle. This implies (remember the rule of thumb) that the muscle on the opposite side (the dorsiflexors, principally *tibialis anterior*) is active. Notice that the magnitude (length) of the vector is quite small, though, suggesting that the joint moment being generated by *tibialis anterior* is low.

By Figure 7.2B, the vector has swung forwards so that it now passes through the ankle joint (roughly indicated by the lateral malleolus), which indicates no *net* muscle activity: either no muscles are active or (more likely) the plantarflexors and dorsiflexors are contracting equally. During this time, the vector is also posterior to the knee, indicating that the extensors (*quadriceps femoris*) must be active.

In Figure 7.2C–D, the vector has now swung in front of the ankle, indicating that the muscles on the posterior side of the joint (the plantarflexors, *gastrocnemius* and *soleus*) are active. The lever arm of the vector increases by Figure 7.2E, implying that the plantarflexors are increasingly active. Meanwhile, notice that the vector is now anterior to the knee, indicating an internal flexor moment is being generated. This could mean that the knee flexors (hamstrings) are active, but notice that the knee is fully extended. The moment is therefore likely to be coming from taut posterior capsule ligaments. By toe-off, Figure 7.2F, the centre of pressure (CoP) has moved under the hallux.

Figure 7.2   Progression of the GRV during normal gait.

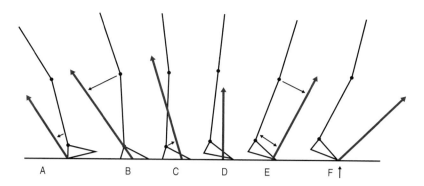

A   B   C   D   E   F ↑

Observational kinetics?

The mathematical process in the symbolical method [algebra] is like running a railroad through a tunneled mountain, that in the ostensive [geometry] is like crossing the mountain on foot. The former causes us, by a short and easy transit, to our destined point, but in miasma, darkness and torpidity, whereas the latter allows us to reach it only after time and trouble, but feasting us at each turn with glances of the earth and of the heavens, while we inhale the pleasant breeze, and gather new strength at every effort we put forth.

Sir William Hamilton*

Geometry and algebra are two ways of looking at the same thing. Both have their advantages. Algebra, such as that used in inverse dynamics, reveals the most accurate and complete picture but can be difficult to visualize. On the other hand, geometrical approaches, like using the GRV to estimate joint moments, often provide a more intuitive and satisfying insight.

Similarly, when evaluating a pathological gait some clinicians start at the trunk and work distally, while others start at the foot and work proximally. Without a force platform, kinetics are difficult to assess, but to the experienced eye there are some subtle clues. The GRV will often (though not always) point in the region of the body's centre of mass (Bruckner 1998), which is dominated by the trunk because of its large mass. Similarly, the CoP must be located some-

Figure 7.3

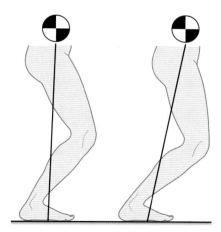

where between the walking base – during single support it must be under the stance foot. Of course, these assumptions are very rough and not always valid, especially when there are large accelerations, but luckily this is rarely the case in slow pathological gaits. Thus by joining an imaginary line between trunk CoM and estimated location of the CoP, one can make a tentative judgement about the line of action of the GRV (Fig. 7.3). Having done this, some assessment of the likely joint moments can be made. If this all sounds very speculative and approximate, that's because it is, but in the clinic it is often all that is available. With *glances of the earth and of the heavens*, the attempt to estimate kinetics may at least encourage the art of observation!

*Olson R 1975 Scottish philosophy and British physics, 1750–1880: a study in the foundations of the Victorian scientific style. Princeton University Press, Princeton, New Jersey
Bruckner J S 1998 The gait workbook. SLACK Inc., Thorofare, New Jersey

Although the GRV approach to determining muscle action is a bit simplistic, it is quite accurate (about ± 1%) at the ankle and fairly accurate (about ± 5%) at the knee (Wells 1981). Since it only takes into account the ground reaction and ignores accelerations, predictions about hip muscle activity tend to be not so reliable, though, especially around initial contact when accelerations are relatively large. Moreover, the technique is limited to qualitative interpretation, and gives no information about muscle activity during swing phase. Nevertheless, it does have the advantage of giving an instant intuitive indication of muscle activity, and has found application in rapid clinical assessment, particularly for prosthetic and orthotic alignment (Stallard 1987).

? MCQ 7.1

If the GRV passes anterior to the ankle and posterior to the knee, which muscles must be active?
(a) *Vasti* and plantarflexors
(b) *Vasti* and dorsiflexors
(c) Hamstrings and plantarflexors
(d) Hamstrings and dorsiflexors

INVERSE DYNAMICS

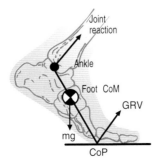

Figure 7.4 Free-body diagram of the foot showing the forces acting on it.

To obtain *quantitative* values for the joint moments (including those during swing phase), a mathematical equivalent, called a *link-segment model*, of the lower limb must be constructed, using Newton's equations (Winter 1990). This approach is called inverse dynamics because it involves working back from the kinematics to deduce the muscle activity that must be responsible for them.

Mathematical modelling can be a bit daunting at first, but it is very powerful in modern gait analysis, so it is important to try to at least understand the principles involved.

In link-segment modelling, the lower-limb segments are disarticulated from each other and each is treated separately as a rigid body. A *free-body diagram* (FBD) is then drawn for each of them, starting with the foot (Fig. 7.4).

Anthropometry

The science of biomechanics has traditionally been divided into two: *rigid body dynamics* and *tissue mechanics*. The former studies the motion of body segments as if they were rigid uniform bodies linked by frictionless joints, while the latter studies the deforming effects of forces on tissues such as bone, ligament, tendon, muscle and skin. The main reason for this divide is that different mathematical equations are used to describe the two types of behaviour. Modern computing techniques are allowing much more sophisticated models to be developed which tend to bridge the gap between the two approaches, but by and large the distinction still applies.

In a basic rigid body analysis, the body is divided into segments (foot, shank, thigh, trunk, etc.). Each of these segments is assumed to have a uniform density (somewhere between that of bone and soft-tissue), with mass concentrated at a single point, the centre of mass. Whilst it is possible to measure the exact size and shape of the segments of an individual, people are, in practice, assumed to be pretty much alike, once scaled for height, weight and (for children) age.

Most of the anthropometric tables (Table 7.1) used were compiled in the heyday of aviation and space research in the 1950s and 1960s. The principles are straightforward: a cadaver is dissected to disarticulate the segments, which are then weighed to determine their mass, m, as a percentage of total body mass (BM). The centre of mass location, l_{CoM}, is determined by finding the point along the length of the segment at which it balances. This is usually expressed as the percentage of segment length from the distal end (joint) of the segment. A third parameter, the radius of gyration, k, describes the distribution of mass within the segment and is measured by observing the way the segment swings when pivoted like a pendulum. This is used to calculate the *moment of inertia* of the segment, I.

Table 7.1   Anthropometric data

Segment	Segment length, l (%BH)	Mass, m (%BM) [Dempster]	Child <14 y mass (kg) [Jensen]	l_{CoM} (%BH) (from distal joint)	l_{CoM} (%BH) Child < 14 y	Radius of gyration k_{CoM}
Head	9.6	7.8	23.8–1.14 × age	50	50	0.5
Trunk	31.6	49.7	42.46–0.06 × age	49.5	40.13 + 0.18 × age	0.4
HAT		68				0.68
Upper arm	16.4	2.7	0.084 × age + 2.2	56.4	−0.028 × age + 55.7	0.3
Forearm	13.7	2.3	0.015 × age + 1.2	55	0.19 × age + 56.1	0.3
Hand	8.2	0.6		50		0.3
Thigh	25.4	9.9	0.364 × age + 6.634	56.7	53.42 + 0.115 × age	0.3
Shank	23.3	4.6	0.122 × age + 3.809	57	55.74 + 0.3 × age	0.3
Foot	11.7	1.4	0.015 × age + 1.87	50	56.49 + 0.186 × age	0.48
Shank-foot	24.6	6.1				0.74

BH, Body Height; BM, Total Body Mass; HAT, Head/Arms/Trunk; Moment of Inertia, $I = m(k_{CoM} \times l_{CoM})^2$

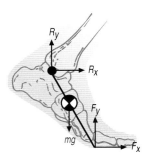

Figure 7.5   Free-body diagram of the foot showing vertical and horizontal force components.

The weight of the foot segment (mg, where m = its mass and g = 9.81 m/s^2) can be considered to act at its centre of mass (CoM), the point marked with the ☻ symbol. This is the point at which the foot would balance if suspended on a knife edge. Its location is usually obtained from experiments done on cadavers (Dempster 1955, Jensen 1986, Stoudt 1981, Plagenhoef et al 1983). Most of this work was done in the pioneering days of aviation and space research in the 1950s and 1960s. The principles are straightforward: a cadaver is dissected to disarticulate the segments, which are then weighed to determine their mass (as a percentage of total body mass) and suspended in order to find the CoM. Regression equations are then derived so that the body segment parameters (BPSs) can be estimated for a given person based on their height and body mass. Nowadays it is possible to estimate the BSPs of an individual more directly by magnetic resonance scanning (Cheng et al 2000), but most laboratories still rely on the cadaver regressions, especially those by Dempster (1955).

As the weight of the foot acts at its CoM, so the GRV acts at its CoP. There is also a third force that acts at the ankle joint, where the foot has been disarticulated from the rest of the lower-limb. This force is called the joint reaction. To simplify the mathematics, the two vectors (the GRV and joint reaction) can be replaced by their horizontal (x) and vertical (y) components (Fig. 7.5).

The forces can then be *resolved* in the two directions by using Newton's $F = ma$.

$$\text{Resolving horizontally: } F_x + R_x = ma_x$$

where a_x is the acceleration of the foot in the horizontal direction. This equation can be rearranged to calculate the unknown ankle reaction force, R_x:

$$R_x = ma_x - F_x$$

Of course, if the foot is stationary (which is pretty much the case during the stance phase of gait) a_x will be close to zero, and R_x will be equal and opposite to F_x. Resolving the vertical forces:

$$F_y + R_y - mg = ma_y$$

$$\text{from which: } R_y = ma_y - F_y + mg$$

Once again, in the static case when there are no accelerations, the ma_y term will be zero, and since the foot mass is relatively small, mg will also be small. Thus, R_y will be approximately equal and opposite to F_y, meaning that the ankle reaction is downward. This is not surprising, since the rest of body weight (apart from the foot segment) is passing through the ankle. Nevertheless, to prevent confusion, it is better in practice to always draw forces on the FBD as acting upward and to the right, letting their signs indicate that their direction is reversed.

ANKLE MOMENT

As well as the reaction forces at the ankle joint, of course, there are muscles acting. These cause the joint to rotate in a dorsiflexor or

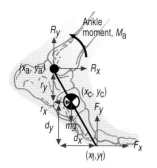

Figure 7.6 The ankle musculature generates a dorsiflexor-plantarflexor moment about the joint.

plantarflexor direction according to whether the *gastrocnemius–soleus* or *anterior tibialis* are contracting. This introduces a moment at the ankle, which is positive in the anti-clockwise direction or negative in the clockwise direction (Fig. 7.6). This moment can be determined in a similar way to the forces, but instead of $F = ma$, the equation for moments is $M = I\alpha$. A moment is calculated as the product of a force and its moment arm about a pivot point or fulcrum. This can be any arbitrary point, but it turns out that using the segment centre of mass (CoM) makes the maths a bit easier.

Put your left index finger on the segment CoM and push with your right index finger along each force. It should be clear that the forces F_x and F_y rotate in the anti-clockwise (+) direction, while R_x and R_y rotate in the clockwise (−) direction. Remember that the moment arm is the perpendicular distance from the line of action of the force to the fulcrum. So, for example, the moment arm of F_x is d_y, while that of F_y is d_x. Thus,

$$M_a + F_y d_x + F_x d_y - R_y r_x - R_x r_y = I\alpha$$

Notice that the moment arm of the segment weight, mg, is zero since it passes directly through the CoM, so it does not appear in the equation. Rearranging this equation,

$$M_a = F_y d_x + F_x d_y - R_y d_x - R_x d_y = I\alpha$$

The distances d_x, d_y, r_x and r_y can be determined from the coordinates of the ankle and toe markers. For example, $d_x = x_f - x_c$ where x_f is the x-coordinate of the foot marker (or the CoP during stance), and x_c is the x-coordinate of the segment CoM. The latter can be calculated by proportion from the anthropometry:

$$x_c = x_f + c_f (x_f - x_a)/100$$

where c_f is the distance of the CoM from the distal (foot) marker expressed as a percentage of foot length.

Finally, the acceleration force, $I\alpha$, is comprised of α, the foot angular acceleration (in radians per second, rad/s²) and another anthropometric term, I, which is called the *moment of inertia* of the foot. This is the rotational equivalent of mass and can also be obtained from the radius of gyration, which is available from anthropometric tables:

$$I = m(kl)^2 \ldots$$

where k = radius of gyration about segment CoM, and l = segment length.

EXERCISE

1. Repeat the derivation of joint moment using the ankle joint as the fulcrum for calculating moments. Was there any difference in the result?
2. Try the exercise again for the foot in the position it is in at initial contact. Confirm that the result does not depend on the orientation of the foot.

KNEE AND HIP MOMENTS

Once the ankle moment and joint reaction forces have been calculated, similar equations for the next proximal segment, the shank (s), can be solved to find the knee (k) joint forces and moment. Finally, the thigh segment (t) model can be solved to find the hip (h) variables:

ANKLE

$$R_x = ma_x - F_x$$

$$R_y = ma_y - F_y + m_f g$$

$$M_a = F_y(CoP - x_f) + F_x(y_c - y_f) - R_y(x_c - x_a) - R_x(y_a - y_c) + I_f \alpha_f$$

KNEE

$$R_x = ma_x - (-R_x)$$

$$R_y = ma_y - (-F_y) + m_s g$$

$$M_k = F_y(x_a - x_s) + F_x(y_s - x_a) - R_y(x_s - x_k) - R_x(y_k - y_s)$$
$$+ I_s \alpha_s - (-M_a)$$

HIP

$$R_x = ma_x - (-R_x)$$

$$R_y = ma_y - (-F_y) + m_t g$$

$$M_h = F_y(x_k - x_t) + F_x(y_t - x_k) - R_y(x_t - x_h) - R_x(y_h - y_t)$$
$$+ I_t \alpha_t - (-M_k)$$

ASSUMPTIONS

The human body is composed of some 212 bones bound and surrounded by soft tissues. To understand such a complex system, certain assumptions, simplifications and approximations must inevitably be made.

Notice that the foot is modelled as a single rigid body – quite an assumption! The reason for this simplistic approach is partly due to the complexity of foot anatomy, which is difficult to model mathematically, but also because until very recently, three-dimensional motion analysis systems have had difficulty tracking the motion of the small bones of the foot. Recently there have been attempts to develop more sophisticated foot models, but these are not yet being used for routine clinical work.

There are several other assumptions:

- That friction between the joint surfaces is negligible. This is probably correct – at least for joints that are not affected by arthritis.
- That all the mass of each segment is concentrated at its centre of mass – certainly not true in reality, but a reasonable mathematical

approximation if the density of the segment is close to uniform. Fortunately, the densities of bone and soft tissue are quite similar.

- That muscles can be represented as torque motors – a close approximation because the lever arms of most muscles are small compared to segment lengths.
- That air drag is negligible – probably safe to assume at typical walking speeds.
- That the estimates of body segment parameters (BSPs) provided by cadaver studies are sufficiently close to the real anthropometry of the person whose gait is being analysed. In practice, the errors from inaccurate BSPs are thought to be very small, at least in normal gait (Pearsall & Costigan 1999).
- More importantly, the joint centre locations as estimated from the skin markers (Holden et al 1997) and model used may be inaccurate (Holden & Stanhope 1998).
- A common source of inaccuracy in practice is misalignment between the force platform location and the laboratory origin (Baker 1997).
- That there is no *co-contraction* of the opposing agonist and antagonist muscles. If this occurs, a *net* moment will be calculated, which will be the difference between the moments generated by the two muscles. Co-contraction probably occurs quite often even in normal gait (Park et al 1999), but it is especially common in patients with spasticity. The possibility of the phenomenon should therefore always be borne in mind when interpreting joint moment curves.
- That muscles cross only one joint (monoarticular), resulting in some error due to forces transmitted by two-joint muscles.

VALIDATION OF INVERSE DYNAMICS

The number of assumptions and approximations involved in performing an inverse dynamics analysis might appear so bewildering as to cast doubt on the whole technique, but fortunately studies have been performed which have validated the results.

A gold standard comparison would be to implant strain gauges (so called 'buckle' transducers) directly into the tendons and measure the forces directly (Komi 1990). Clearly, there are methodological and ethical difficulties in finding volunteers to have such surgery, and so far it has only been performed on the Achilles tendon, which is relatively superficial. Ankle forces and moments are, however, least prone to inaccuracies in inverse dynamics modelling.

A few researchers have implanted hip replacements (endoprostheses) instrumented with strain gauges to measure hip joint forces (Lu et al 1998, Bergmann et al 2001). The data were transmitted in real-time over a radio link and recorded simultaneously while the volunteer underwent conventional 3D motion analysis and inverse dynamics. During gait, the forces and moments estimated by the two approaches were found to agree within ± 12% (Heller et al 2001).

Other researchers have used electromyography to estimate muscle moments and have also found good agreement with those calculated by inverse dynamics in a variety of conditions (Lloyd & Besier 2003). Recently intramuscular pressure has emerged as an alternative technique which correlates very well with joint moment, but it has also so far been limited to study of the ankle musculature (Ballard et al 1998).

DEBATING POINT

Debate the advantages and disadvantages of the following in clinical gait analysis:
– Video vector display for estimating joint moments
– Inverse dynamics for calculating joint moments

JOINT MOMENTS IN NORMAL GAIT

Figure 7.7 shows the typical ranges (mean ± 1 standard deviation) measured for the main joint moments of the lower limb during normal gait. Notice that the convention normally used is opposite to that used for joint angles: *extensor* moments are shown as being positive while flexor moments are negative. The reasoning behind this is that extensor (or plantarflexor) moments are mainly responsible for supporting the body ('anti-gravity'). Indeed, most of the moments are extensor for most of the gait cycle. Flexor activity mainly occurs at the knee, and at the hip around toe-off.

After being briefly dorsiflexor immediately after initial contact, the ankle moment becomes increasingly plantarflexor throughout stance phase, until contralateral initial contact, when it falls quickly to zero in swing phase.

The knee moment shows an extensor followed by a flexor pattern in stance phase, with a final flexor pattern in terminal swing (indicating hamstrings activity). Note that the initial flexor moment immediately after initial contact is most likely an artefact (spurious or erroneous finding) caused by discrepancies in filtering of the ground reaction and kinematics (see chapter 10).

The sagittal hip moment is mostly extensor, except for a brief period shortly after toe-off, when it is flexor (indicating *iliopsoas* activity). In the frontal plane, it is strongly abductor during swing phase (indicating *gluteus medius* activity), and virtually zero during swing.

It is worth pointing out that these are internal moments – for the ankle and the knee they will be approximately equal and opposite to the external moment generated by the GRV. So, for example, if the *internal* moment is positive (extensor) at the knee, this must mean that the GRF is generating an *external* flexor moment, i.e. it must be posterior to the knee joint.

Figure 7.7 The major joint moments during normal gait. Note that while joint angles are usually shown with flexion positive, the convention is reversed for moments, with extensor moments shown as positive. Means ± 1 SD are shown, with units in N m/kg body mass.

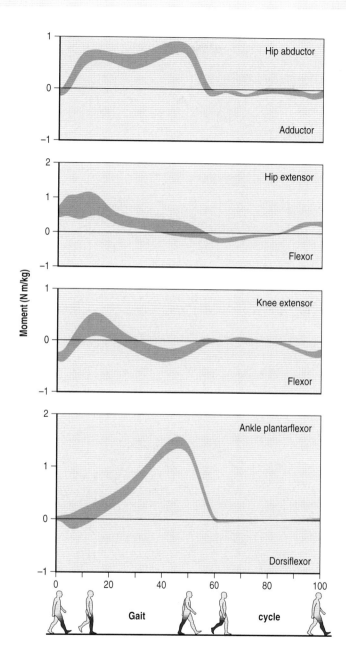

EFFECT OF SPEED

The effect of increasing speed on the joint moments is shown in Figure 7.8. The changes are relatively minor except at the knee, where both the stance phase extensor and flexor moments are increased, together with the flexor moment in terminal swing.

Figure 7.8 Effect of speed on joint moments (data from Stansfield et al 2001, with permission). Mean joint moments at walking speeds of 0.5 m/s (dark red), 1.0 m/s (black) and 1.5 m/s (light red) are shown: the major changes occur at the knee joint, with increased moments during both stance and swing phase.

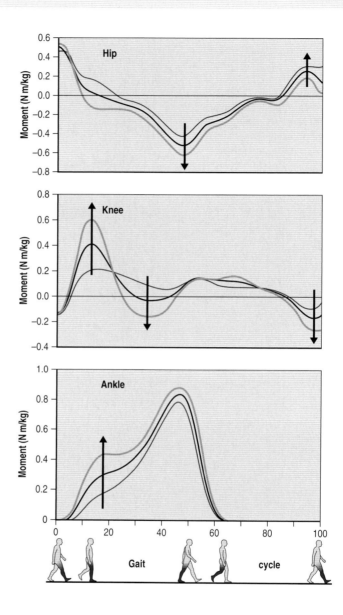

EFFECT OF ASCENDING AND DESCENDING

Whilst most research has been performed on level gait, a few studies have examined walking on slopes (Redfern & DiPasquale 1997) and stairs (Riener et al 2002). These data not only provide insights into the compensations involved, but also contribute to the understanding of the mechanism of falls. Higher shear forces are needed on ramps compared to level walking, making slips more likely (Sun et al 1996, Redfern & DiPasquale 1997). In walking down a slope, this shear is directed posteriorly, directing the GRV backwards, which necessitates increasingly dorsiflexor (less plantarflexor) ankle moment, extensor knee moment and flexor hip moment (Fig. 7.9).

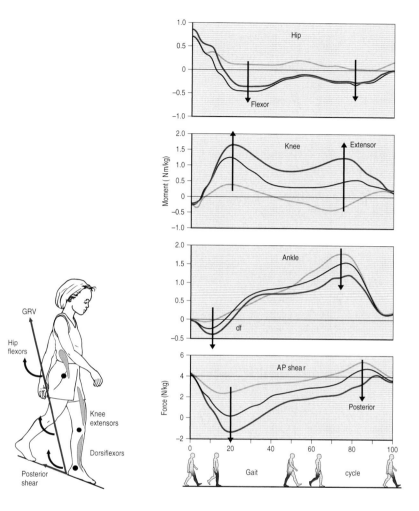

Figure 7.9 Lower-limb joint moments while walking down slopes (data from Redfern & DiPasquale 1997). Mean joint moments at slopes of 0° (dark red), 10° (black) and 20° (light red). The ankle moment becomes progressively more dorsiflexor, while the knee moment becomes dramatically more extensor, as a result of the increasingly posterior AP shear force.

? MCQ 7.2

What would be the effect of walking *up* an incline?

(a) Increased anterior shear, plantarflexor ankle moment, flexor knee and extensor hip moments

(b) Increased posterior shear, dorsiflexor ankle moment, extensor knee and extensor hip moments

(c) Increased anterior shear, plantarflexor ankle moment, flexor knee and flexor hip moments

(d) Increased posterior shear, dorsiflexor ankle moment, extensor knee and flexor hip moments

JOINT FORCES

The joint moment not only produces a rotation of the joint, but also presses the bones together. Figure 7.10 shows why this is so. The joint moment is generated, of course, by the muscle force or tension, T, acting at a distance, the *lever arm* (moment arm), l, from the joint centre (Table 7.2):

Figure 7.10 Origin of bone-on-bone forces in the knee joint.

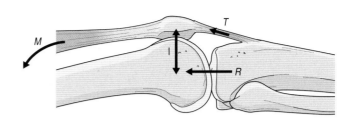

Table 7.2 Moment (lever) arms, in mm, of the major lower-limb muscles (from Hawkins & Hull 1990, Spoor et al 1990, Viser et al 1990). The moment arms of some muscle groups vary quite significantly between individuals and with joint motion (Arnold et al 2000)

Muscle	Hip	Knee	Ankle
Iliopsoas	20–30		
Gluteus maximus	70		
Hamstrings	45–70	40–60	
Rectus femoris	40	60	
Vasti		60	
Gastrocnemius		25	50
Soleus			50

$$\text{Joint Moment}, M = T \times l$$

The muscle tension can thus be calculated:

$$\text{Muscle Tension}, T = \text{Joint Moment}/\text{Lever Arm} = M/l$$

Assuming that the tendon pulls longitudinally (a reasonable approximation in most circumstances), the total bone-on-bone contact force is the sum of this tension and the joint reaction force already calculated:

$$\text{Bone-on-bone Force}, B = T + R$$

Since the lever arm, l, of most muscles is very small (usually a few centimetres), muscle tension is often very large, making the total bone-on-bone force exceed body weight in many situations (Paul 1966, Morrison 1970). This has important consequences, because in conditions such as osteo- and rheumatoid arthritis, pain increases as the affected joint is subjected to higher forces. People with joint pain therefore often adopt a pain-minimizing strategy, using passive mechanisms (the combination of GRV and joint ligaments) to stabilize the joint, thereby avoiding painful muscle contraction.

? MCQ 7.3

What would be the quadriceps muscle tension if the knee joint moment is 25 N m and patellar tendon lever arm 5 cm?
(a) 5 N
(b) 50 N
(c) 500 N
(d) 125 N

In practice, the estimation of bone-on-bone force is complicated by the simultaneous action of several muscles at each joint. Since each has a

Figure 7.11 Peak hip contact forces measured in various activities with an instrumented endoprosthesis (data from Bergmann et al 2001). Such data are extremely useful in the design of implants.

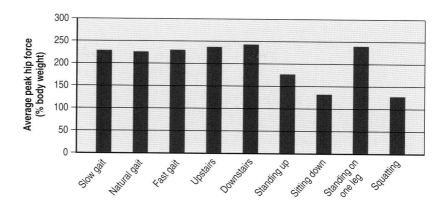

different lever arm, knowing how the moment is shared out between the various muscles is necessary to determine the contribution of each muscle to the bone-on-bone force. This *compartmentalization* problem turns out to be very tricky. Various approaches have been devised to solve it, including mathematical *optimization* techniques, in which the nervous system is assumed to share the force out in the most efficient manner (Crowninshield & Brand 1981, Hatze 2000). Electromyography can also provide some information, although it is often difficult to distinguish the activity of muscles which are close together using surface electrodes – a problem known as *crosstalk*. For these reasons, the estimation of bone-on-bone forces is rarely attempted in routine clinical gait analysis and it is reserved for research purposes – especially in the design of endoprostheses for joint replacement arthroplasty. Direct measurement of hip contact forces has recently become possible using an instrumented endoprosthesis (Fig. 7.11).

KEY POINTS

★ In general (at ankle and knee), muscle activity opposes the action of the ground reaction vector

★ Joint moments are calculated by inverse dynamics from a link-segment model

★ Error propagation generally causes accuracy to fall from ankle to knee to hip joint

★ The joint moment can be used to infer muscle activity at that joint

★ Bone-on-bone forces are generated by a combination of gravity (weight) and muscle action

References

Arnold A S, Salinas S, Asakawa D J, Delp S L 2000 Accuracy of muscle moment arms estimated from MRI-based musculoskeletal models of the lower extremity. Computer Aided Surgery 5:108–119

Baker R 1997 The 'poker' test: a spot check to confirm the accuracy of kinetic gait data. Gait & Posture 5(2):177–178

Ballard R E, Watenpaugh D E, Breit G A et al 1998 Leg intramuscular pressures during locomotion in humans. Journal of Applied Physiology 84(6):1976–1981

Bergmann G, Deuetzbacher G, Heller M et al 2001 Hip contact forces and gait patterns from routine activities. Journal of Biomechanics 34:859–871

Cheng C K, Chen H H, Chen C S et al 2000 Segment inertial properties of Chinese adults determined from magnetic resonance imaging. Clinical Biomechanics 15(8):559–566

Crowninshield R D, Brand R A 1981 A physiologically based criterion of muscle force prediction in locomotion. Journal of Biomechanics 14:793–801

Dempster W T 1955 Space requirements of the seated operator. WADC-TR-55-159, Aerospace Medical Research Laboratories, Ohio

Hatze H 2000 The inverse dynamics problem of neuromuscular control. Biological Cybernetics 82:133–141

Hawkins D, Hull M L 1990 A method for determining lower extremity muscle-tendon lengths during flexion/extension movements. Journal of Biomechanics 23:487–494

Heller M O, Bergmann G, Deuretzbacher G et al 2001 Musculo-skeletal loading conditions at the hip during walking and stair climbing. Journal of Biomechanics 34:883–893

Holden J P, Stanhope S J 1998 The effect of variation in knee center location estimates on net knee joint moments. Gait & Posture 7(1):1–6

Holden J P, Orsini J A, Siegel K L et al 1997 Surface movement errors in shank kinematics and knee kinetics during gait. Gait & Posture 5(3):217–227

Jensen R K 1986 Body segment mass, radius and radius of gyration proportions of children. Journal of Biomechanics 19:359–368

Komi P 1990 Relevance of in vivo force measurements to human biomechanics. Journal of Biomechanics 23:23–34

Lloyd D G, Besier T F 2003 An EMG-driven musculoskeletal model to estimate muscle forces and knee moments in vivo. Journal of Biomechanics 36:765–776

Lu T-W, O'Connor J J, Taylor S J G, Walker P S 1998 Validation of a lower limb model with in vivo femoral forces telemetered from two subjects. Journal of Biomechanics 31:63–69

Morrison J B 1970 The mechanics of the knee joint in relation to normal walking. Journal of Biomechanics 2:51–61

Park S, Krebs D E, Mann R W 1999 Hip muscle co-contraction: evidence from concurrent in vivo pressure measurement and force estimation. Gait & Posture 10(3):211–222

Paul J P 1966 Force actions transmitted by joints in the human body. Proceedings of the Institute of Mechanical Engineers 18(3):8–15

Pearsall D J, Costigan P A 1999 The effect of segment parameter error on gait analysis results, Gait & Posture 9(3):173–183

Plagenhoef S, Evans F G, Abdelnour T 1983 Anatomical data for analyzing human motion. Research Quarterly in Exercise and Sport 54:169–178

Redfern M S, DiPasquale J 1997 Biomechanics of descending ramps. Gait & Posture 6:119–125

Riener R, Rabuffetti M, Frigo C 2002 Stair ascent and descent at different inclinations, Gait & Posture 15(1):32–44

Spoor C W, Vanleeuwen J L, Meskers C G M et al 1990 Estimation of instantaneous moment arms of lower-leg muscles. Journal of Biomechanics 23:1247

Stallard J 1987 Assessment of the mechanical function of orthoses by force vector visualisation. Physiotherapy 73(8):398–402

Stansfield B W, Hillman S J, Hazlewood M E et al 2001 Sagittal joint kinematics, moments, and powers are predominantly characterized by speed of progression, not age. Journal of Pediatric Orthopedics 21:403–411

Stoudt H W 1981 The anthropometry of the elderly. Human Factors 23:29–37

Sun J, Walters M, Svensson N, Lloyd D 1996 The influence of surface slope on human gait characteristics: a study of urban pedestrians walking on an inclined surface. Ergonomics 39(4):677–692

Tait J H, Rose G K 1979 The real time video vector display of ground reaction forces during ambulation. Journal of Medical Engineering & Technology 3(5):252–255

Viser J J, Hoogkammer J E, Bobbert M F, Huijing P A 1990 Length and moment arms of human leg muscles as a function of knee and hip-joint angles. European Journal of Applied Physiology 61:453–460

Wells R P 1981 The projection of ground reaction force as a predictor of internal joint moments. Bulletin of Prosthetics Research 18:15–19

Winter D A 1990 The biomechanics and motor control of human movement, 2nd edn. John Wiley, New York

Chapter 8

Muscles

If you want to know if your brain is flabby, feel your legs.

Bruce Barton

Muscles are the motors of gait, with each precisely specialized to accomplish its task in the gait cycle.

ANATOMY

It's worth revising some basic neuroanatomy and neurophysiology: the main muscles of the lower-limb involved in gait are listed in Table 8.1 and illustrated in Figure 8.1.

Table 8.1   Main muscle groups involved in gait. The knee is constrained to move in the sagittal plane so has no musculature for frontal plane motion. Muscle action in the transverse plane is not considered here

Joint	Sagittal plane	Frontal plane
Hip	Flexor: *Iliopsoas* Extensor: *Gluteus maximus*, Hamstrings	Abductor: *Gluteus medius/minimus* Adductor: *Adductor longus/magnus*
Knee	Flexor: Hamstrings Extensor: Quadriceps (*Vasti + Rectus femoris*)	
Ankle	Dorsiflexor: *Tibialis anterior* Plantarflexors: *Triceps surae* (*Gastrocnemius + Soleus*)	Inverter: *Tibialis anterior, Tibialis posterior* Everter: *Peronei*

Figure 8.1   Major muscles used in gait.

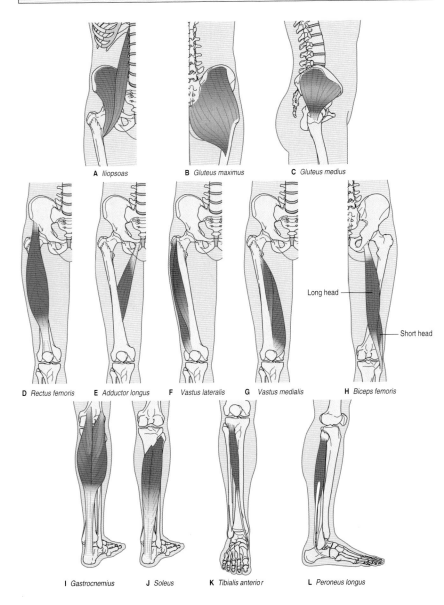

A *Iliopsoas*   B *Gluteus maximus*   C *Gluteus medius*

D *Rectus femoris*   E *Adductor longus*   F *Vastus lateralis*   G *Vastus medialis*   H *Biceps femoris*

Long head

Short head

I *Gastrocnemius*   J *Soleus*   K *Tibialis anterior*   L *Peroneus longus*

POLYARTICULAR MUSCLES

Some muscles span two (biarticular) or more (polyarticular) joints. Examples are *psoas*, hamstrings, *gastrocnemius* and *rectus femoris*. The function of these two-joint muscles has been hotly debated.

One possibility is energy transfer between joints (Lieber 1990, Wells 1998). For example, hamstrings may transfer the energy of knee extension to hip extension during late swing (Prilutsky et al 1998, Kuo 2001). Two-joint muscles may also be better at generating shear forces at the foot than monoarticular muscles (Hof 2001).

? **MCQ 8.1**

Which of these is a polyarticular muscle?
(a) *Psoas*
(b) *Iliacus*
(c) *Soleus*
(d) *Tibialis anterior*

Action at a distance

It's important to realize that muscles can have effects at joints far removed from those they span. A clear example of this is in the control of the knee during standing. If the GRF is behind the knee, making it unstable, there are several ways in which stability can be restored. The most obvious would be to activate the knee extensors (Fig. 8.2A). However, note that contracting the hip extensors (Fig. 8.2B) or ankle plantarflexors (Fig. 8.2C) has the same result. In (B), the thigh and in (C) the shank is pulled backwards, both actions that restore a stable posture by extending the knee and pulling it behind the GRF. Thus, although the *gluteus maximus* and *soleus* are usually thought of as hip extensors or plantarflexors, respectively, in this situation they are both behaving as knee extensors.

In more dynamic activities muscle action can be even more complicated and counter-intuitive. For example, it has been shown that even the *gastrocnemius* can act as a knee extensor in certain situations (Zajac & Gordon, 1989). During

Figure 8.2

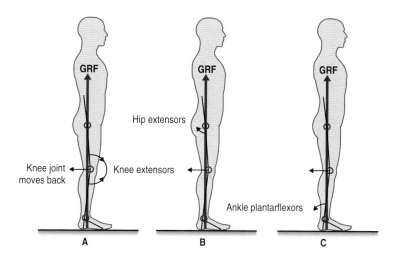

gait, knee stability can even be aided by contributions from the musculature of the *contralateral* limb! The end result of an individual muscle contraction effectively depends on the dynamic state of all body segments, making it difficult to predict the effect of an individual muscle contraction without extensive and accurate biomechanical models (Zajac et al 2003). Polyarticular muscles have especially complex effects (Kuo 2001).

This recent work has revealed the traditional open-chain anatomical classification of muscles to be imprecise at best and occasionally downright wrong. Muscle activation is best thought of as being *task-specific*. In other words, muscles act in whatever combination is appropriate to the task underway.

Kuo A D 2001 The action of two-joint muscles: The legacy of W P Lombard. In: Latash M L, Zatsiorsky V M (eds) Classics in movement science. Human Kinetics, Champaign, IL

Zajac F E, Gordon M F 1989 Determining muscle's force and action in multi-articular movement. Exercise and Sport Science Reviews 17:187–230

Zajac F E, Neptune R R, Kautz S A 2003 Biomechanics and muscle coordination of human walking – Part II: Lessons from dynamical simulations and clinical implications. Gait & Posture 17(1):1–17

NEUROANATOMY

Each muscle contraction starts with the excitation of an upper motor neuron (UMN) in the motor cortex of the brain, which travels down the spinal cord (in the pyramidal tract) to synapse with a lower motor neuron (LMN) in the ventral horn of the spinal cord at the level of the nerve root innervating the muscle (Fig. 8.3).

Note that neurons in the central nervous system (CNS), i.e. brain and spinal cord, have little capacity for repair once damaged, while those in the peripheral nervous system (PNS), i.e. nerve roots and peripheral nerves, will regenerate at a rate of about 1 mm/day (*Wallerian regeneration*) after injury.

Figure 8.3 Motor control schematic, showing sites of common lesions affecting gait. 1 (motor cortex): stroke, head injury; 2 (upper motor neuron): cerebral palsy, spinal cord injury, multiple sclerosis, myelopathy; 3 (anterior horn cell): spina bifida, poliomyelitis, motor neuron disease; 4 (peripheral nerve): sciatica, common peroneal nerve palsy; 5 (muscle): muscular dystrophy, myasthenia gravis.

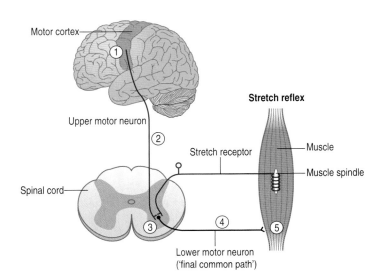

Because the stretch reflex is generally inhibited by descending UMN fibres, lesions in the white matter cause an UMN syndrome, characterized by a spastic paralysis with increased muscle tone and exaggerated reflexes. On the other hand, *denervation* of muscle caused by lesions of the LMN result in flaccid weakness with muscle atrophy.

? MCQ 8.2

Which of these typically causes a flaccid paralysis?
(a) Spinal cord injury
(b) Cerebral palsy
(c) Poliomyelitis
(d) Stroke

EXCITATION–CONTRACTION COUPLING

The action potential arrives at the endplate of a motor unit supplied by the lower motor neuron. The number of fibres in each motor unit varies inversely with the amount of fine control possible, and is around 2000 in most of the lower-limb musculature (Feinstein et al 1955). A motor unit action potential (MUAP), triggered by the release of acetylcholine, causes the release of calcium from the sarcoplasmic reticulum. This calcium binds to a protein called troponin-tropomyosin (T-T system), changing its shape and causing cross-bridges to form between overlapping *sliding filaments* of myosin and actin.

The molecular power source, adenosine triphosphate (ATP), binds to the myosin and generates a power-stroke (Huxley & Simmons 1971). ADP+P moves off the myosin and a new ATP molecule binds to it, allowing it to release the actin, and the cycle begins again in a 'grab and swivel' ratchet mechanism.

Muscle force is generated by summation of the tiny forces generated in each muscle fibre. It is important to realize that force production in each fibre is an all-or-none effect (Hatze 1979). Increase in force arises from *recruitment* of more motor units (spatial summation) and increased firing rate (temporal summation) of motor units (Milner-Brown et al 1973). Not all muscle fibres are the same size – following the *size principle*, the smallest have the lowest threshold and so are recruited first (Henneman et al 1965).

The UMN normally regulates muscle tone by modulating the activity of the monosynaptic stretch reflex (reflex arc). When UMN control is lost (the LMN remaining intact), the stretch reflex becomes hyperactive and the muscle spastic. If the LMN ('final common path' of Sherrington) is transected or destroyed, muscle innervation is lost, resulting in a flaccid paralysis.

FIBRE TYPES

Although all muscle fibres are the same, their properties can be conditioned by the innervating motor neuron (Burke et al 1971). Three characteristic patterns have been described: Type I, Type IIA and Type IIB (Table 8.2). Type I fibres have an aerobic metabolism that relies on a good blood flow, and are capable of generating low to moderate force over long periods (tonic contraction) without fatigue. Type IIB fibres have contrasting and complementary properties, being more dependent on glycolytic anaerobic metabolism, which is faster but susceptible to rapid fatigue. They are also larger diameter and therefore capable of generating higher forces. Type IIA fibres are intermediate between these two extremes, capable of rapid, repetitive action.

In general, fast twitch muscle fibres generate small amounts of energy very quickly whereas slow twitch muscles generate a lot of energy slowly. The recruitment sequence is thought to proceed from I to IIA to IIB as increasing force is required.

The dark (red) meat in chicken legs, used for walking and standing, is mainly composed of slow twitch fibres. The white meat in the breast is largely made up of fast twitch muscle fibres, and used for brief bursts of flight, which requires much energy.

The weakness and disuse atrophy associated with many of the conditions causing gait disorders tend to particularly affect Type I fibres, resulting in a preponderance of fast twitch fibres.

? MCQ 8.3

Which of these properties should a postural muscle have?
(a) Oxidative metabolism
(b) Fast twitch
(c) Large fibres
(d) High MTPase activity

Table 8.2 Contrasting properties of types of muscle fibre. Type I (slow twitch) fibres are specialized for low-intensity, fatigue-resistant activity, while Type IIB (fast twitch) fibres are suited to rapid, high-intensity contractions. An intermediate subtype (Type IIA) has properties midway between these two extremes (fast but relatively fatigue-resistant)

	Type I S (slow)	Type IIA FR (fast resistant)	Type IIB FF (fast fatiguable)
Contraction	tonic	phasic	phasic
Excitation coupling delay	long	short	short
Fibre size	small	intermediate	large
Threshold	low	high	high
Mitochondria	many	intermediate	few
Vascularity	rich	rich	poor
Myoglobin content	rich	rich	poor
Metabolism	aerobic (oxidative)	intermediate	anaerobic (glycolytic)
Myosin ATPase activity	low	low	high
Fatigue	resistant	intermediate	vulnerable
Peak tension	low	intermediate	high
Time to peak force	long (60–120 ms)	short	short (10–50 ms)
Function	tonic (postural)	repetitive phasic	phasic motion
Examples	*soleus, gluteus maximus*	*gastrocnemius*	hamstrings

MUSCLE ARCHITECTURE

Rather than being arranged parallel with the tendon (strap muscle), the fibres in most muscles are set at an angle. This is called *pennation*, and allows the physiological cross-sectional area (PCSA) of the muscle to be increased. This increases the force-generating capacity at a cost of slowing the speed of shortening. Other important differences between muscles include the ratio of tendon and fibre length (Table 8.3).

DYNAMIC ELECTROMYOGRAPHY

The summation of many MUAPs from all the motor units active at a given time results in electrical (*myoelectric*) activity called the electromyogram. This can be picked up over the skin surface over the muscle (sEMG), or by percutaneous (*indwelling*) fine needle electrodes inserted into the muscle belly (Bogey et al 2000).

The EMG signal recorded by surface electrodes is very small – less than 1 mV – so its amplitude must be increased using an *amplifier* in order to record and display it. One potential problem in doing this, however, is that this will also amplify any background electrical *noise* caused by fluorescent lamps, motors or computers in the vicinity of the subject. In the old days, laboratories used to be equipped with Faraday cages to try to isolate the subject from all this noise, but fortunately modern *instrumentation* amplifiers make this unnecessary. This is a form of *differential* amplifier that multiplies the difference between its two input terminals by a large gain (of the order of 1000), whilst having a very small gain for any voltage that is present on both terminals. Electrical noise is rejected, since it is common to both terminals, while the signal is amplified (Fig. 8.4).

The *common mode rejection ratio* (CMRR) is very large for EMG amplifiers – typically 90 dB. The unit dB (*decibel*) is just a shorthand way of expressing the ratio between two quantities:

$$90 \text{ dB} = 20 \log_{10} (\text{Differential Gain/Common Gain})$$
$$\text{rearranging, Differential Gain/Common Gain} = 10^{90/20}$$
$$\text{or } 10^{4.5} = 30{,}000$$

Assuming a differential gain of 1000 this means that the common gain must be 1000/30,000 = 1/30. In other words, the noise will actually be

Table 8.3 Architectural properties of some of the major lower-limb muscles (from Wickiewicz et al 1983)

Muscle	Fibre length (mm)	PCA (mm^2)	Pennation angle (°)	Tendon/ fibre length	Twitch time (ms)
Rectus femoris	68	1250	5	5	
Vastus lateralis	67	3000	5	2.7	
Soleus	30	5800	30	11.3	
Gastrocnemius	48	3000	15	8.9	

Figure 8.4 A differential
amplifier rejects noise present
on both inputs by preferentially
amplifying the difference by a
gain, G.

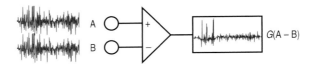

attenuated (reduced in amplitude) by a factor of 30 while the signal (the EMG) is increased 1000-fold.

? MCQ 8.4

What would be the noise attenuation in an amplifier with a CMRR of 100 dB and differential gain of 1000?
(a) 1/10
(b) 1/30
(c) 1/100
(d) 1/1000

Instrumentation amplifiers have greatly simplified EMG recording, but it is important to note that the principle of its operation depends on the noise being equally present on both input leads. In order to best achieve this, the electrodes should therefore be attached as close together as possible (without overlapping). Luckily, the fibres of a motor unit are scattered quite randomly through the muscle, so the signal picked up by a surface electrode is reasonably representative of the whole muscle. The location of the electrodes is therefore not particularly critical, but they are typically placed over the centre of the muscle belly, with the electrodes oriented longitudinally (Basmajian & De Luca 1985). Larger diameter motor units (especially IIB) generate higher potentials than the smaller, slower twitch Type I fibres.

Surface electrodes can be either *passive* or *active*. Passive electrodes are generally made of silver/silver chloride (Ag/AgCl) and are available in sizes of 7–20 mm (Fig. 8.5). They are usually disposable, self-adhesive and contain their own conductive gel. Reusable types are also sometimes used, in which case gel must be applied from a tube before use. They also need to be attached with adhesive tape, making them somewhat messy to use.

Many companies now incorporate a pre-amplifier in an *active* electrode (Fig. 8.6).

Figure 8.5 Disposable, self–adhesive Ag/AgCl electrodes (10 mm conductive area) with snap connector. Dual electrodes are also available (here with an inter-electrode distance 20 mm). Both by Noraxon USA, Inc.

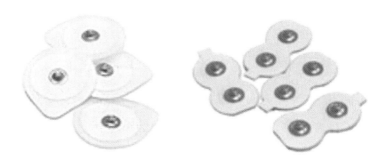

Figure 8.6 Active electrodes. Delsys DE-2.3 active EMG electrode (gain of 1000, bandwidth 20–450 Hz), and Motion Lab Systems MA-311 (CMRR > 100 dB), which is a double differential type.

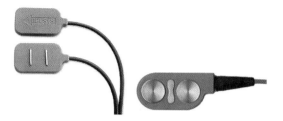

CROSSTALK

Although electrodes are intended to record the EMG of a particular muscle, in practice a certain proportion of the signal (perhaps 10–20%) is likely to have arisen (or 'leaked') from adjacent muscles (De Luca & Merletti 1988). This phenomenon is called *crosstalk*, and is especially likely when the muscle belly is small (e.g. the *peronei*) and close to large muscles (e.g. *gastrocnemius*). It can be avoided to some extent by using a *double differential* technique (Fig. 8.7). This requires an amplifier with three active electrodes (Winter 1990, Winter et al 1994). Differential signals are obtained between each of the outer two electrodes and a central electrode. The final signal is derived from the differential between these two signals.

Sometimes it is impossible to avoid crosstalk or the muscle (e.g. *iliopsoas* or *tibialis posterior*) is simply too deep for surface electrodes to collect an adequate signal. In such cases, *fine-wire* electrodes are necessary. These are introduced into the muscle *percutaneously* (through the skin) using a sterile *trocar* (Fig. 8.8).

Figure 8.7 The double differential technique for reducing crosstalk.

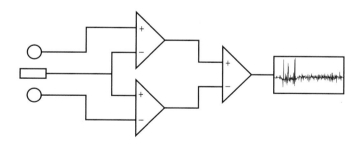

Figure 8.8 Insertion of a fine-wire electrode. The wire is typically 50 μm, nylon insulated nickel-chromium alloy with the last 2 mm bared, and inserted inside a 30 gauge needle (courtesy Motion Lab Systems, Baton Rouge, LA, USA).

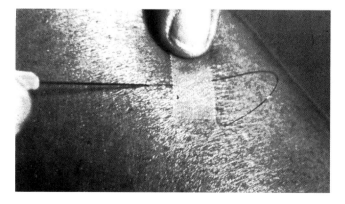

The signal detected by an intramuscular electrode is somewhat different from surface EMG, in that only fibres very close to the tip will be sampled. The precise location of the tip within the muscle is therefore critical. Often it is adjusted until an appropriate signal is achieved, if possible by asking the subject to contract the muscle voluntarily, or by using electrical stimulation to initiate a contraction. Clearly, some experience is essential for good results.

DEBATING POINT

Debate the advantages and disadvantages of the following in clinical electro-myography:
– Surface electrodes
– Fine-needle electrodes

MOTION ARTEFACT

Two other operations are also usually performed on the EMG signal. Firstly, any slight movement of the electrodes (whether surface or intra-muscular) tends to cause a very low frequency *motion artefact*. This is due to changes in the small direct current (DC) offset voltage on each electrode, and so can be greatly reduced by high-pass filtering the signals on each input terminal before they are amplified. The cutoff frequency chosen for the motion artefact filter is somewhat arbitrary but is around 10–40 Hz in most commercial systems. There is a slight trade-off in that higher cutoff values tend to degrade the EMG signal a little, so some journals (e.g. ISEK) insist on a 10 Hz cutoff. For gait analysis this can sometimes fail to elimi-nate all motion artefact and 40 Hz is generally preferred.

ANTI-ALIASING

These days, most EMG signals are sampled by an analogue to digital con-verter (ADC) to be stored in a computer, so a second low-pass filtering stage is also usually included to prevent *aliasing*. This is a distortion of the signal that can take place when it has frequency components which are more than twice the sampling rate of the converter (Nyquist theorem). So, for example, if the final EMG is sampled at 1000 Hz then the anti-aliasing filter should have a cutoff of 500 Hz or less. Together with the high-pass (motion artefact) filter, the anti-aliasing low-pass filter defines the fre-quency response, or *bandwidth*, of the EMG system.

ENVELOPING

Since it is composed of thousands of individual MUAPs, the EMG signal consists of a series of spikes. Sometimes, no further processing of the EMG is performed and this signal is simply interpreted by eye to reveal the on and off periods of muscle activity (Fig. 8.9). Alternatively, the time

Figure 8.9 Raw EMG signal. Periods of muscle activity are often defined clinically by eye (shaded regions). Such an interpretation is somewhat subjective, especially during periods when EMG activity is equivocal (dashed lines) (courtesy Motion Lab Systems, Baton Rouge, LA, USA).

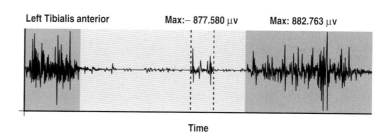

Figure 8.10 Rectified EMG signal (courtesy Motion Lab Systems, Baton Rouge, LA, USA).

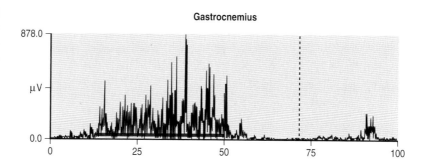

at which the EMG signal rises above, or falls below a threshold set by, for example, two or three standard deviations of the average noise level, can be used to define the periods of muscle activity.

If this is done, it is important to realize that there is an excitation coupling delay between the EMG signal and the force or moment output by the muscle. This delay depends on the fibre-type composition of the muscle (with slower twitch fibres having a slower rise-time), the firing rate (since higher firing rates recruit larger diameter fibres), and the length and properties of the muscle and tendon (which determine the transfer of force from muscle to bone). The total delay between EMG and peak joint moment resulting can be up to a few hundred milliseconds. In practice, few clinicians take this into account. Moreover, since average conduction velocity is about 4 m/s (longer when the muscle is fatigued), the signal will require at least 10 ms just to reach the electrode, making interpretation of the timing of muscle activity from raw EMG fraught with difficulty.

It should also be noted that raw EMG is biphasic, while muscles can only pull, not push, and since the force (twitch) produced by a given muscle fibre lasts much longer than the action potential, the joint moment resulting from a muscle contraction is much smoother than the EMG associated with it. In order to make the EMG signal resemble the force or moment generated, therefore, an operation called *enveloping* needs to be performed.

First, the raw EMG is rectified by a detector, which allows only the positive halves of the biphasic signal through (Fig. 8.10). Finally, a low-pass filter is used to smooth this rectified signal such that it resembles the muscle force (Fig. 8.11).

Figure 8.11   EMG signal after linear enveloping (courtesy Motion Lab Systems, Baton Rouge, LA, USA).

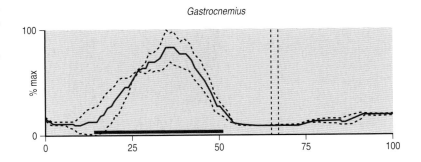

This smooth curve is called the linear envelope of the original signal, and its smoothness depends on the cutoff frequency of the final low-pass filter. In order to make the signal most closely track the muscle force or moment, the cutoff frequency should ideally be matched to the twitch time of the muscle. In practice, most laboratories use a single cutoff frequency for all muscles – usually 3 Hz (Winter 1990), although it has been suggested that a cutoff of 25 Hz preserves important transients evident in gait as compared to isometric preparations (Hof et al 2002).

FOOTSWITCHES

In order to determine the relationship of the EMG to the gait cycle, some means of detecting initial contact and toe-off is required. If the EMG is recorded simultaneously while a 3D motion analysis is being performed, the data can be obtained from the force platform and kinematics. However, the combination of carrying the instrumentation for recording EMG while wearing reflective markers can be somewhat encumbering to some subjects. An alternative in these situations, and for studies where 3D motion analysis is not required, is to use small footswitches attached to the sole. These switches are designed to make contact at specific gait cycle events and their output can be recorded along with the EMG data for later processing. Switches are generally placed over the heel, medial and lateral forefoot, and hallux (Fig. 8.12).

Figure 8.12   Footswitches used in recording EMG during gait (courtesy Motion Lab Systems, Baton Rouge, LA, USA).

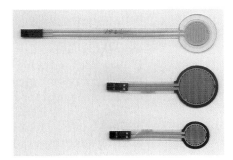

TELEMETRY

There are two basic methods for transmitting the EMG data from the subject to the recording station. One uses a thin cable to carry the signals *multiplexed* onto a single thin wire (Fig. 8.13). The other eliminates cable altogether by transmitting the signals by wireless radio *telemetry*. Each has its advantages: obviously, the wireless method is least encumbering but may introduce noise and dropout due to radio propagation problems. Telemetry systems are often more expensive too.

NORMALIZATION

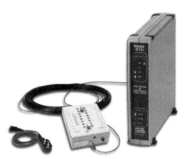

Figure 8.13 MA-300 16-channel EMG system (uses double-differential active electrodes) with 18 m of 2 mm thin coaxial cable (courtesy Motion Lab Systems , Baton Rouge, LA, USA).

Since there are so many factors affecting the amplitude of the EMG signal obtained for a given force or moment, e.g. skin impedance, amount of subcutaneous fat, level of fitness of the subject, some form of normalization procedure is desirable (De Luca 1997). This can be done by asking the subject to generate a maximal isometric force and record the resulting EMG. The root mean square (RMS) is then calculated (in a similar manner to standard deviation) by summing the square of each sample and dividing by the number of samples, and taking the square root:

$$\text{RMS} = \sqrt{\frac{\sum e_i^2}{n}}$$

where $i = 1$ to n samples of the EMG, e.

The amplitude of subsequent recordings can then be divided by this value. Unfortunately there are problems with this approach. First, generating a maximal force can be somewhat subjective and requires a comprehensive anatomical knowledge together with a suitably designed restraining device to ensure that the muscle being tested is the main one being activated. Electrical stimulation using a supramaximal voltage and high frequency can be used to try to ensure a maximal contraction, but it is not clear how such *synchronous* firing, due to this artificial stimulation, compares with the normal *asynchronous* activation by the CNS. The procedure becomes even more problematical in patients with weakness, spasticity or those who lack selective muscle control.

For these reasons, in practice most clinical gait laboratories do not attempt to normalize their EMG recordings.

FACTORS GOVERNING THE RELATIONSHIP BETWEEN EMG AND MUSCLE FORCE

Although EMG amplitude is well correlated with muscle force in a static situation (Milner-Brown & Stein 1975), this relationship breaks down during motion due to the characteristics of the sliding filament mechanism. The length–tension relationship (Hill 1938) dictates an optimal length for each muscle for force generation. When the muscle is longer or shorter than that 'resting length', force generation is compromised (Fig. 8.14).

There is a force–velocity relationship, too (Fenn & Marsh 1935, Hill 1953, Perrine & Edgerton 1978), with muscle force tailing off as the speed of the contraction increases (Fig. 8.15).

In addition to these properties, as muscle contracts, its relationship to the electrodes changes.

Figure 8.14   The length–tension relationship of muscle. Contractile force is maximal at the resting length of the muscle, and decreases markedly when the muscle length is outside the normal operating range.

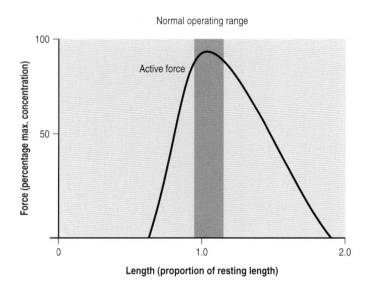

Figure 8.15   Force–velocity relationship. In general, the speed of contraction slows as the muscle is made to contract against a greater load, and vice versa. The greatest force can be maintained at zero velocity (isometric contraction), while the greatest velocity (V_{max}) occurs at zero force.

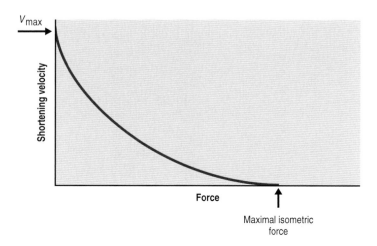

Management of spasticity

Hyperactivity of the stretch reflex, resulting in hypertonia and rigidity, is common in upper motor neuron disorders, such as stroke and cerebral palsy. A number of interventions (Fig. 8.16) have been developed in an attempt to reduce spasticity and/or mitigate its effects, ranging from the *conservative* to the more *aggressive* (surgical).

Drug therapy with baclofen or dantrolene sodium can be effective but these have the side effect of sedation, which often prevents the most effective dose from being used. Intrathecal pumps inject the drug into the spinal fluid around the nerve roots supplying leg muscles, and thus produce the same effect at a lower dosage, but require a cannula to be inserted into the spinal cord. Whilst there is some evidence that neuromuscular electrical stimulation (NMES) of the muscle, its antagonist, or even the cerebellum, can reduce spasticity, results have generally been disappointing. In recent years, injection of botulinum toxin (Botox) into the affected muscles has become popular. It causes reversible paralysis for a period of 6–8 weeks following the injection. Unfortunately, antibodies to the toxin (which is produced by bacteria responsible for food-poisoning) gradually develop which may require the dosage to be increased. Physical therapy techniques such as neurodevelopmental therapy (NDT) or proprioceptive neuromuscular facilitation (PNF) may be effective, but are time-consuming and expensive.

Figure 8.16

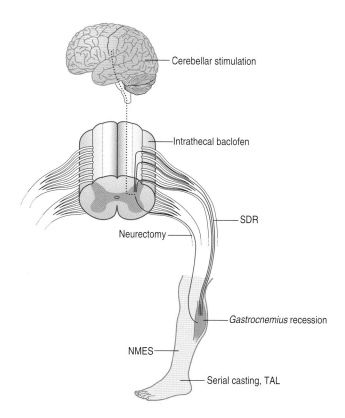

Orthotic approaches include inhibitory ('tone-reducing') braces and serial casting, in which a series of orthoses (usually AFOs) are worn over a period of several weeks or months. The orthosis is set in dorsiflexion, which is steadily increased each time it is reapplied, in an effort to stretch a contracted Achilles tendon.

Selective dorsal rhizotomy (SDR) is a surgical division of the sensory nerve roots, which requires sophisticated intraoperative monitoring to differentiate abnormal from healthy fibres. Selective neurectomy is a procedure in which the motor neuron to a severely spastic muscle is severed.

A good example of the complexities of surgical intervention is the management of ankle equinus. Since the fibre length of the *soleus* is shorter than that of the *gastrocnemius*, the former is more sensitive to Achilles tendon (heel cord) lengthening (TAL), with the result that the ankle collapses into dorsiflexion. This has led some surgeons to prefer the more selective *gastrocnemius* recession, which leaves the *soleus* intact (Baker 1956). Such approaches are, however, limited to correcting only mild to moderate deformities, and recurrence is quite common. Another possibility is proximal recession, in which the origin, rather than insertion, of the biarticular *gastrocnemius* muscle is moved – this tends be reserved for cases in which the *gastrocnemius* causes knee contracture. As a last resort, pantalar (triple) arthrodesis of the ankle is occasionally performed.

The existence of such a vast range of therapies is an indication that none of them is perfectly satisfactory. The management of spasticity is consequently one of the most controversial topics in the rehabilitation of gait disorders.

Baker L D 1956 A rational approach to the surgical needs of the cerebral palsy patient. Journal of Bone and Joint Surgery 38A:313–323

NORMATIVE EMG

The combination of these factors makes EMG measurements a poor guide to muscle force during movement. Figure 8.17 shows the typical linear envelopes recorded in normal gait, alongside the joint moment recorded by inverse dynamics.

Whilst the patterns of excitation generally resemble the shape of the joint moment curves, it should be noted that, for the reasons outlined above, the amplitude of the EMG does not accurately reflect the joint moment. There are also some interesting differences which illustrate the complementary roles of the two measurement approaches (Table 8.4). For example, the knee flexor moment during mid-stance is likely due to tension in the posterior capsule ligaments (which are electrically silent) as the knee is fully extended at this time. On the other hand, activity of the *tibialis anterior* in swing is not reflected in the moment curve because the moment required to lift the foot is negligible – the EMG is large because the muscle is superficial and a signal easily obtained.

It is possible under controlled conditions to use kinematic measurements to correct the EMG, such that a linear relation between EMG amplitude

Figure 8.17 Electromyography of normal gait alongside the corresponding joint moment as calculated by inverse dynamics. The moment curves have also been scaled (and filled in) to match the EMG envelopes, and the flexor moments have been inverted. There is a broad agreement between the patterns of both methods of estimating muscle activity, with a few exceptions. For example, the knee flexor moment during mid-stance is likely due to tension in the posterior capsule ligaments (which are electrically silent) as the knee is fully extended at this time. Meanwhile, activity of the *tibialis anterior* in swing is not reflected in the moment curve because the moment required to lift the foot is negligible (data from Winter & Yack 1987, Wooton et al 1990, Hof et al 2002).

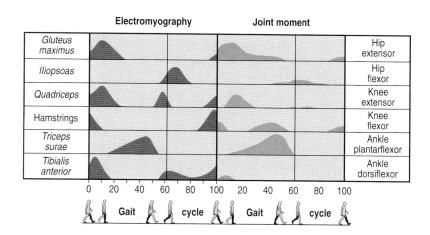

and force is obtained (Hof & van den Berg 1981a,b,c, White & Winter 1993, Lloyd & Besier 2003). However, in practice this is rarely attempted because it requires a number of time-consuming calibration procedures to estimate the various muscle parameters, many of which are subject-dependent. Instead, EMG tends to be used for 'on/off' information on muscle activity, to confirm inappropriate (e.g. spastic) contractions. Bar graphs summarizing this information (Fig. 8.18) are often used for this purpose.

It has been shown that the EMG of a given muscle in normal gait can be derived from a small subset of patterns, providing evidence for the central pattern generator theory of locomotor control (Hof et al 2002). These basic patterns appear to be modified by a 'speed controller' in the CNS to adapt muscle action accordingly.

Table 8.4 Some contrasting characteristics of joint moment and EMG when used to estimate muscle activity. The two techniques are often complementary and can provide a more complete picture when used together

Characteristic	Joint moment	EMG
Results	Quantitative	Qualitative (on/off) or semi-quantitative
Agonist/antagonist co-contraction	Measures net moment	May suffer crosstalk
Taut ligaments (end range of motion)	Cannot differentiate between muscle and ligament	Unaffected
Error sources	Incorrect marker attachment, malalignment between force platform and kinematic origin	Incorrect electrode placement, electrical noise

Figure 8.18 Normative gait muscle activity 'on/off' times illustrated by EMG bars (adapted by permission from Sutherland D H 1984 Gait disorders in childhood and adolescence. Lippincott Williams & Wilkins, Baltimore, MD). L.H., Long head; S.H., short head.

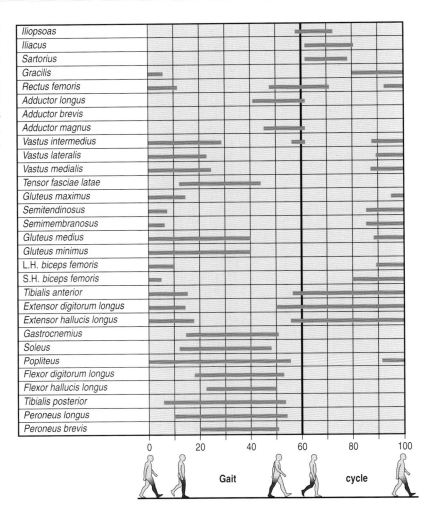

Moment vs EMG

Here's an interesting experiment to illustrate the complex relationship between EMG amplitude and joint moment (Hof & van den Berg 1981a,b,c).

When standing on tiptoes (Fig. 8.19), the GRF (half body weight, assuming the subject stands symmetrically) passes through the toes, so the external moment is easy to calculate – simply the GRF multiplied by the moment arm of the GRF at the ankle joint. As the ankle is plantarflexed further, this moment arm decreases as the ankle joint moves anteriorly closer to the line of action of the GRF. Since body weight hasn't changed, this must mean that the external moment has fallen. Of course, the external moment is matched by an equal internal moment from the plantarflexors, so this must also have fallen. Yet the RMS EMG level is found to rise dramatically – how can this be?

The solution is found in the length–tension curve of the muscles. As the ankle plantarflexes, the *gastrocnemius* and *soleus* shorten. When this happens the neural input (EMG) has to rise in order to maintain tension in the Achilles tendon. Even though the moment generated by the plantarflexors falls, the EMG measured progressively rises.

Figure 8.19

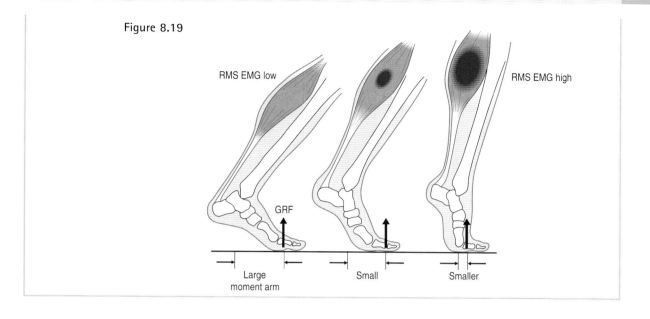

EFFECT OF FATIGUE

Another useful parameter of the EMG is its power spectrum (frequency content), which is usually calculated by a Fast Fourier Transform (FFT). As the muscle fatigues, the mean power frequency (MPF) or median frequency (MF) of the EMG falls (Fig. 8.20) (Merletti & Roy 1996). This drop in frequency also correlates with a reduction in force generation (Mannion & Dolan 1996).

PASSIVE CONNECTIVE TISSUE PROPERTIES

As well as the contractile component, muscle is also composed of fibrous connective tissue in the fascial sheaths (*parallel elastic* component) and the tendon (*series elastic* component). Both these components influence the time course of force generation, as well as having non-linear force–length characteristics of their own (Chapman 1985). These become especially important when the muscle is inactive, or stretched significantly beyond its resting length (Fig. 8.21).

Exactly how much energy can be stored in the elastic elements of muscle and tendon is a subject of some debate (Hof & van den Berg 1986, Ingen Schenau et al 1990). Whilst it can be substantial during running, especially in animals such as horses and kangaroos (Alexander & Bennet-Clark 1977, Biewener & Roberts 2000), energy storage is probably insignificant during human walking, except perhaps at the ankle.

Figure 8.20   Power spectra of soleus EMG before and after 40 standing heel-rise repetitions. The median frequency of the spectrum shifts down as the muscle is fatigued.

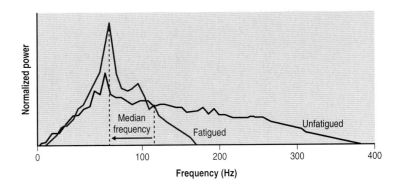

Figure 8.21   Simple muscle model, incorporating a contractile, parallel elastic (fascia) and series elastic (tendon) elements. The passive force due to these components (particularly the parallel elastic element) adds to the active force when the muscle is stretched.

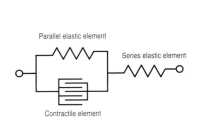

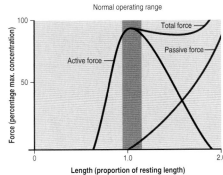

MUSCLE LENGTH ESTIMATION

In spastic conditions, such as cerebral palsy, muscles can be shortened either statically (due to contracture) or dynamically (due to a hyperactive stretch reflex). Although it is difficult to measure the length of the muscle directly, it can be estimated from a kinematic model (Fig. 8.22) (Eames et al 1995, 1997, Delp et al 1996, Lengsfeld et al 1997).

The length of muscle fascicles can also be measured in vivo by ultrasound (Fukunaga et al 1997, 2001) (Fig. 8.23). Fibre length has been shown to shorten with age (Gajdosik et al 1999).

KEY POINTS

★ Muscles may be mono- or poly-articular

★ Muscle tone is maintained by the stretch reflex, which is overactive in spastic paralysis

★ Muscle fibres can be slow/fatigue-resistant, fast/fatigue-sensitive or intermediate types

Figure 8.22 Lower-limb muscle lengths (percentage of resting length) over the gait cycle estimated from a 3D musculoskeletal model (courtesy of Dr Richard Baker, University of Melbourne, Australia).

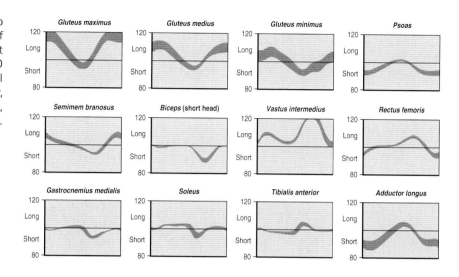

Figure 8.23 Muscle fibres visualized by ultrasound (courtesy Dr A Shortland, One Small Step gait laboratory, Guy's Hospital, London, UK).

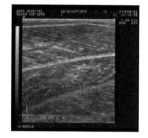

★ A differential amplifier is used to record electromyography from the muscle

★ The EMG may be interpreted raw, or following rectification and smoothing (linear envelope)

★ The relationship between EMG and muscle force is non-linear and depends on many factors

References

Alexander R M, Bennet-Clark H C 1977 Storage of elastic strain energy in muscle and other tissues. Nature 265:114–117

Basmajian J V, De Luca C J 1985 Muscles alive, 5th edn. Williams and Wilkins, Baltimore, MD

Biewener A A, Roberts T J 2000 Muscle and tendon contributions to force, work, and elastic energy savings: a comparative perspective. Exercise and Sport Science Review 28:99–107

Bogey R A, Perry J, Bontrager E L, Gronley J K 2000 Comparison of across-subject EMG profiles using surface and multiple indwelling wire electrodes during gait. Journal of Electromyography and Kinesiology 10:255–259

Burke R E, Levine D N, Zajac F E 1971 Mammalian motor units: physiological histochemical correlation in three types of motor units in cat gastrocnemius. Science 174:709

Chapman A E 1985 The mechanical properties of human muscle. Exercise and Sports Sciences Reviews 13:443–501

De Luca C J 1997 The use of surface electromyography in biomechanics. Journal of Applied Biomechanics 13:135–163

De Luca C J, Merletti R 1988 Surface myoelectric crosstalk among muscles of the leg. Electroencephalography and Clinical Neurophysiology 69:568–575

Delp S L, Arnold A S, Speers R A, Moore C 1996 Hamstrings and psoas lengths during normal and crouch gait: implications for muscle-tendon surgery. Journal of Orthopaedic Research 14:144–151

Eames N, Baker R, Cosgrove A 1995 Estimating gastrocnemius length from joint rotation measurements. Gait & Posture 3(4):277–278

Eames N W A, Baker R J, Cosgrove A P 1997 Defining gastrocnemius length in ambulant children. Gait & Posture 1(6):9–17

Feinstein B, Lindegård B, Nyman E, Wohlfart W 1955 Morphologic studies of motor units in normal human muscles. Acta Anatomica 23:127–142

Fenn W O, Marsh B S 1935 Muscular force at different speeds of shortening. Journal of Physiology 85:277–297

Fukunaga T, Ichinose Y, Ito M, Kawakami Y, Fukashiro S 1997 Determination of fascicle length and pennation in a contracting muscle in vivo. Journal of Applied Physiology 82(1):354–358

Fukunaga T, Kubo K, Kawakami Y et al 2001 In vivo behaviour of human muscle tendon during walking. Proceedings of the Royal Society of London B 268:229–233

Gajdosik R L, Linden D W V, Williams A K 1999 Influence of age on length and passive elastic stiffness characteristics of the calf muscle-tendon unit of women. Physical Therapy 79:827–838

Hatze H 1979 A teleological explanation of Weber's law and the motor unit size law. Bulletin of Mathematical Biology 41:407–425

Henneman E, Somjen G, Carpenter D O 1965 Functional significance in cell size in spinal motoneurons. Journal of Neurophysiology 28:560–580

Hill A V 1938 The heat of shortening and the dynamic constants of muscle. Proceedings of the Royal Society B 126:136-195

Hill A V 1953 The mechanics of active muscle. Proceedings of the Royal Society of London (Biology) 141:104–117

Hof A L 2001 The force resulting from the action of mono- and biarticular muscles in a limb. Journal of Biomechanics 34:1085–1089

Hof A L, van den Berg J W 1981a EMG to force processing I: an electrical analogue of the Hill muscle model. Journal of Biomechanics 14:747–758

Hof A L, van den Berg J W 1981b EMG to force processing II: estimation of parameters of the Hill muscle model for the human triceps surae by means of a calf ergometer. Journal of Biomechanics 14:759–770

Hof A L, van den Berg J W 1981c EMG to force processing III: estimation of model parameters for the human triceps surae muscle and assessment of the accuracy by means of a torque plate. Journal of Biomechanics 14:771–785

Hof A L, van den Berg J W 1986 How much energy can be stored in human muscle elasticity? Human Movement Science 5:107–114

Hof A L, Elzinga H, Grimmius W, Halbertsma J P K 2002 Speed dependence of averaged EMG profiles in walking. Gait & Posture 16(1):78–86

Huxley A F, Simmons R M 1971 Proposed mechanism of force generation in striated muscle. Nature 233:533–538

Ingen Schenau van G J, Bobbert M F, Haan A de 1990 Does elastic energy enhance work and efficiency in the stretch-shortening cycle? Journal of Applied Biomechanics 13(4):389–415

Kuo A D 2001 The action of two-joint muscles: the legacy of W P Lombard. In: Latash M L, Zatsiorsky V M (eds) Classics in movement science. Human Kinetics, Champaign, IL

Lengsfeld M, Pressel T, Stammberger U 1997 Lengths and lever arms of hip joint muscles: geometrical analyses using a human multibody model. Gait & Posture 6(1):18–26

Lieber R L 1990 Hypothesis: biarticular muscles transfer moments between joints. Developmental Medicine and Child Neurology 32:456–458

Lloyd D G, Besier T F 2003 An EMG-driven musculoskeletal model to estimate muscle forces and knee moments in vivo. Journal of Biomechanics 36:765–776

Mannion A F, Dolan P 1996 Relationship between myoelectric and mechanical manifestations of fatigue in the quadriceps femoris muscle group. European Journal of Applied Physiology 74:411–419

Merletti R, Roy S 1996 Myoelectric and mechanical manifestations of muscle fatigue in voluntary contractions. Journal of Orthopaedic and Sports Physical Therapy 24:342–353

Milner-Brown H S, Stein R B 1975 The relation between the surface electromyogram and muscular force. Journal of Physiology 246:549–569

Milner-Brown H S, Stein R B, Yemm R 1973 The orderly recruitment of human motor units during voluntary isometric contractions. Journal of Physiology 230:359–370

Perrine J J, Edgerton V R 1978 Muscle force-velocity and power-velocity relationships under isokinetic loading. Medicine and Science in Sports 10(3):159–166

Prilutsky B I, Gregor R J, Ryan M M 1998 Coordination of two-joint rectus femoris and hamstrings during the swing phase of human walking and running. Experimental Brain Research 120:479–486

Sutherland D H 1984 Gait disorders in childhood and adolescence. Lippincott Williams & Wilkins, Baltimore, MD

Wells R P 1998 Mechanical energy costs of human movement: an approach to evaluating the transfer possibilities of two-joint muscles. Journal of Biomechanics 21:955–964

White S C, Winter D A 1993 Predicting muscle forces in gait from EMG signals and musculotendon kinematics. Journal of Electromyography and Kinesiology 2:217–231

Wickiewcz T L, Roy R R, Powell P L, Edgerton V R 1983 Muscle architecture of the human lower limb. Clinical Orthopedics and Related Research 179:275–283

Winter D A 1990 Biomechanics and motor control of human movement, 2nd edn. Wiley, New York

Winter D A, Yack H J 1987 EMG profiles during normal human walking: stride-to-stride and inter-subject variability. Electroencephalography and Clinical Neurophysiology 67:402–411

Winter D A, Fugelvand A J, Archer S E 1994 Crosstalk in surface electromyography: theoretical and practical estimates. Journal of Electromyography and Kinesiology 4:15–26

Wooton M E, Kadaba M P, Cochran G V B 1990 Dynamic electromyography II. Normal patterns during gait. Journal of Orthopedic Research 8(2):259–265

Chapter 9

Gravity and centre of mass

Giant steps are what you take
Walking on the moon
I hope my legs don't break
Walking on the moon

Sting

OBJECTIVES

- Know how to calculate the total body centre of mass
- Know the general characteristics of the trajectory of the centre of mass during normal gait
- Know the determinants of gait and their limitations
- Understand how energy is exchanged to increase walking efficiency
- Understand how a force platform can be used to monitor body centre of mass
- Appreciation of the relationship between centre of mass, centre of pressure and base of support

In the same way that each segment has a CoM, the body as a whole also has a CoM, at which all its mass can be considered concentrated. Thus, we could replace all the body segments with just one large mass situated at the CoM. Its position can be calculated by taking moments about an arbitrary origin (Fig. 9.1).

$$x_{CoM} = (x_1 m_1 + x_2 m_1 + x_3 m_1 + \ldots x_n m_n)/M$$

$$y_{CoM} = (y_1 m_1 + y_2 m_1 + y_3 m_1 + \ldots y_n m_n)/M$$

$$z_{CoM} = (z_1 m_1 + z_2 m_1 + z_3 m_1 + \ldots z_n m_n)/M$$

Figure 9.1 Determination of the total body centre of mass (CoM). The CoM of each body segment (◔) exerts a moment about an arbitrary origin (0,0,0). The sum of these moments can be replaced by a single total body mass at the total body CoM (◕), which in normal gait is situated in the pelvis.

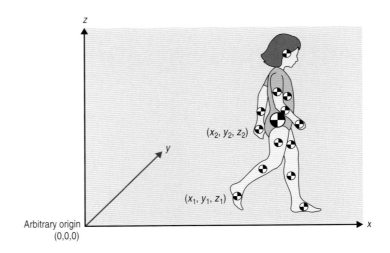

where (x_1, y_1, z_1) are the coordinates of the first body segment etc., and M = total body mass.

Clearly, some body segments (especially the trunk) have more mass and thus have more influence on the location of the CoM: it is the weighted average of the mass of all the body segments.

In general, during standing the CoM is located in the pelvis, at approximately the level of the second sacral vertebra (S2), or 55% of body height from the floor. During gait, the body behaves as an inverted pendulum, with the CoM falling during each double support phase, and rising during each single support (Fig. 9.2).

Notice that, since there are two double support phases and two single support phases during each gait cycle, the CoM oscillation has a frequency of twice the stride frequency. The amplitude of the motion is

Figure 9.2 Inverted pendulum model of gait, showing how CoM rises during single support and falls during double support. The amplitude of the displacement, *h*, is proportional to step length, *S*.

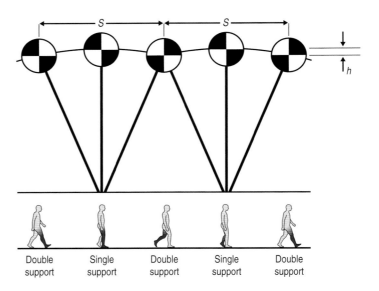

related to step length, so also tends to increase with speed (Gard & Childress 1999).

When is the body CoM highest in the gait cycle?
(a) Initial contact
(b) Mid-stance
(c) Double support
(d) Toe-off

Oscillations of similar amplitude also take place in the mediolateral (ML) and anteroposterior (AP) directions (Fig. 9.3). Note that in the former case the frequency is equal to the stride frequency, tracking the shift in weight over the supporting limb. In the AP direction, there is a relative forward movement of the CoM with the swing limb shortly after each toe-off, and backward motion during early single support, when the contralateral limb is trailing. This *relative* motion should not be confused with the *absolute* AP motion of the CoM, which is always forwards. At no time does the body move backwards with respect to the room – the CoM is simply moving backwards *within* the body. This is a subtle (and tricky!) but important distinction.

Figure 9.3 Height-normalized excursion of the body CoM (mean ± 1 SD) in the three directions in a sample of six normal adults aged 22–35 years, and 10 children aged 6–17 years (Eames et al 1999).

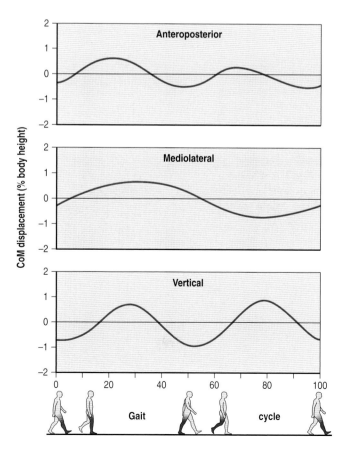

THE DETERMINANTS OF GAIT

Since gravity acts as a downward force on objects, lifting them up requires work to be done (or energy input). This potential energy (PE) can be calculated as:

$$PE = mgh$$

where m = mass of the object, g = gravitational acceleration (9.81 m/s^2) and h is the height through which the object is raised. A strong correlation (r^2 = 0.91) has been observed between the amplitude of the vertical displacement of the CoM and energy consumption (Kerrigan et al 1995).

One of the great pioneers of gait analysis, Verne Inman, thought that the driving aim of gait was to minimize vertical and horizontal motion of the CoM, so as to maximize efficiency. PE would have to be used to raise the body each cycle, which would be wasteful. Inman theorized that CoM motion would be reduced by increasing the effective lower-limb length during double support and decreasing it during single support. Six mechanisms, or *determinants* were described (Saunders et al 1953).

1. Pelvic rotation – the pelvis rotates forwards (internally) on the leading leg to increase its effective length. Of course, it also rotates externally on the contralateral side to simultaneously increase the length of the trailing limb (Fig. 9.4).

Figure 9.4   Effect of pelvic rotation in increasing the effective lower-limb length. (With permission from Saunders J B, Inman V, Eberhart H. The major determinants in normal and pathologic gait. JBJS 1953: 35: 3: 543–58; Figs 2, 3, 4 and 5 © The Journal of Bone and Joint Surgery, Inc.)

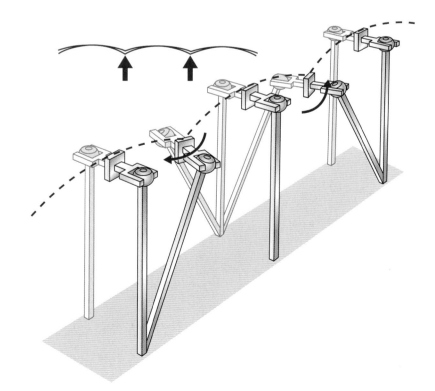

2. Pelvic obliquity – the pelvis lists downward to increase the effective leg length of the trailing limb (Fig. 9.5).

   There is a problem with this determinant. A quick look at the pelvis kinematics (Fig. 9.6) shows that the timing is not right – the pelvis does list downwards, but too late to help raise the CoM.

3. Stance phase knee flexion – the knee flexes during single support to effectively shorten the stance limb (Fig. 9.7).

   Once again, this sounds plausible until the timing is examined: stance knee flexion occurs too early (during double support) to provide the necessary shortening (Fig. 9.8), and the knee has already extended again by the time the CoM trajectory is highest in mid-stance (about 30% cycle).

4. Ankle rockers – the plantarflexion at toe-off was said to increase the effective length of the trailing limb at initial contact. In addition, heel-rise during the trailing support phase may be a much more important source of lift during double support (Kerrigan et al 2000).

5. Rotation of leg segments – internal rotation/pronation tends to shorten the limb during stance, while external rotation/supination lengthens it during toe-off.

6. Physiological genu valgum – the normal slight abduction of the knee (*genu valgum*) was claimed to reduce excessive lateral motion of the CoM by bringing the feet closer together and so reducing the walking base or step width (Fig. 9.9).

Figure 9.5   Effect of pelvic list (obliquity) in increasing trailing limb length. (With permission from Saunders J B, Inman V, Eberhart H. The major determinants in normal and pathologic gait. JBJS 1953: 35: 3: 543–58; Figs 2, 3, 4 and 5 © The Journal of Bone and Joint Surgery, Inc.)

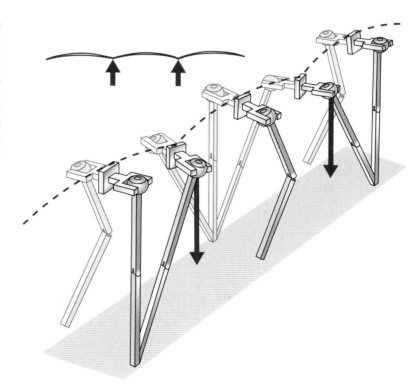

Figure 9.6 Pelvic list is too late to help raise the CoM.

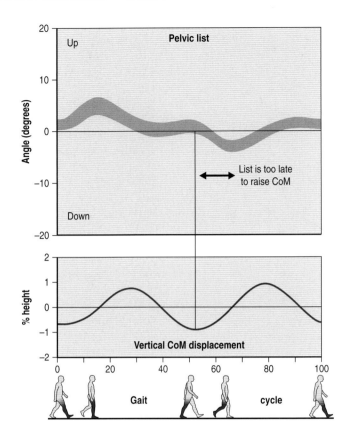

Figure 9.7 Effect of stance phase flexion in lowering the CoM. (With permission from Saunders J B, Inman V, Eberhart H. The major determinants in normal and pathologic gait. JBJS 1953: 35: 3: 543–58; Figs 2, 3, 4 and 5 © The Journal of Bone and Joint Surgery, Inc.)

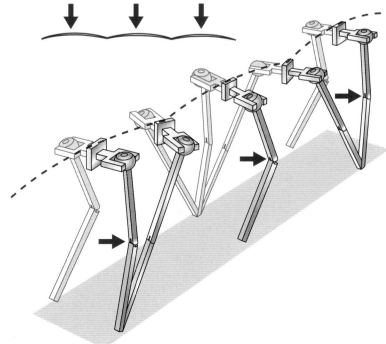

Figure 9.8 Stance phase knee flexion occurs too early to help lower the CoM during mid-stance.

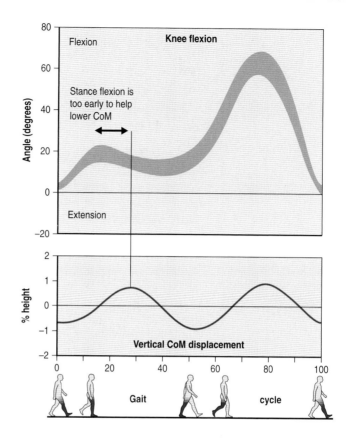

Figure 9.9 Effect of the physiological genu valgum angle at the knee in reducing excessive lateral motion of the CoM by decreasing step width. (With permission from Saunders J B, Inman V, Eberhart H. The major determinants in normal and pathologic gait. JBJS 1953: 35: 3: 543–58; Figs 2, 3, 4 and 5 © The Journal of Bone and Joint Surgery, Inc.)

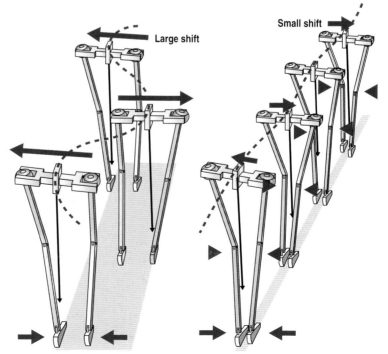

? MCQ 9.2

Which action would increase effective lower-limb length?
(a) Ipsilateral hip internal rotation at initial contact
(b) Ipsilateral pelvic list at initial contact
(c) Contralateral internal pelvic rotation at initial contact
(d) Contralateral knee flexion during mid-stance

Despite being a pillar of understanding of gait for many years, the determinants of gait have now been thoroughly discredited (Gard & Childress, 1997, 1999, 2001, Della Croce et al 2001, Kerrigan et al 2001). Problems have arisen not only with the timing of many of the mechanisms supposedly aimed at reducing CoM displacement, but also the premise that a larger CoM excursion is necessarily deleterious to energy consumption. CoM motion increases with step length, and therefore with increased speed.

From penguins and pregnancy to African women and astronauts

Penguins are notoriously inefficient walkers, expending twice as much energy as any other animal of the same size over the same distance. It used to be assumed that this was due to their waddling gait (Fig. 9.10), but a recent study (Griffin & Kram 2000) showed that it actually helps conserve energy. The rocking motion enables potential and kinetic energy to be exchanged with a recovery rate of up to 80% – among the highest of any land animal. Without the side-to-side and forward–backward motion, penguins would be less efficient. This is very important because penguins such as the Emperor may walk over 100 miles from their nests to the sea after fasting for 4 months during the long Antarctic winter.

Penguins have made an evolutionary tradeoff. Their short legs help reduce heat loss while incubating the eggs in winter, and make them better swimmers, but make walking less efficient. The cost of generating muscular force to support body weight is an important determinant of

Figure 9.10   (Reproduced by permission of Dr Tim M Griffin, Duke University Medical Center, Durham, NC, USA).

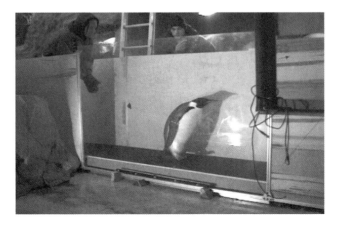

the metabolic cost of walking. Energy consumption is inversely proportional to the duration of stance phase, and since short-legged animals are in contact with the ground for a shorter time than long-legged animals at the same speed, their muscles need to generate more power, which is less efficient.

The results have implications not only for penguins, but also for anyone with a condition that causes an increase in lateral motion, such as obesity and pregnancy (Foti et al 2000). Women of the Kikuyu and Luo tribes in Kenya have the remarkable ability to carry a basket on their head weighing up to 70% of body weight (Heglund et al 1955). It turns out that their potential-kinetic recovery rate is 80%.

The optimal walking speed depends on the value of *g*. On the moon (where gravity is less than one-fifth that on earth), the optimal walking speed is so slow that it becomes useless – hence the reason for the bouncing moonwalk adopted by Apollo astronauts (Fig. 9.11) (Minetti 2001).

Figure 9.11

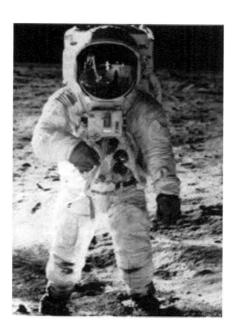

Foti T, Davids J R, Bagley A 2000 A biomechanical analysis of gait during pregnancy. Journal of Bone and Joint Surgery 82:625–632

Griffin M, Kram R 2000 Biomechanics: penguin waddling is not wasteful. Nature 408:929

Heglund N C, Willems P A, Penta M, Cavagna G A 1995 Energy-saving gait mechanics with head-supported loads. Nature 375:52–54

Minetti A E 2001 Walking on other planets. Nature 409:467–469

ENERGY EXCHANGE

In formulating the determinants, Inman and colleagues assumed that all the energy used to raise the CoM would be wasted, but in fact much of it is recovered when the CoM falls. The PE released from this fall is converted into another type of energy – kinetic energy (KE) – which does work on the body by increasing velocity by a small amount, v:

$$KE = (mv^2)/2$$

During the next rise (contralateral single support) this KE is then converted back into PE (accompanied by a small decrease in speed), and so on (Fig. 9.12).

The recovery rate during walking is about 65%, so only about 35% of the energy needs to be replenished each cycle (Cappozzo et al 1976, Cavagna et al 1976). PE/KE energy exchange is not perfect because maximum PE and KE are not equal. Moreover, the recovery rate depends not only on the relative magnitudes of the potential and kinetic energy curves, but also on the phase difference, α, between the time when one is at a maximum and the other at a minimum:

$$\alpha = 360° \times (\Delta t / T)$$

where T is the stride time. When $\alpha = 0°$ the curves are perfectly out of phase and the gait is most efficient.

The optimal speed at which energy recovery is maximal turns out to be about 0.6 m/s in 2-year-olds, increasing to 1.6 m/s in adults – close to the natural walking speeds at those ages. At speeds greater than the optimal speed, the recovery rate decreases, with correspondingly more muscle work needed, especially in children. The recovery rate does not account for simultaneous positive and negative work by the legs during double support (Donelan et al 2001).

A lot of energy appears to be associated with the transition between inverted pendulum phases, which we call step-to-step transition costs. The CoM needs to be redirected from one inverted pendulum arc to the next, and that requires negative work by the leading leg. Positive work is needed to offset this loss, and much (but not all) of this occurs when pushing off with the trailing leg (Kuo 2001).

OTHER WAYS TO MEASURE CoM MOTION

Simultaneous tracking of all 12 major body segments in 3D can be rather laborious because of the number of markers needed, so other methods of estimating CoM motion have been devised.

Figure 9.12 Typical energy exchanges occurring during normal gait (adapted from Griffin et al 1999).

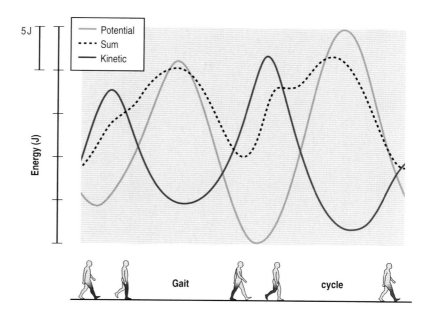

The CoM can be assumed to be located at a fixed point in the pelvis, and tracked using a single marker on, for example, the sacrum, or three markers to define the centre of the pelvis (Kerrigan et al 1995). This of course ignores the effect of the motion of body segments on the location of the CoM (Whittle 1997). In general, the amplitude of the centre of the pelvis displacement is somewhat larger than that of the true body CoM, especially in children and in pathological gait (Eames et al 1999), but the approximation isn't too bad for normal adults.

More accurate methods rely on the use of Newton's second law to derive the CoM displacement from force recordings (Shimba 1984, Crowe et al 1993, Whittle 1997, Saina et al 1998). The acceleration of the CoM is simply equal to the GRF divided by body mass (M), remembering to subtract body weight from the vertical force (Fig. 9.13).

$$a_{AP} = F_{AP}/M$$

where F_{AP} is the anteroposterior shear force,

$$a_{ML} = F_{ML}/M$$

where F_{ML} is the mediolateral shear force, and

$$a_{vertical} = (F_{vertical} - Mg)/M$$

where $F_{vertical}$ is the vertical load and Mg = body weight.

Note that body mass (M) needs to be measured carefully in order for the acceleration to be accurate.

Figure 9.13 Relationship between GRF and CoM acceleration.

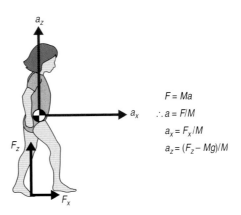

$$F = Ma$$
$$\therefore a = F/M$$
$$a_x = F_x/M$$
$$a_z = (F_z - Mg)/M$$

MCQ 9.3

What is the vertical acceleration of the CoM if the vertical GRF is 1000 N and body mass 75 kg (assume $g = 10$ m/s^2)?
(a) 1 m/s^2
(b) 1.25 m/s^2
(c) 3.33 m/s^2
(d) 10.33 m/s^2

The velocity of the CoM can be derived from the acceleration by integration:

$$v = \int a \, dt$$

where v is the velocity of the CoM.

Numerically (i.e. on a computer), integration can be done simply by a cumulative sum of each sample multiplied by the sampling interval (Δt), which is the reciprocal of the frame rate (e.g. $1/50$ s = 20 ms for a frame rate of 50 Hz). Using Σ to represent the sum, this can be written as:

$$v = \Sigma \, a\Delta t + v_0$$

The constant, v_0, is the initial velocity of the CoM (start of the cumulative sum).

Unfortunately, this is not known. For the vertical velocity, it can be calculated if it is assumed that the mean velocity (over one or more steps) is zero. This must be true, of course, otherwise the subject would lift off or disappear into the floor. Thus:

$$v - v_0 = \Sigma \, a\Delta t$$
$$\bar{v} - v_0 = 0$$

where $\bar{v}$ is the mean velocity. This means that:

$$v_0 = -\bar{v}$$

In practical terms, this means first integrating with the initial velocity set to zero, calculating the mean velocity, $\bar{v}$, then integrating again using $-v$ as the initial velocity.

The displacement of the CoM, d, can finally be found by integrating the velocity:

$$d = \Sigma\, v\Delta t + d_0$$

In this case, d_0 is the initial height of the CoM from the floor. Usually this is not important, since it is the amplitude of the CoM displacement that is of interest.

The advantages of estimating the motion of the CoM in this way are that no kinematic analysis is needed – no expensive cameras are required and no markers need be attached to the subject. Moreover, since it does not rely on anthropometric estimates, it is potentially more accurate. The method is also particularly useful for long-term recordings with in-shoe force or pressure sensors.

DEBATING POINT

Debate the advantages and disadvantages of these techniques for measuring CoM:

– Full-body kinematics
– Integration of forces
– Low-pass filtering of the CoP

RELATIONSHIP BETWEEN CoM AND CoP

It is important to be clear about the difference between CoM and CoP. The CoM is the point at which all the mass of the body appears to be concentrated. Body weight is the force (Mg) which acts vertically down from this point. Some of the GRV is the reaction to this weight, but it has additional components due to any acceleration of the CoM. In quiet standing, the accelerations are very small, so the CoP falls almost directly under the CoM and the GRV is close to vertical.

Indeed, this observation is the basis for yet another method for estimating the CoM motion (postural sway) for balance assessment. By low-pass filtering the CoP signal at a very low cutoff frequency (0.5 Hz), a good approximation of the CoM is obtained (Benda et al 1994). This technique is used by commercial posturography equipment, such as *Balance Master* and *Equitest* (NeuroCom International, Clackamas, OR) (Fig. 9.14).

During walking, however, the accelerations are much larger, and so the CoP rarely falls directly under the CoM. The GRV is also rarely vertical, being tilted by the shear forces caused by accelerations (Ma) of the CoM. Thus, the variables are 'decoupled' whenever there are significant accelerations (Winter 1994).

Figure 9.14 SMART Balance
Master, NeuroCom
International, Inc.,
Clackamas, OR.

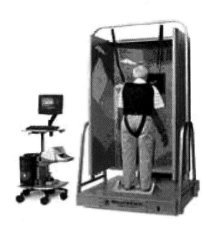

DYNAMIC STABILITY

The projection of the body CoM onto the floor is generally termed the centre of gravity (CoG), and reflects the CoM trajectory (Fig. 9.15). The peak lateral displacement occurs during the stance phase on that side, with the CoP travelling just lateral to the CoG. In this way each foot effectively nudges the CoG toward the mid-line or *plane of progression* – recall that the ML shear force is always directed medially (an action which is accentuated in ice- or roller-skaters).

Just before each foot contact there is a period of time in which the CoG is briefly ahead of the trailing (stance) foot before the leading (swing) foot has landed (Kirtley et al 2000). This illustrates an important difference between *dynamic* and *static* stability. In order for a body to be statically stable, the CoG must remain inside the base of support (BoS), but dynamic stability (i.e. during movement) can be preserved despite short periods in which the body is unsupported. Awareness of the limits of stability is important if falls are to be avoided, leading a group of Canadian researchers to develop a ribbed insole, *SoleSensor*

Figure 9.15 The pathway of the projection of the CoM onto the floor (centre of gravity, CoG) weaves about the plane of progression between the CoP travelling through the footprints from heel to hallux. The dotted parts of the CoG trajectory indicate periods in which it is briefly outside the base of support.

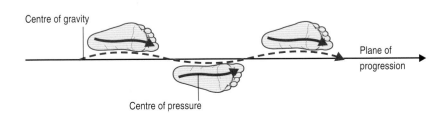

(Fig. 9.16), to provide a warning whenever the centre of pressure approaches the edge of the foot – similar to the way a rumble strip warns motorists that they are straying too close to the edge of the road.

Figure 9.16   The SoleSensor insole provides a tactile warning of instability whenever the centre of pressure approaches the edge of the foot.

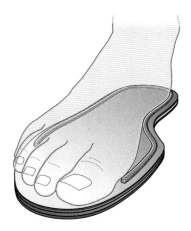

Harmonic analysis

The frequency spectrum of the CoM motion can be revealed by a mathematical procedure called *harmonic analysis*, or *Fourier analysis*. Simply speaking, the Fourier transform converts a signal from the time to frequency domain, in a similar manner to the way light is split into its components (spectrum or rainbow) by a prism (Fig. 9.17) or droplets of water. The most dominant frequency shows up as a large spike at a position along the horizontal axis corresponding to its frequency. Any other frequencies (called harmonics) show up as smaller peaks at different positions according to their frequency (colour).

Figure 9.17

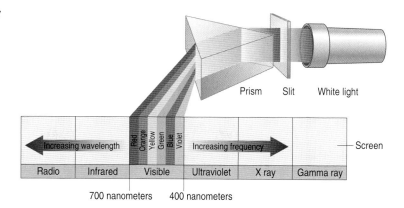

Since there are two steps to every gait cycle, the vertical CoM trajectory has a frequency exactly twice that of the stride frequency, so the second harmonic (at twice the stride frequency) would be expected to have the largest amplitude (Fig. 9.18).

Figure 9.18

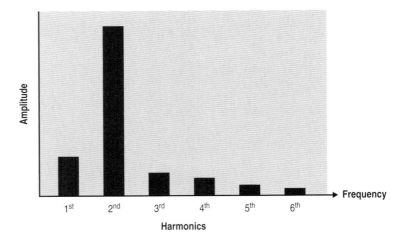

This observation has been used to define a *purity index* that is calculated by the ratio of the second harmonic to the sum of the remaining harmonics. A gait that has a purely sinusoidal CoM trajectory will have a purity index of 1.0, implying optimal interchange between potential and kinetic energy. Values less than 1.0 are claimed to indicate a lack of coordination between the energy exchanges, presumably resulting in loss of efficiency.

There are so many assumptions implicit in the derivation of this index that it is unlikely to be a valid measure. Nevertheless, it does raise interesting questions about just what does make gait efficient.

Alexander R McN, Jayes AS 1980 Fourier analysis of forces exerted in walking and running. Journal of Biomechanics 13:383–390
Murphy N 2002 Behind CoM'nalysis. Company brochure, Tekscan, Inc., Boston, MA

KEY POINTS

★ Body centre of mass is a weighted average of the masses of all the body segments

★ It can be measured by whole body kinematics or integration of the ground reaction force

★ Body centre of mass rises and falls and shifts from side to side during the gait cycle

★ Efficiency of gait is improved by interchange between potential and kinetic energy

★ Dynamic balance depends on the relationship between body centre of mass and base of support

References

Benda B J, Riley P O, Krebs D E 1994 Biomechanical relationship between center of gravity and center pressure during standing. IEEE Transactions on Rehabilitation Engineering 2(1):3–10

Cappozzo A, Figura F, Marchetti P 1976 The interplay of muscular and external forces in human ambulation. Journal of Biomechanics 9:35–43

Cavagna G A, Thys H, Zamboni A 1976 The sources of external work in level walking and running. Journal of Physiology (London) 262: 639–657

Crowe A, Schiereck P, de Boer R, Keessen W 1993 Characterisation of gait of young adult females by means of body centre of mass oscillations derived from ground reaction forces. Gait & Posture 1:61–68

Della Croce U, Riley P O, Lelas J L, Kerrigan D C 2001 A refined view of the determinants of gait. Gait & Posture 14:79–84

Donelan J M, Kram R, Kuo A D 2001 Mechanical and metabolic determinants of the preferred step width in human walking. Proceedings of the Royal Society of London, Series B 268:1985–1992

Eames M H A, Cosgrove A, Baker R 1999 Comparing methods of estimating the total body centre of mass in three-dimensions in normal and pathological gaits. Human Movement Science 18(5):637–646

Gard S A, Childress D S 1997 The effect of pelvic list on the vertical displacement of the trunk during normal walking. Gait & Posture 5:233–238

Gard S A, Childress D S 1999 The influence of stance-phase knee flexion on the vertical displacement of the trunk during normal walking. Archives of Physical Medicine and Rehabilitation 80:26–32

Gard S A, Childress D S 2001 What determines the vertical displacement of the body during normal walking? Journal of Prosthetics and Orthotics 13(3):64–67

Griffin M, Tolani, N A, Kram R 1999 Walking in simulated reduced gravity: mechanical energy fluctuations and transduction. Journal of Applied Physiology 86:383–390

Kerrigan D C, Viramontes B E, Corcoran P J, LaRaia P J 1995 Measured versus predicted vertical displacement of the sacrum during gait as a tool to measure biomechanical gait performance. American Journal Physical Medicine and Rehabilitation 74:3–8

Kerrigan D C, Della Croce U, Marciello M, Riley P O 2000 A refined view of the determinants of gait: significance of heel rise. Archives of Physical Medicine and Rehabilitation 81:1077–1080

Kerrigan D C, Riley P O, Lelas J L, Della Croce U 2001 Quantification of pelvic rotation as a determinant of gait. Archives of Physical Medicine and Rehabilitation 82:217–220

Kirtley C, Smith A W, Ng K P et al 2000 Relationship of body center of mass to the base of support. 3rd Australian and New Zealand Society of Biomechanics Conference, Gold Coast, Australia, 31st Jan to 1st Feb

Kuo A D 2001 A simple model predicts the step length-speed relationship in human walking. Journal of Biomechanical Engineering 123: 264–269

Saina M, Kerrigan D C, Thirunarayan M A, Duff-Raffaele M 1998 The vertical displacement of the centre of mass during walking: a comparison of four measurement methods. Journal of Biomechanical Engineering 120: 133–139

Saunders J B, Inman V T, Eberhart H D 1953 The major determinants in normal and pathological gait. Journal of Bone and Joint Surgery 35A:543–558

Shimba T 1984 An estimation of centre of gravity from force platform data. Journal of Biomechanics 17:53–60

Whittle M W 1997 Three-dimensional motion of the centre of gravity of the body during walking. Human Movement Science 16:347–355

Winter D A 1994 A.B.C. Anatomy, Biomechanics of balance during standing and walking. Waterloo Biomechanic, Waterloo, Ontario

Chapter 10

Power

Nothing is more likely to impede investigation than the premature acceptance of an 'explanation'.

Prof. H Schiller

CHAPTER CONTENTS

OBJECTIVES

- Understand how joint power is calculated
- Know how to interpret power in physiological terms
- Awareness of the major passive power flows in the limb during the gait cycle
- Appreciation of how power and other biomechanical variables can be used to elucidate the role of muscle contractions, particularly in ankle push-off

The variables discussed up to this point have basically been descriptive – they simply document what is happening during gait. For example, the kinematics document the motion itself, while the moment reveals which muscle group is active. In order to determine the purpose of these muscle contractions, a further approach is necessary: that of power analysis. The flow of power through the limb provides insights into the source and destination of the power responsible for driving the gait pattern. Perhaps for that reason, it is also probably the most controversial technique used in biomechanics.

Power analysis can be confusing, not least because of the often imprecise and inconsistent terminology used by many researchers. It is important to understand the various types of power, how each is derived and what it means (Table 10.1).

Of all these measures, most commercial motion analysis systems report only the first, which is a shame. Joint power, whilst certainly being useful, reveals only a small part of the total picture (Quanbury et al 1975). A complete understanding of power flow is analogous to lifting up the bonnet of a car (Fig. 10.1).

Table 10.1   Terminology used for power analysis. Note that some terms use the joint angular velocity, whereas others use the segment angular velocity. The term 'passive flow' describes the flow of power through the joint itself, while 'active flow' is used for power transferred through the muscles spanning the joint

Name	Derivation	Equation	Interpretation
Joint or muscle power	Joint moment × joint angular velocity	$M\omega_{joint}$ or $M(\omega_{proximal} - \omega_{distal})$	Power generation or absorption by muscle at the joint
Passive flow	Joint reaction force × joint linear velocity	Fv_{joint}	Power flow into a segment through a joint
Active flow	Joint moment × segment angular velocity	$M\omega_{segment}$	Power flow into a segment from a muscle
Total joint power flow	Sum of the passive and active power flow at a joint	$Fv_{joint} + M\omega_{proximal} + M\omega_{distal}$	Shows direction and magnitude of power flow at a joint
Segmental power	Sum of the passive and active power flow at each end of the segment	$Fv_{proximal} + M\omega_{proximal} + Fv_{distal} + M\omega_{distal}$	Total power flow into segment
Instantaneous segment power (or rate of energy change)	Change in segment energy with time, dE/dt	$d(mgh_{segment} + \frac{1}{2}mv^2_{segment} + \frac{1}{2}I\omega^2_{segment})/dt$	Total power of a segment at a given time
Power balance	Instantaneous power – power flow	$dE/dt - Fv_{proximal} - M\omega_{proximal} - Fv_{distal} - M\omega_{distal}$	Should be zero if power calculations are correct

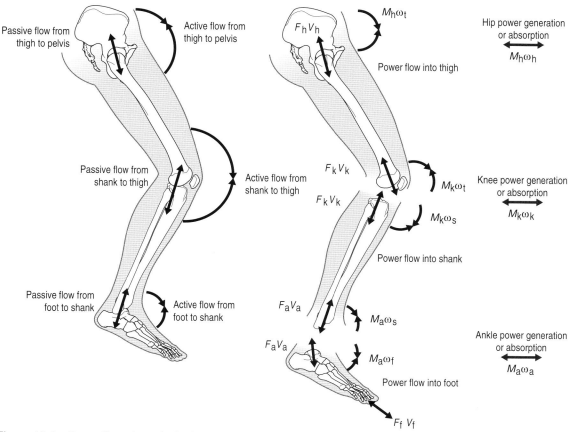

Figure 10.1 Power flow through the lower-limb. Passive flows take place (in either a proximal or distal direction) across the joint surfaces (straight arrows), while active flows transfer power through the muscles and tendons (circular arrows). Flow can be into or out of the ends of the segments. In addition, the muscles generate or absorb power at each joint ($M\omega$ products, shown on the right). Of these, only the latter are generally reported by commercial gait analysis packages.

FUNCTIONS OF MUSCLES

Muscles are fundamentally capable of two functions (Zajac et al 2002):

- Generate or absorb power (concentric or eccentric contraction)
- Redistribute power between segments.

The latter function has been somewhat neglected until recently.

CONCENTRIC, ECCENTRIC AND ISOMETRIC CONTRACTION

During gait, muscle is capable of three basic functions:

1. Shortening against a load (concentric contraction)
2. Lengthening against a load (eccentric contraction)
3. Maintaining constant length against a load (isometric contraction).

During a concentric contraction the muscle generates power, while in eccentric activity it absorbs power. The amount of power can be calculated by multiplying the muscle force (tension) by the shortening velocity:

$$\text{Power} = \text{Force} \times \text{Velocity}$$
$$P = Fv$$

The unit of mechanical power is the watt (W), which is the same as the electrical unit by that name. To get a feel for how much power muscles typically generate, Table 10.2 lists some common devices with their typical power ratings. Clearly, muscle contractions can generate sizeable amounts of power.

In eccentric activity, the muscle lengthens rather than shortens. This has the effect of absorbing power like the brakes on a car. Imagine lifting a weight and then lowering it to the floor. Concentric contraction is used to lift the weight, but lowering it is an eccentric action.

The dynamics of eccentric contraction is least understood, partly because there are safety issues in testing muscle against imposed forces. However, it is known that the force output is larger during eccentric compared to concentric contractions for the same level of EMG.

? MCQ 10.1

What is the power generated by a muscle contracting at 2 m/s against a 100 N load?

(a) 2 W
(b) 50 W
(c) 100 W
(d) 200 W

JOINT POWER

Another way to determine the type of muscle contraction is to look at the angular velocity of the joint. Suppose a flexor muscle is active. If the angular velocity is also flexor (i.e. the muscle is shortening), then the contraction must be concentric. On the other hand, if the joint is rotating in

Table 10.2 Typical power ratings for various mechanical and electrical devices along with some muscle powers

Device	Typical power (W)
Mobile phone	1
Laptop computer	10
Domestic light bulb	100
Ankle power during gait	200
Desktop computer	500
Hip power during a 100 m sprint	1000 (1 kW)
Porsche 911 sports car	320 hp* = 240 kW

*1 hp (horsepower) = 746 W.

the opposite direction (i.e. the muscle is lengthening) the contraction is eccentric. If there is no movement of the joint (zero velocity), the contraction is isometric.

In joint terms, the amount of power can be calculated by multiplying the joint moment by the angular velocity of the joint:

$$\text{Power} = \text{Moment} \times \text{Angular Velocity}$$
$$P = M\omega$$

Angular velocity is normally expressed in degrees per second (deg/s), but in this case it must be in rad/s, where 1 rad = 57.3° (or approximately 60°). So, for example, 120 deg/s is equivalent to about 2 rad/s.

? MCQ 10.2

What is the power generated by a joint that extends through 60° in 0.5 s against a moment of 10 N m?
(a) 5 N m
(b) 20 N m
(c) 75 deg/s
(d) 750 N m

At the joint, this power is calculated by the moment multiplied by the angular velocity of the segments being moved, the sign ($\pm$) indicating generation (+) or absorption (−):

$$\text{Power generation or absorption at joint} = M\omega_{\text{joint}}$$

When the moment and angular velocity act in the same direction, the muscle is performing a concentric contraction. When they are in opposite directions (e.g. a flexor moment when the joint is extending), an eccentric contraction is occurring. If the angular velocity is zero, there is no power generated or absorbed: in other words an *isometric* contraction.

NORMATIVE JOINT POWERS

Although power is probably the single most informative biomechanical variable, it is not without its detractors. This is because a lot of mathematics goes into its calculation, with a correspondingly large opportunity for errors and artefacts to creep in.

To start with, power is a *scalar* quantity, unlike directional *vectors* such as angle and moment. This means that it makes no mathematical sense to divide joint power into sagittal, frontal and transverse plane components. So, although there can be a hip flexion angle and a hip abductor moment, there is only one hip power (Fig. 10.2). Some researchers have broken this rule and described powers in the sagittal and frontal planes, which does seem to make *clinical* sense (Fig. 10.3).

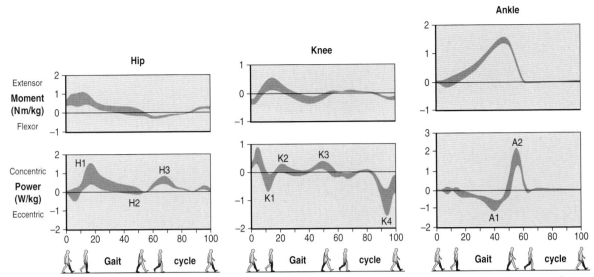

Figure 10.2 Normative joint powers summed across the three axes of rotation (sagittal, frontal and transverse). The shaded region indicates mean ± 1 SD. Moments are also shown so that the source of each power burst can be determined: for example, H1 is a concentric contraction of the hip extensors, while A1 is an eccentric contraction of the plantarflexors.

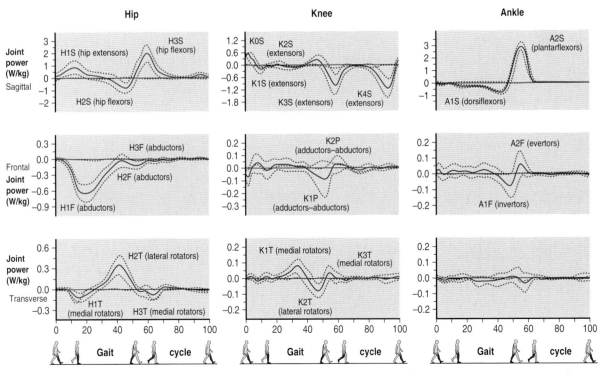

Figure 10.3 Normative joint powers separated into the three orthogonal planes (sagittal, frontal and transverse). Labels indicate the source of each power burst (determined from the joint moment). Dashed lines indicate mean ± 1 SD (modified from Sadeghi et al 2000, by permission of the American Physical Therapy Association). Although this approach may be technically incorrect, it provides more clinical information than the total joint powers.

Another problem can be seen in the knee power curve. Although the power bursts are labelled K1 to K4, there is another peak before K1, immediately after initial contact. It turns out that this is an artefact caused by discrepancies in filtering when calculating the joint moment by inverse dynamics.

ACTIVE POWER FLOW

Note that joint power, ω_{joint} is the same as $(\omega_{proximal} - \omega_{distal})$, so the equation could be written:

$$Power = M\,(\omega_{proximal} - \omega_{distal})$$

$$or\ Power = M\omega_{proximal} - M\omega_{distal}$$

In other words, the power flowing through the muscle has two components – one part delivered to, or drained from, the proximal segment, and one delivered to, or drained from, the distal segment. These are termed the *active* flows to the segments because they arise directly from the muscles attached to the segments at that joint.

When the proximal flow exactly equals the distal flow $(M\omega_{proximal} = M\omega_{distal})$ there is no power generated or absorbed. In other words, the muscle must be contracting isometrically, and is merely transferring power from one segment to the other. On the other hand, in a situation where one segment is fixed (e.g. the foot flat on the floor) there will be power generation/absorption but no transfer. In most cases, some combination of transfer and generation/absorption occurs.

? **MCQ 10.3**

At a certain point in the gait cycle, the shank rotates forward at 2 rad/s while the foot is flat on the floor (plantigrade). Calculate the power generation/absorbed and transferred by the muscle if there is a plantarflexor moment of 50 N m.

(a) 50 W generation + 100 W transfer
(b) 50 W absorption + 0 W transfer
(c) 100 W generation + 0 W transfer
(d) 100 W absorption + 0 W transfer

PASSIVE POWER FLOW

Power can also be transferred through the joint itself, and these *passive* flows turn out to be very significant in gait (Winter & Robertson 1978). They are calculated by the product of the joint reaction force and the linear velocity of the joint:

$$Passive\ Flow = F_{joint}\,v_{joint}$$

In two dimensions, the forces and velocities have two components, so:

$$Passive\ Flow = F_x v_x + F_z v_z$$

where x is the anteroposterior direction, and z is the vertical. In a full 3D analysis, there is also a mediolateral component ($F_y v_y$). Note that the sign indicates the direction of the flow, either into the proximal segment ($+$) or into the distal segment ($-$). This has important implications for understanding gait, because it reveals the purpose of muscle action.

SEGMENT POWER

Each segment will have power flow in or out at each end, so the total power flow into (or out of) the segment will be the sum of all the proximal and distal passive and active flows:

$$\text{Total Segment Power} = F_{\text{proximal}} v_{\text{proximal}} + M_{\text{proximal}} \omega_{\text{segment}} \\ + F_{\text{distal}} v_{\text{distal}} + M_{\text{distal}} \omega_{\text{segment}}$$

Another definition of power is change in segment energy with time, and segment energy can be calculated by adding up the potential and kinetic energies of the segment:

$$\text{Total Segment Energy} = \text{Potential Energy} + \text{Kinetic Energy}$$

The potential energy is proportional to the vertical height, h_{CoM}, of the segment CoM:

$$\text{Segment Potential Energy} = mgh_{\text{CoM}}$$

The kinetic energy has a *translational* component from the linear velocity of its CoM:

$$\text{Translational Kinetic Energy} = \tfrac{1}{2}mv_{\text{CoM}}^2$$

There is also a *rotational* component:

$$\text{Rotational Kinetic Energy} = \tfrac{1}{2}I\omega_{\text{segment}}^2$$

So,

$$\text{Total Segment Energy} = mgh_{\text{CoM}} + \tfrac{1}{2}mv_{\text{CoM}}^2 + \tfrac{1}{2}I\omega_{\text{segment}}^2$$

Notice that the terms in this equation can all be derived from kinematic data or anthropometry – no inverse dynamics is needed. Segment power can now be calculated from the change in energy with time:

$$\text{Segment Power} = dE_{\text{segment}}/dt$$

For this reason, this measure of segment power is usually termed *instantaneous power*, or *rate of energy change*.

From soldiers to toys: pendulum swings in the history of gait energetics	*One rapid but fairly sure guide to the social atmosphere of a country is the parade-step of its army. The goose-step, for instance, is one of the most horrible sights in the world, far more terrifying than a dive-bomber.* George Orwell, *The Lion and the Unicorn* (1941)

Locomotion research was the key to military success in the 18th and 19th centuries (Mosher Flesher 1997). Rather than waste time aiming their inaccurate muskets, soldiers formed tight ranks, shot in the general direction of the enemy and then dropped back to reload while the row behind them advanced. Frederick the Great's soldiers were taught to stand erect and swing their legs stiffly as they marched. Thanks to such goose-stepping tactics, Prussia defeated France in 1763.

By the early 19th century, guns were more accurate, allowing soldiers to take aim. Skirmishes resulted, which required flexibility rather than rigid marching. This change probably inspired three German brothers, Ernst, Wilhelm and Eduard Weber, to develop a new theory of walking based on passive, natural phenomena. Using Hanoverian soldiers as subjects, they postulated that the body was maintained erect by ligament tension, with little or no muscular exertion. Walking was merely a matter of falling forward, arrested by each advancing limb, swinging as a passive pendulum – so-called *pendulum theory*.

This theory was challenged by another German team, Christian Wilhelm Braune (who incidentally was the son-in-law of Ernst Weber) and Otto Fischer. In doing so, they became the first to calculate joint moments and reaction forces. They could only do this during swing phase because there was no way to measure ground reaction forces at that time. Nevertheless, the novel experimental techniques and laborious manual calculations which were required were an impressive effort, and they succeeded in disproving the pendulum theory, showing that gravitational force was not enough to explain the swing of the legs.

Herbert Elftman was responsible for fully determining the forces and energy changes in the leg during walking in 1939. He built the first force platform, which used springs and levers to record the forces and moments acting on the foot by moving pointers recorded simultaneously on the film. The results revealed that walking is very much an active process, requiring the contraction of many muscles to guide the limbs in swing as well as supplying energy that is lost by inexact conversion between potential and kinetic energy (Latash & Zatsiorsky 2001).

Interestingly, passive walking models have recently undergone something of a revival, with much interest in so-called *passive-dynamic* robots (McGeer 1990) (Fig. 10.4), some examples of which are now available in toy shops.

Figure 10.4 (Reproduced by permission of Dr A Ruina, Cornell University, Ithaca, NY, USA. Photographer: Michael Coleman.)

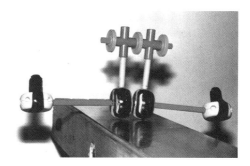

Orthoses have also been developed for paraplegic locomotion which exploit this principle (Fig. 10.5) (Kirtley 1992). No doubt Christian and Otto are turning in their graves while the Webers chuckle!

Figure 10.5

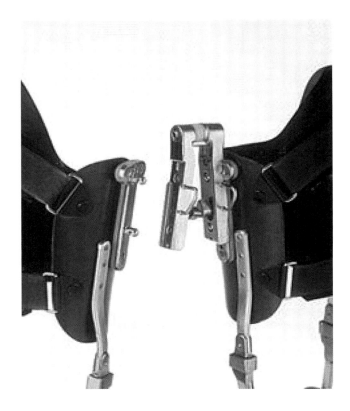

Latash M L, Zatsiorsky V M (eds) 2001 Classics in movement science. Human kinetics, Champaign IL
McGeer 1990 Passive dynamic walking. International Journal of Robotics Research 9:62–82
Mosher Flesher M 1997 Repetitive order and the human walking apparatus: Prussian military science versus the Webers' locomotion research. Annals of Science 54(5):463–487
Kirtley C 1992 Principles & practice of paraplegic locomotion. Australian Orthotic Prosthetic 7(2):4–7

POWER FLOW DURING GAIT

The flow of power through the limbs during gait is quite complex (Fig. 10.6). At heel-strike (A), the flow is generally from proximal to distal as the impact with the floor absorbs the power of the limb. Later in stance (B), the flow reverses (from distal to proximal), and leg power increases rapidly, primarily as a result of power generation at the ankle. Notice, though, that very little power flows through the hip joint until toe-off (C). During early swing (D) there is very little muscle activity (curved arrows) but some passive power flows distally

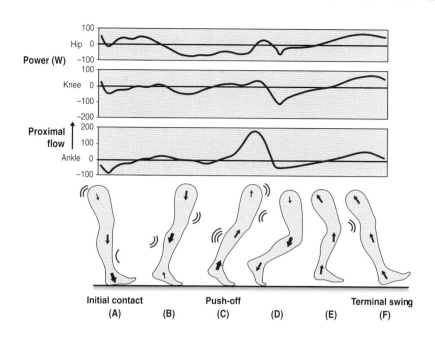

Figure 10.6 Power flow during the gait cycle. Graphs show total flow (passive + active) at each joint. The size of the arrows is roughly proportional to the magnitude of the power flow, and major power generation (convex) and absorption (concave) are indicated by arcs over the active muscle group. Note especially the huge power generation by the *gastrocnemius-soleus* during push-off, which flows to the shank and thigh and is then transferred to the trunk during swing phase (modified from Winter & Robertson 1978, data from Winter 1990).

through the joints. By mid-swing (E) the flow has again reversed (distal to proximal) with significant absorption at the knee, as power leaves the leg in the direction of the trunk, and this continues until the end of swing (F).

In general, extensor muscles remove energy from the lower-limb and add it to the trunk, while flexors (together with gravity) produce the opposite effects. Push-off is an exception to this rule, since the plantarflexors add energy to both lower-limb and trunk. Moreover, opposite power synergies (knee extensor with gravity, hip flexor with ankle plantarflexor) balance power flows through the segments (Siegel et al 2004).

VALIDATION OF POWER ANALYSIS

Since power is a variable that integrates both kinematic and kinetic data, there are a lot of opportunities for error to creep into the calculations. Two methods have been devised to attempt to verify the accuracy of power calculations:

- Power balance
- 'Six-degree-of-freedom' models.

The estimate of segment power obtained by rate of energy change should equal the total segment power already calculated by summing power flows, so this provides a means by which to check the accuracy of the calculations (Winter 1990):

$$\text{Power balance} = \frac{dE_{\text{segment}}}{dt} - (Fv_{\text{proximal}} + M\omega_{\text{proximal}} + Fv_{\text{distal}} + M\omega_{\text{distal}})$$

If all is well, the power balance of a segment should be approximately zero.

Another possible source of error is the identification of joint centres of rotation. This is normally done by predictions based on simple anthropometry, so inaccuracies are quite possible, even *likely*, especially in patients with deformities. One way around this is to avoid attempting to identify the joint centre – so-called *six-degree-of-freedom* joints. This means that the bones are tracked in 3D with no assumption as to location of the joint. If this is done, errors in the translational and rotational terms cancel (Buczek et al 1994).

APPLICATION OF POWER ANALYSIS

Determining the biomechanical role of a muscle group is often not as straightforward as it might at first appear, and may be counter-intuitive. Whilst there is no completely conclusive method, evidence can be gained from a variety of sources in order to build up a picture of what is going on (Table 10.3).

A good example is the action of ankle plantarflexors in gait. Joint moment and EMG show that these are active throughout most of stance phase, with activity increasing to a maximum at about 50% cycle (Fig. 10.7). So what is this activity for?

There are three plausible explanations (Meinders et al 1998):

1. Support (maintaining the height of the centre of mass of the body or trunk)

Table 10.3 Sources of evidence that can be used to determine the role of a muscle

Evidence	Information gained
Joint moment (torque)	Net balance between agonist and antagonist
Electromyography	Timing of muscle action
Joint (muscle) power	Power generated or absorbed by muscle
Segment power	Increase or decrease timed with muscle activity
Power flow	Direction of power flow
Effect of speed	Sources of increased power
Experiments – local anaesthetic nerve block	Effect of paralysing the muscle
Natural experiments – amputation	Effect of loss of the muscle (and joint)

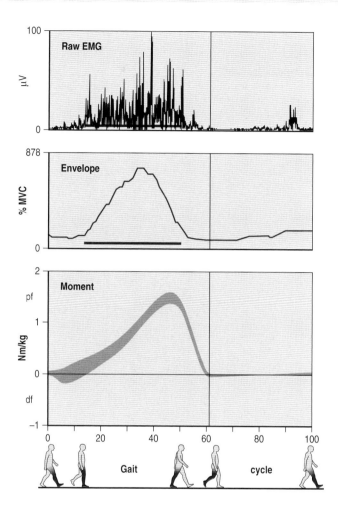

Figure 10.7 Plantarflexor activity during normal gait, as revealed by rectified raw and linear envelope *gastrocnemius* electromyography and joint moment. Note the gradual increase of activity until around 50% gait cycle. Enveloped EMG is normalized to maximum voluntary contraction (MVC). Plantarflexor (pf) joint moment is shown positive, dorsiflexor (df) negative, and normalized to body mass.

2. Propulsion of the leg
3. Forward progression of the trunk.

The EMG and joint moment alone cannot discern between these three possibilities, so more evidence is needed.

Joint power (Fig. 10.8) reveals that there are two distinctive phases of plantarflexor action: an initial eccentric (power-absorbing) contraction, A1, followed by a stronger concentric (power-generating) contraction, A2 (Winter 1983).

To use a car analogy, the plantarflexors are being used first as a brake, and then as an accelerator. The next question, then, is exactly what are they braking and accelerating?

Some clues can be gained by looking at the segment powers (see Fig. 10.6), which show how much power is flowing into or out of the segments. Whilst the source or destination of these changes is not directly visible, one can tentatively infer whether the plantarflexors are a candidate by comparing the shape of the segment powers with that of the ankle joint power (Fig. 10.8).

Figure 10.8 Power generation and absorption at the ankle joint, showing two distinct phases of plantarflexor activity: a negative (A1) burst which absorbs power, followed by a positive burst (A2) that generates power. Notice that the A2 burst is timed to coincide with rapid plantarflexion of the ankle just prior to toe-off.

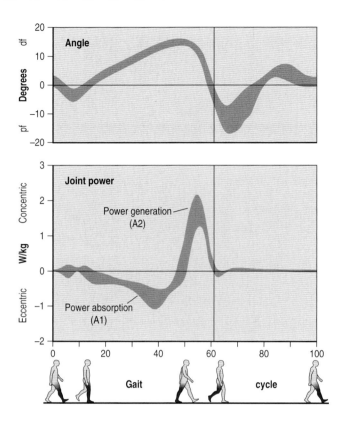

EFFECT OF SPEED

As speed increases, all the major power bursts (both concentric and eccentric) increase in size (Fig. 10.9). However, there is a greater percentage change at the hip compared to the ankle (Chen et al 1997), with hip pull-off (H3, *iliopsoas*) contributing relatively more energy at higher speeds (Fig. 10.10).

These findings suggest a dual role for the ankle push-off power burst. As well as providing energy for swing initiation, the plantarflexors also have an important support function. The trunk (HAT) segment is low at this time, and so some of the energy from the A2 power burst goes into lifting it (Riley et al 2001). This support role likely does not increase with increasing speed, so the A2 energy consequently does not need to rise. Pull-off (H3) has only one role, however – that of swing initiation, and as speed increases the swing limb must be brought forward faster.

OTHER EVIDENCE

An alternative approach to elucidating muscle function is to study what happens when its function is impaired. This can occur naturally, due to

Figure 10.9 Effect of speed on joint powers. Arrows indicate the direction of change in the mean of the major power bursts at walking speeds of 0.5, 1.0 and 1.5 m/s (data from Stansfield et al 2001, with permission).

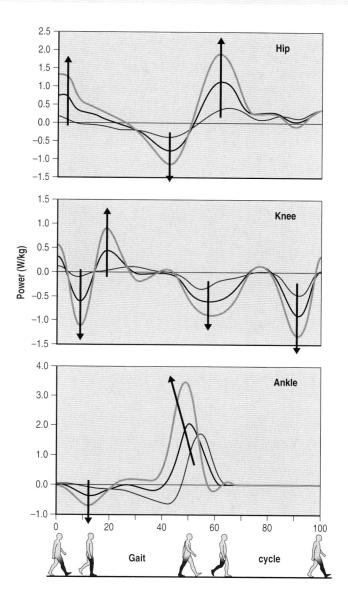

paralysis (Simon et al 1978, Lehmann et al 1980, 1985), excision (Murray et al 1978, Kramers-de Quervain et al 2001), ankle arthrodesis (Mazur et al 1979, Beischer et al 1999, Wu et al 2000) or amputation (Winter & Sienko 1988), or it can be induced artificially by a local anaesthetic nerve block (Sutherland & Cooper 1980).

Gait abnormalities associated with impaired plantarflexor function include a *calcaneal limp* pattern, with increased dorsiflexion in late stance (Sutherland & Cooper 1980). Speed, stride length and contralateral step length are reduced (Simon et al 1978, Mazur et al 1979, Lehmann et al 1985). Indeed, it has been suggested that these variables

Figure 10.10 Change in the relative contribution of each joint to swing initiation. Ankle push-off is the main source of energy, but as speed increases hip pull-off provides a progressively larger contribution (data from Chen et al 1997).

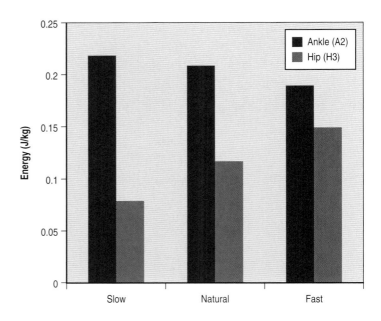

are useful clinical measures of A2 push-off power (Kirtley 2001). Moreover, below-knee amputees (who have no plantarflexor function) have greatly reduced A2 power generation (Winter & Sienko 1988). In the elderly, it seems to be a marker for non-age related functional deterioration (McGibbon & Krebs 1999).

Patients generally seem to compensate by increasing the duration of hip extensor and *quadriceps* activity during stance and increasing hip flexor activity around toe-off. Although normal level gait is possible, more pronounced deficits appear in more demanding tasks such as fast or uphill walking (Kramers-de Quervain et al 2001).

DEBATING POINT

Research and collect evidence for each of the following propositions:
– The main role of ankle push-off is swing limb propulsion
– The main role of ankle push-off is forward progression of the trunk
– The main role of ankle push-off is support of the trunk

AXIAL POWER FLOW AT THE ANKLE

Power flow can be used to elucidate the direction of control at joints. For example, functional foot orthoses (FFOs) are often used to exploit the torque converter effect discussed in chapter 3, on the assumption that frontal plane motion of the foot will cause rotation of the tibia. Power flow at the ankle (proximal to distal, i.e. tibia to foot) during walking actually suggests that the foot is driven by the tibia (Fig. 10.11A). Rather than reducing tibial rotation stress on the knee joint by controlling eversion, orthoses may therefore actually *increase* stresses by impeding the natural dissipation of power – rather like pressing on the brake and accelerator at the same time, to use a car analogy (Bellchamber & van den Bogert 2000). In running (Fig. 10.11B), the flow of power is not as consistent as in walking, and it is conceivable that certain runners with distal-to-proximal power flow might benefit from FFOs. These findings may explain the variable effectiveness of foot orthoses noted in several studies (Kilmartin & Wallace 1994, Eng & Pierrynowski 1994, Cornwall & McPoil 1995), and potentially provide a means with which to identify those who are more likely to benefit from orthotic intervention. Further research also needs to determine whether the direction of power flow is affected by foot and knee disorders.

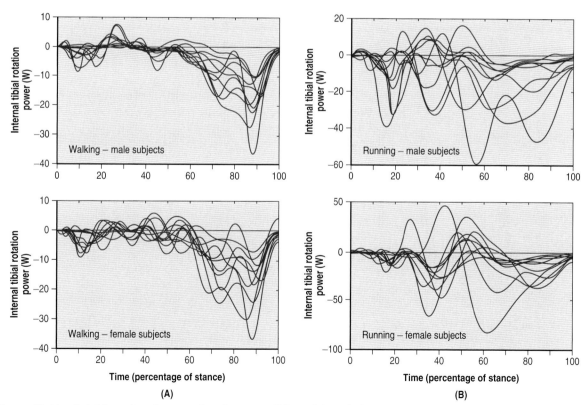

Figure 10.11   Axial (rotational) power flow between tibia and foot during normal walking and running in 10 men and 10 women. Foot to tibia flow is shown as positive, while tibia to foot flow is negative. During walking (A) the flow is almost completely in the tibia to foot direction, meaning that the foot 'follows' the tibia. In running (B) the pattern is not as consistent, with some subjects demonstrating periods of positive (foot to tibia) flow between 20–60% stance phase, which may be amenable to orthotic intervention (data from Bellchamber & van den Bogert 2000).

ENERGY STORAGE AND EXCHANGE

Although (in contrast to kangaroos) there is little evidence that significant energy can be stored in human soft tissue (Alexander & Bennet-Clark 1977, Ker et al 1987), energy can be stored in moving body segments (Caldwell & Forrester 1992). There are two mechanisms for this:

- 'Pendulum' type exchange between potential and kinetic energy within segments (as discussed previously).
- 'Whip' type exchange between linear and rotational kinetic energy within segments.

The large amount of power injected into the shank-foot at push-off raises its energy level during swing and this energy is then transferred to the trunk to propel it forward (Dillingham et al 1992). This is an example of whip-type energy exchange.

MEASURES OF ENERGY EXPENDITURE

The amount of work done (*mechanical cost*) by the body can be estimated by integrating the potential (mgh) and kinetic $\frac{1}{2}(mv^2 + I\omega^2)$ energies of each body segment over the gait cycle (Cavagna et al 1963). The head, arms and trunk (HAT segment) are usually grouped together as one segment. When the resting (minimum) potential energy is subtracted, the total is about 50 J over each gait cycle.

Alternatively, the power generated (ignoring eccentric contractions) at each joint can be summed over the gait cycle to calculate the total body work (TBW) or total lower-limb work (TLW), if the upper-limbs are ignored. This requires inverse dynamics (with a force platform) whereas mechanical cost can be computed from kinematic data alone (Winter 1979).

TBW is larger, and the difference between the TBW and mechanical cost provides a measure of the 'power competition' which occurs when muscles work against each other – a common cause of inefficiency in pathological gait (Caldwell & Forrester 1992).

METABOLIC ENERGY EXPENDITURE

Energy expenditure (or power consumption) can be measured indirectly from the rate of oxygen consumption ($\dot{V}O_2$), using either a Douglas bag or breath-by-breath gas analyser (Winter 1978). Neither of these two methods is very pleasant for the subject, who has to wear a facemask, but modern telemetric systems (Fig. 10.12) have made it much more practical (Crandall et al 1994, Wideman et al 1995).

The results can then transformed into watts (Brockway 1987), assuming aerobic metabolism by substituting 1 ml O_2 = 21 J. Oxygen consumption ($\dot{V}O_2$) for normal gait is about 14 ml/kg/min, or an energy expenditure E_w of $(14 \times 21/60)$ = 5 W/kg, i.e. about 350 W for a typical

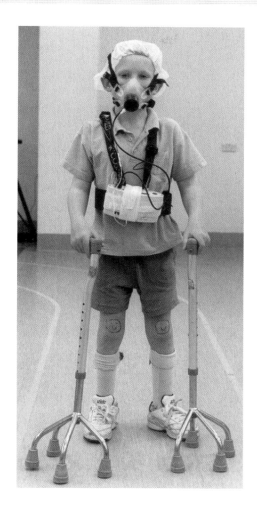

70 kg adult (using watts rather than ml O_2/min facilitates interpretation in terms of mechanical power). Incidentally, quiet standing alone consumes about 3.5 ml/kg/min, or 1 W/kg (Waters & Mulroy 1999).

Oxygen consumption and energy expenditure rise with the square of the walking speed, v (in m/s), but the relationships are close to linear at walking speeds below 1.67 m/s (Waters & Mulroy 1999).

$$\dot{V}O_2 \text{ (in ml/kg/min)} = 2.6\,v + 7.5$$
$$E_w \text{ (in W/kg)} = 2.6\,v + 0.9$$

To eliminate the effect of speed, an *oxygen cost* can be calculated by dividing the oxygen consumption by the walking speed (Moore et al 2001, Unnithan et al 1999). The units of this will be (ml/kg/min)/(m/s), and if the consumption is converted to ml/kg/s by dividing by 60, the seconds cancel out – leaving ml/kg/m. So, an oxygen *consumption* of 14 ml/kg/min at 1.5 m/s would be an oxygen *cost* of 14/1.5/60 = 0.16 ml/kg/m, or an *energy cost* per metre, E_m, of $0.16 \times 21 = 3$ J/kg/m.

The advantage of a cost function is that it allows comparisons to be made across different speeds. Furthermore, the energy cost of using a wheelchair is about 3 J/kg/m (the same as walking), so if walking cost is substantially greater than this, the wheelchair will be preferred (Williams et al 1983).

With increasing power output, the body eventually reaches an *aerobic capacity* or *limit* ($\dot{V}O_{2\,max}$), at which sufficient oxygen can no longer be supplied for metabolic needs. At this point anaerobic metabolism begins, which incurs an oxygen debt that must be repaid after the exercise is over. Lactate and other anaerobic metabolites accumulate and fatigue rapidly ensues. Healthy people have a $\dot{V}O_{2\,max}$ of about 40 ml/kg/min (or 9 W/kg), so during normal gait a person is typically working at about 35% of aerobic capacity. $\dot{V}O_{2\,max}$ can be increased by training, and declines with both age (by about 0.4 ml/kg/min/year) and obesity – overweight people have been found to walk at around 56% aerobic capacity (Mattsson et al 1997). It should be emphasized that wheelchair locomotion is fast and efficient (Beekman et al 1999) so will often be preferred by patients unless gait is competitive in terms of energy consumption.

WALKING EFFICIENCY

The term 'efficiency' is often mentioned in the assessment of gait, yet is difficult to define in physical terms. Theoretically, it can be calculated by:

$$\text{Walking efficiency} = \text{Total work done}/\text{Metabolic expenditure}$$

Depending on which measure of work is used, walking efficiency appears to be around 15–25% (Cavagna & Kaneko 1977). Another measure (Perry 1992) can be defined as:

$$\text{Walking efficiency} = (100 \times \text{Oxygen cost of healthy person})/ \text{Oxygen cost of patient}$$

Factors which may be responsible for reducing efficiency include co-contraction by muscle agonists and antagonists (Unnithan et al 1996).

PHYSIOLOGICAL COST INDEX

A useful clinical measure of the energy cost of gait makes use of the dependence of heart rate (HR, or pulse rate, PR) on oxygen consumption. By subtracting the resting heart rate from its value during walking the number of additional beats per minute (bpm) in response to the exercise is obtained. An increase consumption of 1 ml/kg/min results in approximately 3 bpm rise in heart rate (Rose et al 1989). By dividing by the walking speed, a *physiological cost index* (PCI) is derived (Butler et al 1984, Rose et al 1991):

$$\text{PCI} = (\text{Walking heart rate} - \text{Resting heart rate})/\text{Walking speed}$$

The units are bpm per minute per second, i.e. bpm/m/s, which are roughly indicative of oxygen cost (oxygen cost = PCI/180 ml/kg/m), and for that reason it is sometimes referred to as *energy cost*. Of course, there are other influences on heart rate apart from exercise, such as anxiety, drugs (coffee, heart and asthma medication) and fitness level, so the PCI needs to be used with caution (Boyd & Fatone 1999). The heart rate should be taken over several (at least eight) 25 m laps. However, the simplicity of the measure makes it suitable for tracking progress during rehabilitation and evaluating the efficacy of therapeutic interventions.

LABORATORY: ENERGY COST OF WALKING

1. Measure out a reasonably long distance (e.g. 10 m).
2. Ask subjects not to drink tea or coffee or take any other drugs in the 4 hours before the lab.
3. Allow the subjects to rest and relax before beginning the test.
4. Record subjects' resting PR: the easiest way is to count the number of beats in 15 s and multiply by four to derive the rate in bpm.
5. Ask them to walk 10 circuits of the course (total distance 200 m) at natural, slow and fast speeds. Record the times when they start and stop the last circuit.
6. Record subjects' final PR.
7. Estimate subjects' oxygen consumption (ml/kg/min) from (Final PR − Resting PR)/3.
8. Convert to energy expenditure (W/kg) by multiplying by 21/60.
9. Calculate the walking speed over the last circuit (distance/time).
10. Calculate PCI from (Final PR − Resting PR)/Walking speed.
11. Derive energy cost, E_m in J/kg/m ($21 \times PCI/180$). Does E_m stay constant as speed varies?
12. Plot the relationship between walking speed and energy expenditure (E_w). How closely does it fit the equation: $E_w = 2.6\,v + 0.9$?
13. Calculate the mean and CV of the energy cost. How do they compare with the expected values for level walking (3 J/kg/m ± 5%)?

DEBATING POINT

Research and debate the advantages and disadvantages of these techniques for assessing energy expenditure during gait:
– Centre of mass motion
– Oxygen cost from breath-by-breath gas analysis
– Calculation of total body work
– Physiological cost index

These boots are not made for walking

Shoes have a number of functions, including protection from the elements and walking surface, aesthetics and fashion. Although most people wear shoes almost all their waking hours, people are usually studied in the gait laboratory barefoot, because markers can then be attached to the foot rather than the shoe. Wearing no footwear also helps standardize the analysis because there is no shoe to consider.

To determine the effect of footwear on gait, holes can be drilled into the shoe to allow markers to be attached to the skin of the foot. The main effect of wearing shoes is to restrict the foot's movement. For example, in barefoot walking the longitudinal distance between the calcaneus and first metatarsal

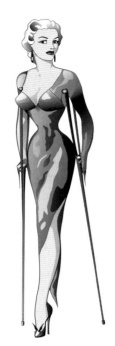

shortens in late stance as a result of the windlass effect on the plantar fascia. This behaviour is prevented when walking in shoes. Similarly, the variation in foot width seen in barefoot walking (the foot being wider during loading) is also inhibited by shoes. Whether such a stiffening of the foot has any deleterious effect on its function or development is unknown, but they are commonly blamed for causing hallux abducto valgus deformity. The wearing of high-heel shoes (Fig. 10.13) impairs plantarflexor function, and prevents the normal supination at push-off, resulting in reduced swing knee flexion. Moreover, rapid fatigue of the *peroneus longus* increases the vulnerability to inversion injuries.

Lee K H, Shieh J C, Matteliano A, Smiehorowski T 1990 Electromyographic changes of leg muscles with heel lifts in women: therapeutic implications. Archives of Physical Medicine and Rehabilitation 71(1):31–33

Opila-Correia K A 1990 Kinematics of high-heeled gait. Archives of Physical Medicine and Rehabilitation 71(5):304–309

Gefen A, Megido M, Itzchak Y, Arcan M 2002 Analysis of muscular fatigue and foot stability during high-heeled gait. Gait & Posture 15:56–63

Esenyel M, Walsh K, Walden J G, Gitter A 2003 Kinetics of high-heeled gait. Journal of the American Podiatric Medical Association 93(1):27–32

Figure 10.13

KEY POINTS

★ Joint power is calculated by the joint moment multiplied by the joint angular velocity

★ Positive power indicates concentric contraction, negative power indicates eccentric activity

★ Power can also be transferred passively between segments via bones and muscles

★ The flow of power can be used to determine the functional role of a muscle contraction

★ Energy consumption can be measured by total work done or by metabolic measures

References

Alexander R Mc, Bennet-Clark H C 1977 Storage of elastic strain energy in muscle and other tissues. Nature 265:114–117

Beekman C E, Miller-Porter L, Schoneberger M 1999 Energy cost of propulsion in standard and ultralight wheelchairs in people with spinal cord injuries. Physical Therapy 79(2):146–158

Beischer A D, Brodsky J W, Pollo F E, Peereboom J 1999 Functional outcome and gait analysis after triple or double arthrodesis. Foot and Ankle International 20(9):545–553

Bellchamber T L, van den Bogert A J 2000 Contributions of proximal and distal moments to axial tibial rotation during walking and running. Journal of Biomechanics 33:1397–1403

Boyd R S, Fatone T 1999 High or low-technology measurements of energy expenditure in clinical gait analysis. Developmental Medicine and Child Neurology 41:676–682

Brockway J M 1987 Derivation of formulae used to calculate energy expenditure in man. Human Nutrition Clinical Nutrition 41:463–471

Buczek F L, Kepple T M, Siegel K L, Stanhope S J 1994 Translational and rotational Joint power terms in a six degree-of-freedom model of the normal ankle complex. Journal of Biomechanics 27(12):1447–1457

Butler P, Engelbrecht M, Major R E et al 1984 Physiological cost index of walking of normal children and its use as an indicator of physical handicap. Developmental Medicine and Child Neurology 26:607–612

Caldwell G E, Forrester L W 1992 Estimates of mechanical work and energy transfers: demonstration of a rigid body power model of the recovery leg in gait. Medicine and Science in Sports and Exercise 24(12):1396–1412

Cavagna G A, Kaneko M 1977 Mechanical work and efficiency in level walking and running. Journal of Physiology 268:647–681

Cavagna G A, Saibene F P, Margaria R 1963 External work in walking. Journal of Applied Physiology 18:1–9

Chen I H, Kuo K N, Adriacchi T P 1997 The influence of walking speed on mechanical power during gait. Gait & Posture 6(3):171–176

Cornwall M W, McPoil T G 1995 Footwear and foot orthotic effectiveness research: a new approach. Journal of Orthopaedic and Sports Physical Therapy 21:337–344

Crandall D G, Taylor S L, Raven P B 1994 Evaluation of the Cosmed K2 portable telemetric oxygen uptake analyzer. Medicine and Science in Sports and Exercise 26(1):108–111

Dillingham T R, Lehmann J F, Price R 1992 Effect of lower limb on body propulsion. Archives of Physical Medicine and Rehabilitation 73:647–651

Elftman H 1939 Forces and energy changes in the leg during walking. American Journal of Physiology 125:339–356

Eng J J, Pierrynowski M R 1994 The effect of soft foot orthotics on three-dimensional lower-limb kinematics during walking and running. Physical Therapy 74:836–844

Ker R F, Bennet M B, Bibby S R et al 1987 The spring in the arch of the human foot. Nature 325:147–149

Kilmartin T E, Wallace W A 1994 The scientific basis for the use of biomechanical foot orthoses in the treatment of lower limb sports injuries – a review of the literature. British Journal of Sports Medicine 28:180–183

Kirtley C 2001 The importance of ankle push-off in healthy and pathological gait. British Journal of Podiatry August: 259–268

Kramers-de Quervain I A, Läuffer J M, Käch K et al 2001 Functional donor-site morbidity during level and uphill gait after a gastrocnemius or soleus muscle-flap procedure. Journal of Bone and Joint Surgery 83A(2):239

Lehmann J F, Ko M J, de Lateur B J 1980 Double-stopped ankle-foot orthosis in flaccid peroneal and tibial paralysis: evaluation of function. Archives of Physical Medicine and Rehabilitation 61:536–541

Lehmann J F, Concon S M, de Lateur B J, Smith J C 1985 Gait abnormalities in tibial nerve paralysis: a biomechanical study. Archives of Physical Medicine and Rehabilitation 66:80–85

Mattsson E, Evers Larsson U, Rössner S 1997 Is walking for exercise too exhausting for obese women? International Journal of Obesity 21(5):380–386

Mazur J M, Schwartz E, Simon S R 1979 Ankle arthrodesis. Long-term follow-up with gait analysis. Journal of Bone and Joint Surgery 61(7):964–975

McGibbon C A, Krebs D E 1999 The effects of age and functional limitations on leg joint power and work during stance phase of gait. Journal of Rehabilitation Research and Development 36(3):173–182

Meinders M, Gitter A, Czerniecki J M 1998 The role of ankle plantar flexor muscle work during walking. Scandinavian Journal of Rehabilitation Medicine 30:39–46

Moore C A, Nejad B, Novak R A, Dias L 2001 Energy cost of walking in low lumbar myelomeningocele. Journal of Pediatric Orthopedics 21(3):388–391

Murray M P, Guten G, Sepic S B et al 1978) Function of the triceps surae during gait. Journal of Bone and Joint Surgery 60A:473–476

Perry J 1992 Gait analysis: normal & pathological function. Slack, Thorofare, NJ

Quanbury A O, Winter D A, Reimer G D 1975 Instantaneous power and power flow in body segments during walking. Journal of Human Movement Studies 1:59–67

Riley P O, Croce U D, Kerrigan D C 2001 Propulsive adaptation to changing gait speed. Journal of Biomechanics 34(2):197–202

Rose J, Gamble J G, Medeiros J M et al 1989 Energy cost of walking in normal children and in those with cerebral palsy. Comparison of heartrate and oxygen uptake. Journal of Pediatric Orthopedics 9:276–279

Rose J, Gamble J G, Lee J et al 1991 The energy expenditure index: a method to quantitate and compare walking energy efficiency for children and adolescents. Journal of Pediatric Orthopedics 11:571–578

Sadeghi H, Allard P, Duhaime M 2000 Contributions of lower-limb muscle power in gait of people without impairments. Physical Therapy 80(12):1188–1196

Siegel K L, Kepple T M, Stanhope S J 2004 Joint moment control of mechanical energy flow during normal gait. Gait & Posture 19(1):69–75

Simon S R, Mann R A, Hagy J L, Larsen L J 1978 Role of the posterior calf muscles in normal gait. Journal of Bone and Joint Surgery 60A:465

Stansfield B W, Hillman S J, Hazlewood M E et al 2001 Sagittal joint kinematics, moments, and powers are predominantly characterized by speed of progression, not age. Journal of Pediatric Orthopedics 21:403–411

Sutherland D H, Cooper L D 1980 The role of the plantarflexors in normal walking. Journal of Bone and Joint Surgery 62A:354

Unnithan V B, Dowling J J, Frost G, Bar-Or O 1996 Role of cocontraction in the O_2 cost of walking in children with cerebral palsy. Medicine and Science in Sports and Exercise 28(12):1498–1504

Unnithan V B, Dowling J J, Frost G, Bar-Or O 1999 Role of mechanical power estimates in the O_2 cost of walking in children with cerebral palsy. Medicine and Science in Sports and Exercise 31(12):1703–1708

Waters R L, Mulroy S 1999 The energy expenditure of normal and pathologic gait. Gait & Posture 9:207–231

Wideman L, Stoudemire N M, Pass K A et al 1995 Assessment of the Aerosport TEEM 100 portable metabolic measurement system. Medicine and Science in Sports and Exercise 28(4):509–515

Williams L O, Anderson A D, Campbell J et al 1983 Energy cost of walking and of wheelchair propulsion by children with myelodysplasia: comparison with normal children. Developmental Medicine and Child Neurology 255:617–624

Winter D A 1978 Energy assessments in pathological gait. Physiotherapy Canada 30:183-191

Winter D A 1979 A new definition of mechanical work done in human movement. Journal of Applied Physiology 46:79–83

Winter D A 1983 Biomechanical motor patterns in normal walking. Journal of Motor Behavior 15(4):302–330

Winter D A 1990 Biomechanics and motor control of human movement, 2nd edn. Wiley, New York

Winter D A, Robertson D G 1978 Joint torque and energy patterns in normal gait. Biological Cybernetics 29:137–142

Winter D A, Sienko S E 1988 Biomechanics of below-knee amputee gait. Journal of Biomechanics 21:361

Wu W L, Su F-C, Cheng Y-M et al 2000 Gait analysis after ankle arthrodesis. Gait & Posture 11:54–61

Zajac F E, Neptune R R, Kautz S A 2002 Biomechanics and muscle coordination of human walking. Part I: Introduction to concepts, power transfer, dynamics and simulations. Gait & Posture 16:215–232

PART II

Practice

Part II Practice

Introduction

TEAM–BASED REHABILITATION

The practice of gait analysis in the clinic is based on the biomechanical principles discussed in Part I, but is also heavily influenced by more established clinical approaches. These two perspectives are not necessarily inconsistent, but the difference in the terminology can sometimes be quite confusing. Rehabilitation is still a young, evolving specialty, with a multidisciplinary philosophy that is often in marked contrast to the traditional medical model of disease and treatment. The scientific foundations of many of the traditional strategies adopted over many decades of clinical experience are still being elucidated.

A modern rehabilitation team will usually consist of a doctor (e.g. a physiatrist, specializing in rehabilitation; a neurologist, specializing in nervous diseases; a rheumatologist, specializing in joint diseases; or an orthopaedic surgeon), rehabilitation nurse (who is also often the care coordinator), physiotherapist, occupational therapist, podiatrist, prosthetist-orthotist, neuropsychologist, speech pathologist, social worker, rehabilitation engineer, as well as the family of the person undergoing rehabilitation. To be effective, therefore, the modern rehabilitation practitioner needs to be comfortable with the language and methods used by a variety of professions, aiming to integrate biomechanical principles into management wherever possible, but also with an appreciation of medical and psychosocial models.

CLASSIFICATION OF GAIT DISORDERS

The approach used to classify gait disorders varies according to its purpose. For example, physicians (especially neurologists) tend to focus on the anatomical *level* of the lesion (Table B1). On the other hand, those directly involved in rehabilitation (e.g. therapists and physiatrists) are more interested in the biomechanical causes of the abnormalities (Watelain et al 2003).

This book is aimed at understanding general principles useful in analysing any gait disorder. Nevertheless, it is important to be aware of the main pathologies and their typical characteristic clinical presentations.

STROKE

In an average year, around 0.2% of the population has a stroke (Roth & Harvey 1996). It is the most common of all neurological deficits and the leading cause of gait impairment in rehabilitation facilities. Sometimes called cerebrovascular accident (CVA), stroke is due to thromboembolism (in 80% of cases) or haemorrhage (20%) of an artery supplying

Table B1 A gait classification based on the level of the impairment, often used by neurologists

High-level	Cautious gait
	Subcortical dysequilibrium
	Frontal dysequilibrium
	Isolated gait ignition failure
	Frontal gait disorder
	Psychogenic gait disorder
Mid-level	Hemiplegic gait
	Diplegic gait
	Paraplegic gait
	Cerebellar ataxic gait
	Parkinsonian gait
	Choreic gait
	Dystonic gait
Low-level	Peripheral musculoskeletal problems:
	• arthritic gait
	• antalgic gait
	• myopathic gait
	• peripheral neuropathic gait
	Peripheral sensory problems:
	• sensory ataxic gait
	• vestibular ataxic gait
	• visual ataxic gait

the cerebral cortex of the brain. There is about a 10% recurrence rate per year, and 50% of patients remain dependent on others for their care after 6 months, with 20% unable to walk and another 20% severely disabled. It is the third leading cause of death in developed countries, with smoking, hypertension, hypercholesterolaemia and diabetes being the main risk factors. Recovery is most marked in the first 3 months, with little further improvement after 12 months.

? | **MCQ B1**

Based on an incidence of 0.2%, how many people suffer a stroke in the UK (population 60 million) every year?
(a) 60,000
(b) 120,000
(c) 1.2 million
(d) 12 million

Strokes can be classified into four subtypes that help to predict outcome (Table B2). For example, TACI strokes have a negligible chance of good functional outcome with high mortality, while patients in the PACI and POCI groups are more likely to have an early recurrent stroke but have a better chance of a good functional outcome. People in the LACI group usually remain significantly disabled (Bamford et al 1991).

One of the major effects is *hemiparesis* – weakness on one side of the body (lower/upper-limb and face). The word *hemiplegia* implies a more

Table B2   Oxford classification of stroke subtypes (Bamford et al 1991)

Type	Incidence	Diagnosis	Independence at 1 year
Total anterior circulation infarct (TACI)	17%	Weakness (± sensory deficit) of at least 2 of face/arm/leg; homonymous hemianopia higher cerebral dysfunction	5%
Partial anterior circulation infarct (PACI)	24%	Restricted motor/sensory deficit (e.g. one limb, face and hand); higher cerebral dysfunction alone	55%
Lacunar circulation infarct (LACI)	25%	Small infarctions (arteriolar) in basal ganglia, internal capsule or brainstem. Can be motor (commonest) or sensory, and ataxic	60%
Posterior circulation infarct (POCI)	24%	Brainstem, cerebellar or occipital lobes, cranial nerve palsy, hemianopia, coma, drop attacks, vertigo, nausea, vomiting, cranial nerve palsies, ataxia	60%

dense (severe) paralysis, although in practice the two terms are often used interchangeably. It is important to understand that the hemiparesis occurs contralateral to the side of the lesion because the pyramidal tracts carrying the voluntary motor pathways cross over (*decussate*) at the level of the midbrain. Thus, a left-sided stroke will cause a right-sided hemiparesis and vice versa – somewhat confusing! Along with the hemiparesis, there is often a unilateral sensory loss on the same side as the weakness, and loss of vision to that side (*hemianopia*).

Depending on the side of the lesion, a variety of higher brain functions can also be impaired (Table B3). For example, the speech centre (Broca's area) is normally located in the left cerebral hemisphere (even in left-handers), so difficulty speaking (*dysphasia*) is common in those with a right hemiparesis. On the other hand, those with a left hemiparesis often have more subtle language problems, such as difficulty with emotions and humour (*dysprosodia*), along with perceptual problems, such as neglect of the paretic side (*agnosia*), problems in sequencing and coordinating movements (*apraxia*), and other frontal lobe functions (e.g. insight and judgement – denial and over-confidence are common problems). Awareness of these two common stroke syndromes is essential for appropriate rehabilitation.

There is a selective loss of muscle control with the emergence of primitive patterned movements. Typically there is increased extensor tone in the affected lower-limb, with equinovarus and stiff knee. Vaulting and circumduction are frequent compensations for the reduced clearance. Muscle imbalance and spasticity may result in joint contractures.

ARTHRITIS

Arthritis affects nearly one in six people, making it the leading cause of disability. By the year 2020, as the baby boom generation ages, an estimated 20% of the population will have significant arthritis. The commonest joints to be affected are the hip and knee, so gait is frequently impaired.

Table B3 Common syndromes (collections of symptoms and signs) accompanying a stroke in each cerebral hemisphere

Hemiparesis	Left	Right
Lesion	Right hemisphere	Left hemisphere
Speech	Unaffected	Dysphasia, communication problems
Perception	Left-sided neglect (agnosia)	Intact
	Apraxia	Intact
Learning	Does not learn from mistakes	Learns by imitation and making mistakes
Insight and judgement	Impaired – impulsive, disorganized	Intact
Confidence	Can be over-confident	Cautious in unfamiliar situations

Rheumatoid arthritis (RA) is a chronic inflammation of the joint lining (synovium), typically causing acute flare-ups of pain, stiffness, warmth, redness and swelling, along with a gradual degeneration of the articular cartilage and bone. Joint deformities (e.g. *genu varum*) are common. RA is a systemic disease, however, and loss of appetite (*anorexia*), fever (*pyrexia*), loss of energy (*anergia*) and anaemia are also common. Onset is usually in middle-age, but a juvenile chronic form (JCRA) can begin in childhood (Lechner et al 1987). Although the cause is unknown, RA is classified as an autoimmune disease because the immune system appears to be disordered, and a *rheumatoid factor* can be detected in the bloodstream in 80% of cases. There is some genetic basis, with people positive for the marker HLA-DR4 being more at risk for RA, and twice as many women (36 per 100,000) as men (14 per 100,000) have rheumatism (Suarez-Almazor & Foster 2001).

In osteoarthritis (OA) the cartilage and joint degeneration occur without inflammation (leading some to prefer the name *osteoarthrosis*). Most commonly affecting middle-aged and older people, it affects the knees, hips, feet and spine, causing pain that is relieved by rest and made worse by movement and weight-bearing. In primary ('wear and tear') OA, there seems to be no obvious cause (though it is likely that cartilage repair is in some way impaired), whereas in secondary OA there is a history of joint injury (e.g. sports injury, accidents, repetitive work-related trauma). About 75% of people aged 65 and over have some arthritis of the weight-bearing joints.

The natural history of arthritis, as with all degenerative diseases, is of a slow decline in function with time (Fig. B1). However, the rheumatoid form is especially characterized by flare-ups (relapses) and periods of relative improvement (remissions). This pattern can make the assessment of interventions difficult, since it is often not clear whether an improvement is simply due to chance. Patients are also often tempted by a range of alternative treatments because they may happen to take one just before a remission and thereby credit it with the improvement.

Figure B1   Natural history in OA and RA. While functional level declines in both diseases, OA is characterized by a steady decline in function, while in RA the picture is more variable, with alternating periods of relapse and remission. This needs to be taken into consideration when evaluating the effect of interventions.

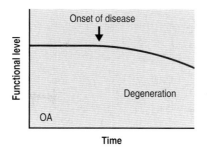

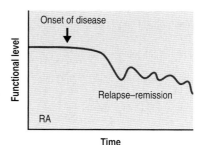

Five major foot deformities are seen in RA (Dimonte & Light 1982):

- Hallux abducto valgus (HAV)
- Hyperpronation
- Metatarsal head depression
- Hammer and claw toes
- Tendocalcaneal bursitis and plantar spur formation.

Patients with RA tend to have a hindfoot valgus deformity with excessive subtalar joint eversion motion in stance phase, coupled with excessive internal tibial rotation (Woodburn et al 2002, 2003).

CEREBRAL PALSY

Cerebral palsy (CP) is a *perinatal* disorder (occurring before, during or shortly after birth) of *idiopathic* aetiology (meaning that no cause has yet been elucidated). Incidence is about 2 per 1000 live births (Barnhart & Liemohn 1995). Although it is more common in babies with low birth weight and prematurity (birth before 32 weeks), there seems to be a background incidence that improvements in obstetric care have failed to eliminate entirely.

While the neurological damage is non-progressive (meaning that the brain lesion does not get any worse), secondary problems (muscular contractures and abnormal bone growth) often cause deterioration in function as the child ages. Nevertheless, about 70% of people with CP can walk (Campos da Paz et al 1994, Damiano & Abel 1996), and a plethora of therapeutic interventions in recent years have made understanding CP gait one of the main challenges in clinical gait analysis today.

There are three basic types: *spastic* (around 70%), involving the pyramidal tracts and causing either hemiplegia (Winters et al 1987) or diplegia (bilateral involvement, with lower-limbs affected more than upper-limbs); *athetoid* or *dyskinetic* (20%), which affects the extrapyramidal system, causing involuntary movements; and *ataxic* (10%), involving the cerebellum and resulting in balance problems. Some cognitive function impairment is present in approximately 40%.

The natural history of cerebral palsy is not entirely clear. Almost all children undergo some form of therapy, so it is difficult to observe their natural progress. The effects of growth further complicate the picture. Two studies in which two gait analyses were performed several years apart showed a decline in function (Johnson et al 1997, Bell et al 2002). This is thought to be due to a combination of two processes. Spastic muscles become tighter as the long bones grow, and while muscle strength increases according to the square of its diameter (cross-sectional area), body weight (or volume) increases according to the cube (Gage 1991). Thus the child becomes progressively weaker with growth.

There are three fundamental problems in CP: weakness, spasticity, and loss of selective motor control with retained primitive reflexes and postural reactions. Equinus, excessive knee and hip flexion, early heel-rise, foot-drop and excessive limb flexion during swing are common gait deviations. In weaker patients excessive pronation, excessive dorsiflexion, knee and hip flexion (crouch gait) and toe drag occur.

TOE–WALKING

Although toe-walking can be a sign of calf spasticity, it is also often seen in healthy children during the first few years of walking. Toe-walking may have certain advantages, in simplifying control of the foot (Gage 1991).

 DEBATING POINT

Research and debate the following:
– Toe-walking is a normal variant of childhood gait with no deleterious sequelae
– Toe-walking is a clinical condition that should be treated

SPINA BIFIDA (MYELOMENINGOCELE/ MYELODYSPLASIA)

Spina bifida (SB) has an incidence of 1 in 1000 births (Sarwark 1996). It is due to incomplete closure of the neural tube around the 20th day of pregnancy, due, at least in part, to a lack of folic acid in the diet. Vitamin supplementation in early pregnancy has reduced the incidence somewhat in recent years, and many nations now fortify bread with folate. Approximately 90% of these lesions occur in the midlumbar, lumbosacral and sacral regions, which compromise gait. Many children born with SB also have hydrocephalus, the accumulation of fluid in the brain, which can be controlled by a ventriculo-peritoneal shunt.

The weakness in SB is often characterized by muscle imbalance. For example, the *gluteus maximus* and *gluteus medius* are commonly weak compared to *iliopsoas* and adductors because the nerve supply of the latter arises above the lesion. Innervation of the ankle dorsiflexors and plantar flexors is also from L5–S1, so these muscle groups are typically weak too. The gait is characterized by exaggerated pelvic and hip motion, knee flexion and ankle dorsiflexion ('crouch gait'). Orthoses (AFO/FRO, KAFO and HKAFO) are frequently prescribed, with quite good results.

SPINAL CORD INJURY

There are approximately 30 to 50 spinal cord injury cases per million each year with mild to severe injuries. The average age of injury is 26 years, with men more often injured than women. Eighty per cent of the spinal cord injured population is under the age of 45 (Waters et al 1995). Injuries occur most commonly in regions of maximal spinal curvature: cervicothoracic (C5–7), midthoracic (T4–6) and thoracolumbar (T12–L1). Table B4 provides a list of the nerve supplies of the important muscle groups (myotomes) of the lower limb. In complete paraplegia, all of these groups are paralysed, although low-level (thoracolumbar) lesions often retain some weak hip flexion from trunk musculature. In addition, higher-level lesions may have impaired trunk control. As a result, gait analysis and therapy tend to be focused on those with a low-level or incomplete lesion (e.g. the

Table B4 Myotomes of the lower-limb. These are best remembered with the mnemonic '2,3,4' (hip flexion L2-3, extension L4-5; knee flexion L3-4, extension L5-S1, ankle dorsiflexion L4-5, plantarflexion S1-2)

Joint	Motion	Key muscles
Hip	Flexion/Adduction/Medial rotation: L2-3	*Iliopsoas*
	Extension/Abduction/Lateral rotation: L4-5	*Gluteus maximus, medius*
Knee	Extension: L3-4	*Quadriceps*
	Flexion: L5-S1	Hamstrings
Ankle/Foot	Dorsiflexion: L4-5	*Tibialis anterior*
	Plantarflexion: S1-2	*Gastrocnemius*, soleus
	Inversion: L4	*Tibialis posterior*
	Eversion: L5-S1	*Peroneii*

unilateral weakness of a Brown–Sequard quadriplegia), who can often walk with the assistance of an AFO or KAFO.

MULTIPLE SCLEROSIS

Multiple sclerosis (MS), sometimes called *demyelination*, is a disorder in which the myelin sheath of upper motor neuron degenerates, leaving *plaques* of scar tissue in the CNS. It commonly affects the cerebellum, causing ataxia, and the spinal cord (*transverse myelitis*), resulting in a spastic paralysis. The incidence of MS is highest in higher latitudes (up to 150/100,000) and lowest in equatorial regions (less than 5/100,000), with the Orkney and Shetland Islands having the highest rates in the world. Deficiency of vitamin D (which is made by the skin in response to sunlight) has been recently postulated as a causative factor. The natural history of MS (like RA) has a relapse–remission pattern that can be frustrating for both patient and clinician. The effect of therapeutic interventions is often difficult to discern due to the underlying variability of the condition.

AMPUTATION

In general, amputations are performed to remove a 'dead, bad or useless limb'. Approximately 80% of all lower-limb amputations fall into the first category (dead, i.e. necrotic, limbs). This ischaemia (arterial insufficiency, peripheral vascular disease or dysvascularity) due to narrowing of arteries (atherosclerosis) is caused by cholesterol plaques, which build up over time as a result of factors such as smoking, a diet rich in fat, diabetes and hypertension. 'Bad' limbs include tumours, such as osteosarcoma or melanoma, and rare infections (e.g. necrotizing fasciitis), while 'useless' includes traumatic amputations (as a result of motor vehicle accidents, machinery or warfare) and severe congenital deformities. Advances in prosthetics have greatly improved the quality of life of lower-limb amputees, and have also often stimulated the understanding of normal locomotion. Nevertheless, there are still many challenges, not only in prosthetic component design and optimal alignment, but also in socket-making and stump pressure care.

MUSCULAR DYSTROPHY

Duchenne muscular dystrophy is reported in one of 5000 live male births (Nelson 1996). It is a sex-linked genetic disorder (only affecting boys), which causes degeneration of muscle cells. The disorder is usually diagnosed between the ages of 1 and 5 years, and by 12 years of age, the child often progresses to wheelchair dependence and bed care. Unfortunately, death usually occurs in late adolescence or early adulthood due to pulmonary and cardiac complications. Common observed gait deviations include Trendelenberg, toe-walking, lumbar lordosis, knee instability and recurvatum, and balance problems.

POLIOMYELITIS

Although the last epidemics of polio occurred in the late 1950s, and new cases are now rare thanks to universal vaccination, there are approximately 1.6 million polio survivors worldwide (Bruno et al 1994). More men than women were affected. The virus attacks and destroys the anterior horn cells of the spinal cord, causing paralysis, flaccidity and atrophy.

Knee hyperextension (recurvatum) and foot-drop are common, and contractures occur due to imbalance between agonist and antagonist muscle groups. Fatigue often limits range. Orthoses (AFO, KAFO) and walking aids are popular.

Recovery varies considerably among patients, from permanent disability to nearly full recovery. In recent years, post-polio syndrome has developed in approximately 80% of all polio survivors with an onset from 10 to 50 years post-infection (Aston 1992). The most common complaint is increased fatigue. Post-polio syndrome was once thought to be caused by a reactivation of the polio virus but now appears to be due to overuse of the remaining muscle fibres.

The mystery of polio

The earliest pictorial record of poliomyelitis can be found on a 3000-year-old Egyptian tablet (Fig. B2). *Ruma*, a gatekeeper at the temple of Astarte, is shown with a withered right leg, bringing fruit, wine, and a gazelle to the goddess he believed saved his life.

Polio was actually quite uncommon until the turn of the 20th century. Large epidemics of other virus diseases, such as smallpox, yellow fever, influenza, and measles, are recorded throughout history, but it seems that something happened to suddenly make the polio virus more virulent. Otherwise known as *infantile paralysis* because of its predilection for young children, the term poliomyelitis derives from the Greek words for the grey matter, which the virus infects. Its more evocative name, *Paralysis of the Morning*, succinctly describes the typical onset in a child who goes to bed healthy but is unable to get up in the morning.

In 1789, Underwood's *Diseases of Children* attributed it to 'teething and foul bowels' (it is, in fact, a food- and water-borne infection) and noted that where both lower extremities are paralysed 'nothing has seemed to do any good but irons to the legs, for the support of the limbs, and enabling the

Figure B2

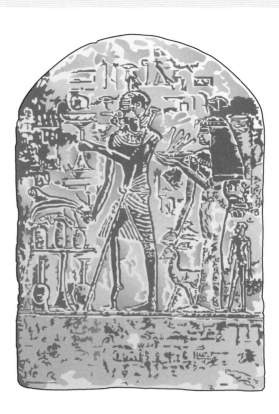

patient to walk'. Such was to be the treatment thereafter, until the last epidemics in the 1950s, before the Salk and later Sabin vaccines virtually wiped the disease out. The World Health Organization hopes that polio will shortly become only the second disease (after smallpox) to be completely eliminated from the globe.

The vaccines were developed too late for one famous president of the United States, Franklin D Roosevelt, who contracted polio in 1923. Robert Graham's sculpture of him in the wheelchair he himself designed was unveiled at the FDR memorial in Washington DC in 2000. Throughout his three wartime terms of office he managed to largely conceal his paralysis from the public – such was the stigma of disability in the 1940s.

Gould T 1997 A summer plague: polio and its survivors. Yale University Press, Yale

TRAUMATIC BRAIN INJURY

Traumatic brain injury (TBI) is commonly a result of road traffic accidents (RTA). Although the characteristic presentation includes a similar pattern of paralysis to stroke (hemiparesis), in TBI the presentation is often more diverse and complex, with higher level deficits.

PARKINSON'S DISEASE

About 1% of people over the age of 50 have Parkinson's disease. It is a degenerative disease of the dopamine-producing cells of the basal ganglia, which is part of the extrapyramidal system. It is usually idiopathic, but may be induced by drugs such as phenothiazine antipsychotics. Unlike pyramidal disorders, strength is relatively preserved, and instead there is rigidity, *bradykinesia* (slow movement) and tremor. Gait is impaired by postural instability and is typically *festinating* in character, with forward trunk flexion and short steps of rapid cadence. Difficulty with gait initiation (freezing) can occur, which can sometimes be helped by drawing lines on the floor.

FALLS

Falls are the leading cause of accidental death in older persons. They are also a significant cause of injury, loss of function, and a marker for functional decline. Around 1% of the elderly fracture a hip when they fall, 5% sustain another fracture, 5% a serious soft tissue injury, and 2% are hospitalized. Fractured neck of femur is a leading cause of morbidity and mortality, with 200,000 occurring each year, costing more than US$1 billion in treatment. About 20% of fallers with hip fracture die within 6 months. Another 20% are admitted to nursing homes. There is currently a great deal of interest in attempting to identify those at risk of falling in the hope that preventative interventions may be made. So far, no single risk factor has emerged, although muscle strength, balance, foot clearance and heel contact velocity, and medication (particularly benzodiazepine sedatives) have all been implicated.

SYSTEMIC DISEASES

The effects of several systemic diseases are manifest in the foot and so deserve special attention.

Diabetes mellitus is a disorder of the regulation of glucose and fat metabolism. Normally, insulin is produced by the islet (beta) cells of the pancreas in response to hyperglycaemia, to stimulate movement of glucose and fat from the blood to the liver and muscles. In type I (juvenile-onset, insulin-dependent diabetes mellitus, or IDDM) diabetes, the islet cells are destroyed (probably due to an abnormal autoimmune reaction to a virus infection) and insulin production is inadequate. In the type II (late-onset, non-insulin-dependent diabetes mellitus, or NIDDM) form, the islet cells are intact, but insulin resistance prevents it from having its normal effect. In general, type I diabetes requires insulin injections to control blood glucose, whereas type II diabetics can usually achieve control with diet, weight reduction, exercise and oral hypoglycaemic medication. In recent years these generalizations have become somewhat blurred, with type II diabetes sometimes being diagnosed in younger people and often requiring insulin for control. These changes may be as a result of the increasing level of sugar and fat consumption in the population, along with a sedentary lifestyle and associated obesity. Such factors have led to an epidemic of diabetes in recent years in developed countries (Fig. B3), which shows signs of spreading to developing countries. Currently around 6% of people in developed countries have diabetes, but the number of diabetics worldwide is set to double by 2030 to 366 million, with the greatest relative increase in prevalence expected in the Middle East, sub-Saharan Africa and India (Wild et al 2004).

The feet of people with diabetes are prone to ulcer formation, due to a combination of sensory neuropathy and vascular insufficiency. Such ulcers are slow to resolve, often healing with scarring, which may predispose to further ulceration. Since a foot ulcer is the initiating factor in 85% of diabetes-related amputations, there is a need for early detection of those at risk (Perry 2002). Callus formation (hyperkeratosis) is a frequent finding in diabetic feet, with a prevalence of 4.4% to 10.5%, and is a significant marker for the development of foot ulceration. Approximately 15% of all patients with diabetes will have foot ulcers during their lifetimes and amputation is necessary in

Figure B3 Rising incidence of diabetes in the UK (number of new cases per 100,000 of the population).

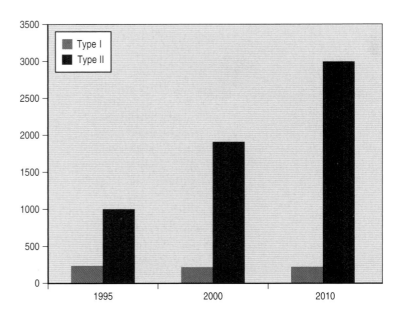

around 2% (Hunt & Gerstein 2003). The hyperkeratosis is a result of hypertrophy under the influence of intermittent compression. Therefore, the callus is either a reaction to abnormal pressure or an abnormality of the area to handle normal pressure. Callus buildup can increase the foot pressure by as much as 30% (Young et al 1992). Peripheral neuropathy is present in more than 80% of diabetic patients with foot ulceration.

Diabetes is the most common cause of *Charcot neuroarthropathy*. Peripheral neuropathy of the sensory afferents makes the involved joints insensate and gives rise to repetitive microtrauma with fractures, dislocations and deformity. This may be complicated by increased osteopenia due to autonomic neuropathy and muscle imbalance secondary to motor neuropathy (Young et al 1992). Glycosylation of collagen in tendons and ligaments may also result in reduced motion of joints in the feet of diabetics (Fernando et al 1991).

FOOT PAIN

Around 10% of people may experience plantar heel pain (Crawford & Thomson 2004). One study shows that 83% of 459 subjects over the age of 60 years of age had foot pain. A study of foot and shoe problems in the Netherlands found that 60% of women and 30% of men suffered from forefoot problems.

FLAT FEET

Most people are born with 'flat feet' but they usually correct over the first decade (Smith 1992, Capello & Song 1998). While a unilateral flat foot suggests some abnormal bone or joint pathology (congenital or acquired), significance of the much commoner bilateral condition (*pes planus* or *planovalgus*) excites much debate and controversy. Apart from acquired causes (e.g. rheumatoid or osteoarthritis, rupture of the *tibialis posterior* tendon, diabetic neuropathy and neuromuscular diseases such as cerebral palsy, muscular dystrophy and spina bifida), the vast majority are *idiopathic* (of undetermined cause).

The foot is flat because the longitudinal arch is flattened with excessive subtalar pronation, but there are still no universally accepted clinical or radiographic definitions of flat foot (Taylor et al 2001, Evans et al 2003). A variety of static measures (arch angle, navicular height, rearfoot angle), footprint indices (valgus, arch index, Denis, Brucken), radiographic measures (calcaneal inclination, arch height to length ratio, rearfoot–forefoot) and pseudo-dynamic measures (great toe extension test, navicular drop/drift, Jack's manoeuvre) have all enjoyed popularity from time to time (Rose et al 1985, Razeghi & Batt 2002). That so many approaches to diagnosis have been devised underscores the deficiencies of each. They are poorly correlated with each other and reliability between practitioners is also poor (Williams & McClay 2000).

Flat feet (along with big feet and 'bad' posture) have been used throughout history as a general aesthetic marker of inferiority, perhaps because the foot is the only part of the body that is horizontal (Zerbe 1985). The eugenics movement of the early 20th century held that Jewish people had flat feet (Gilman 1990), and during World War II thousands of men with asymptomatic flat feet were rejected from military service. Recent studies by the US (Cowan et al 1993) and Australian armies (Rudzki 1997) have found no significantly increased risk of injury in flat-footed recruits, and, in fact, high-arched feet have been found to be much more problematic (Ilahi & Kohl 1998). The transverse tarsal joint seems to compensate for the over-compliant arch during push-off (Inman et al 1994). Moreover, flat feet do not appear to be any more painful than normal feet (Hogan & Staheli 2002).

Despite all these reassuring data, there is still a tendency to over-diagnose and treat flat feet. In a Spanish study of primary school children the incidence was only 2.7%, but four times that number received treatment with orthopaedic footwear or insoles (García-Rodríguez et al 1999). Such interventions may not only be ineffective but can also be uncomfortable and embarrassing for the child (Staheli 1999). On the other hand, a Taiwanese study found impaired temporal–spatial parameters (reduced walking speed and stride length) in children with flat feet, which may be due, at least in part, to increased ligamentous laxity in Chinese populations (Lin et al 2001). There is a wide range of normality in the developing child, which makes diagnosis especially problematic in this age group.

The data on flat feet are thus somewhat confusing and incomplete, and are likely to remain so until satisfactory methods for measuring foot kinematics are developed (Razeghi & Batt 2002).

DEBATING POINT

Research and evaluate the evidence for and against the following:
– That flat foot is a condition that can be reliably diagnosed
– That flat foot has deleterious effects on biomechanical function in gait
– That the biomechanics in flat foot can be corrected by orthotic intervention

TALIPES EQUINOVARUS (TEV)

TEV is a combination of ankle plantarflexion (equinus) together with inversion (varus) and metatarsus adductus. Idiopathic *clubfoot* (as distinguished from the teratologic type associated with cerebral palsy and other neuromuscular diseases) occurs in 1–2 per 1000 live births, and is often bilateral. Surgery is usually necessary but there is often residual stiffness, weakness and hypoplasia (Kuo et al 1997).

CHARCOT–MARIE–TOOTH (CMT) DISEASE

CMT is a genetic disorder with autosomal dominant inheritance. Onset is delayed until the second or third decade of life, with a distal weakness characterized by normal reflexes. A characteristic 'stork leg' appearance is seen, caused by muscle atrophy, resulting in flail calcaneocavus and cavovarus foot deformities, with clawing of the toes. Pressure is increased under the lateral midfoot and forefoot, with decreased pressures under the 1st and 2nd toes. Forefoot loading is initiated earlier in the cycle, with increased pressure–time integrals under the lateral heel and lateral forefoot and premature heel-rise.

METATARSUS ADDUCTUS

This condition is a congenital medial deviation of the forefoot at the tarsometatarsal joints. It is present in 3% of live births, possibly due to intrauterine positioning, and gives rise to in-toeing. Flexible types resolve by the teens, but dynamic metatarsus primus varus (caused by contraction of the *abductor hallucis*) should be excluded.

THE ROLE OF GAIT ANALYSIS

The role of gait analysis in clinical decision-making has been hotly debated over the past 15 years or so (Lee et al 1992, Gage 1994, Watts 1994, Banta 1999, Morton 1999). Fundamentally, applications fall into three basic categories:

- Diagnosis
- Monitoring
- Research.

Like any special test, it should be used with discretion in making a diagnosis. The standard clinical approach, relying on a comprehensive history and examination (including an observational gait analysis) to generate diagnostic hypotheses, should be followed. An instrumented gait analysis (depending on available technology) can then be used to confirm or refute these hypotheses. Unfortunately, in many cases gait analysis is performed 'blindly' in the hope that it will provide the diagnosis on its own. This is bad practice, in the same way that a battery of blood tests is often imprudently used to 'screen' for pathology. To see the importance of carrying out a good history and examination, it is necessary to understand *Bayes' theorem*.

Bayes' theorem

Every test has a *sensitivity* and a *specificity*. The sensitivity of the test is the proportion of patients having a particular disorder in whom the test result is positive, while the specificity is the proportion of those without the disorder in whom the test result is negative. A perfect test would be one with a 100% sensitivity and specificity, i.e. one that gives a positive result for all those with the disorder, and a negative result for the healthy people without the disorder. In the real world, there is no such thing as a perfect test, of course, and so sensitivity and specificity values are in practice less than 100%.

The *positive predictive value* (PPV) is the probability that an abnormality is present when the test is positive, and is calculated as:

PPV = number of true-positives/total number of positives

The number of true-positives can be estimated from the sensitivity if the prevalence of the abnormality (the percentage of people in the population with the disorder) is known:

Number of true-positives = sensitivity × prevalence

So, if the test is 95% sensitive (0.95) and the prevalence is 10%, the number of true positives will be (0.95 × 10) = 9.5%. The *total* number of positives is equal to these true-positives plus any false-positives. The latter can be calculated from the specificity of the test:

Number of false-positives = (1 − specificity) × (1 − prevalence)

So, if the test is 90% specific, there will be (1 − 0.9) × (1 − 0.1) = 9% false-positives. Thus,

PPV = 9.5/(9.5 + 9) or about 50%

In other words, a positive test result only means that there is a 50% chance that the patient has the disorder. If the prevalence is raised to 50%, however, the PPV becomes

(0.95 × 50)/(0.95 × 50 + 0.1 × 50) = 90%

so it is clear that the result depends not only on the sensitivity and specificity of the test, but, more importantly, on the prevalence of the disorder in the population – often termed the *prior probability*.

This is *Bayes' theorem* (named after the English vicar who first came up with it), and it is responsible for causing many controversies in the decision of whether to introduce a screening test. Some examples in recent times include mammography, blood cholesterol and stool testing for colon cancer.

The PPV of these tests when used for mass screening is marginal, with lots of false-positives, and many epidemiologists have concluded that they should not be used. On the other hand, when a test is used to confirm a diagnostic *hypothesis*, the prior probability is boosted by history taking and clinical examination, which filter out most of the healthy people. The PPV of many gait analysis tests is very low indeed, so a comprehensive history and examination are therefore essential components of the gait analysis process.

At present many health insurance companies regard instrumented gait analysis as investigational, with insufficient evidence to support improved health outcomes or benefits from its use. This situation can be expected to change with refinements in the technology and, more especially, appropriate use.

Monitoring uses include the tracking of the progress of a disorder over time, and evaluating the efficacy of treatment, such as drugs, physical therapy, prosthetic or orthotic interventions, or surgery (pre/post comparisons). In such applications, it may be appropriate to track a single or small number of carefully selected *outcome measures* appropriate to the disorder being monitored.

To be useful, especially considering the often considerable investment of time and money required for a comprehensive gait analysis, tests should result in a change to either the management or prognosis of a disorder (Brand & Crowinshield 1981, Cooper et al 1999, Cottalorda 1999). So far, it has to be said that relatively few studies have demonstrated such an effect, especially at multiple centres. In addition a good test should meet the following requirements (Schwartz & Heath 1933):

- Ease
- Rapidity
- Free from error
- Validity (it should measure what it claims to measure)
- Accuracy
- Repeatability and stability (providing consistent results)
- Must not significantly affect the gait that it measures
- Must provide information not able to be directly observed by a skillful clinician
- Be independent of mood, motivation and pain
- Clearly distinguish between normal and abnormal
- Be reportable in some clinically understandable form
- Be cost-effective.

It is arguable how well current gait analysis procedures and technology meet this specification.

GAIT CYCLE CLASSIFICATIONS

Traditionally, the gait cycle has been divided into five stance phase periods and three swing phase periods (Perry 1992, Adams & Perry 1994). This is known as the *Ranchos* classification after the Ranchos Los Amigos hospital in Los Angeles, where it was developed (Fig. B4).

An alternative classification (Sutherland et al 1988) substitutes three periods of stance: initial double support, single limb stance, and second double support (Fig. B5). A more functional classification divides the cycle based on the tasks being performed during each sub-phase (Fig. B6).

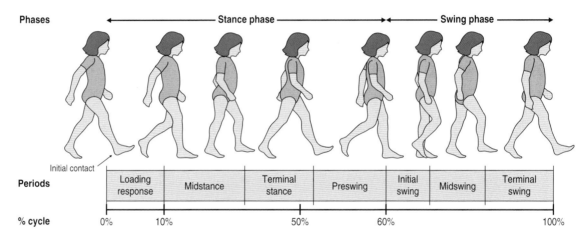

Figure B4   Traditional gait cycle subdivisions developed at Ranchos Los Amigos hospital (Perry 1992).

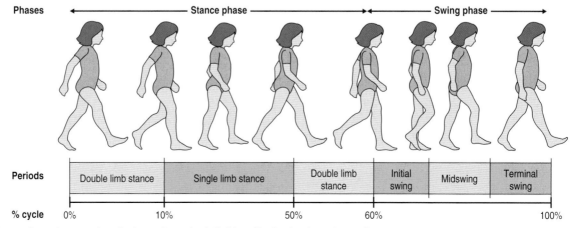

Figure B5   A more descriptive gait cycle definition (Sutherland et al 1988).

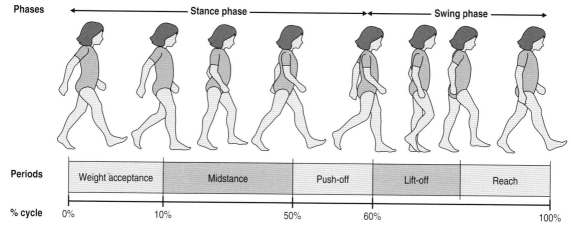

Figure B6   A more functional gait cycle definition (Winter 1985).

Although perhaps useful for documentation purposes, such divisions of the gait cycle cannot be reliably distinguished without technological assistance (Fish & Nielsen 1993), so have limited application in clinical practice.

In view of recent work, which has elucidated the main subtasks of gait (Neptune et al 2001), the following gait cycle classification is suggested, which has the added advantage of simplicity (Fig. B7).

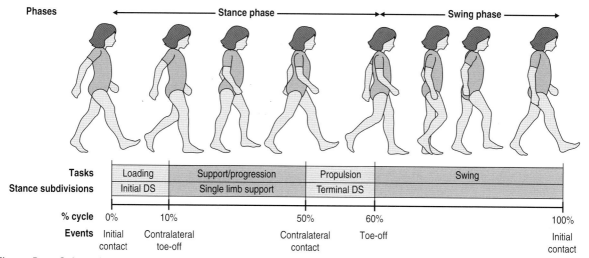

Figure B7   Gait cycle classification adopted in this book. The three fundamental functions (loading, support/progression and propulsion/swing, associated with the three ankle rockers) are clearly defined by gait events.

BRIEF SUMMARY OF THE KEY TASKS OF GAIT

The three main subtasks of gait (which correspond to the three ankle rockers) are:

- 1st Rocker: Loading
- 2nd Rocker: Support/Progression (Single Limb Support)
- 3rd Rocker: Propulsion/Swing.

It can be seen that these tasks are defined by clearly defined gait events (initial contact, contralateral toe-off, contralateral contact and toe-off), and also correspond to the stance subdivisions (initial double support, single limb support and terminal double support/swing phase) so are relatively easy to identify. Moreover, by focusing on the tasks that the locomotor system is performing, attention is automatically centred on biomechanical abnormalities.

Loading

Loading begins with initial contact on the lateral border of the heel. The foot pronates to provide a compliant interface (mobile adaptor) with the floor, while the dorsiflexors and knee extensors act eccentrically to absorb energy. Contact is made by the 5th metatarsal with the ground as the foot continues rolling medially until the metatarsals become fully loaded at the conclusion of the contact phase.

Support/progression

The ankle plantarflexors lock the ankle, providing a knee extensor moment via the plantarflexor–knee extensor couple. The trunk progresses over the stance limb by a combination of hip extensor activity and energy recovered from the swing limb. During this phase the foot supinates, converting from a mobile adaptor into a rigid lever. The hip abductors also prevent collapse of the pelvis (Trendelenberg) on the unsupported swing side.

Propulsion/swing

A powerful plantarflexor contraction throws the shank-foot up and forwards, flexing the knee. Push-off efficiency is enhanced by the rigid platform provided by the supinated foot and taut plantar fascia via the windlass effect. Immediately following this, pull-off from the hip flexors swings the limb forward, with *rectus femoris* controlling heel-rise. Swing phase is characterized by damping muscle contractions which control the swinging limb: heel-rise is limited by *rectus femoris* damping during push-off, while knee extension is terminated by eccentric hamstrings action to slow the foot ready for the next contact, and a new cycle.

The following chapters discuss these tasks in more detail and explore how they are impaired by disease.

References

Adams J M, Perry J 1994 Gait analysis: clinical application. In: Rose J, Gamble J (Eds) Human walking, 2nd edn. Williams and Wilkins, Baltimore

Aston J W 1992 Post-polio syndrome: an emerging threat to polio survivors. Postgraduate Medical Journal 92:249–260

Bamford J, Sandercock P, Dennis M et al 1991 Classification and natural history of clinically identifiable subtypes of cerebral infarction. Lancet 22(337):1521–1526

Banta J 1999 Gait analysis: past, present, and future. Developmental Medicine and Childhood Neurology 41(6):363

Barnhart R C, Liemohn W P 1995 Ambulatory status of children with cerebral palsy: a retrospective study. Perception and Motor Skills 81:571–574

Bell K J, Õunpuu S, DeLuca P A, Romness M J 2002 Natural progression of gait in children with cerebral palsy. Journal of Pediatric Orthopedics 22:677–682

Brand R A, Crowinshield R D 1981 Comment on criteria for patient evaluation tools. Journal of Biomechanics 14:655

Bruno R L, Cohen J, Galski T, Frick N M 1994 The neuroanatomy of post-polio fatigue. Archives of Physical Medicine and Rehabilitation 75:498–504

Campos da Paz A, Burnett SM, Braga LW (1994) Walking prognosis in cerebral palsy: a 22-year retrospective analysis. Developmental Medicine and Child Neurology 36:130–134

Capello T, Song K M 1998 Determining treatment of flatfeet in children. Current Opinions in Pediatrics 10:77–81

Cooper R A, Quatrano L A, Stanhope S J 1999 Gait analysis in rehabilitation medicine: A brief report. American Journal of Physical Medicine and Rehabilitation 78(3):278–280

Cottalorda J 1999 Gait analysis: matching the method to the goal. Reviews of Rheumtism (Engl Ed.) 66(7–9):367–369

Cowan D N, Jones B H, Robinson J R 1993 Foot morphologic characteristics and risk of exercise-related injury. Archives of Family Medicine 2(7):773–777

Crawford F, Thomson C 2003 Interventions for treating plantar heel pain. Cochrane Database of Systematic Reviews (3):CD000416

Damiano D L, Abel M F 1996 Relationship of gait analysis to gross motor function in cerebral palsy. Developmental Medicine and Child Neurology 38:389–396

Dimonte P, Light H 1982 Pathomechanics, gait deviations, and treatment of the rheumatoid foot. Physical Therapy 62:1148–1156

Evans A M, Copper A W, Scharfbillig R W et al 2003 Reliability of the foot posture index and traditional measures of foot position. Journal of the American Podiatry Medical Association 93(3):203–213

Fernando D J S, Masson E A, Veves A, Boulton A J M 1991 Relations of limited joint mobility to abnormal foot pressure and foot ulceration. Diabetes Care 14:8–11

Fish D J, Nielsen J-P 1993 Clinical assessment of human gait. Journal of Prosthetics and Orthotics 5(2):39–48

Gage J R 1991 Gait analysis and cerebral palsy. Blackwell, Oxford, UK & Cambridge University Press, Boston/New York

Gage J R 1994 Editorial. The role of gait analysis in the treatment of cerebral palsy. Journal of Pediatric Orthopedics 14:701–702

García-Rodríguez A, Martín-Jiménez F, Carnero-Varo M et al 1999 Flexible flat feet in children: a real problem? Pediatrics 103:84

Gilman S L 1990 The jewish body: a footnote. Bulletin of the History of Medicine 64(4):588–602

Hogan M T, Staheli L T 2002 Arch height and lower limb pain: an adult civilian study. Foot and Ankle International 23(1):43–47

Hunt D, Gerstein H 2003 Foot ulcers and amputations in diabetes. Clinical Evidence 9:651–659

Ilahi O A, Kohl H W 1998 Lower extremity morphology and alignment and risk of overuse injury. Clinical Journal of Sport Medicine 8(1):38–42

Inman V T, Ralston H J, Todd F 1994 Human locomotion. In: Rose J, Gamble J G (eds) Human walking, 2nd edn. Williams and Williams, Baltimore

Johnson D C, Damiano D L, Abel M F 1997 The evolution of gait in childhood and adolescent cerebral palsy. Journal of Pediatric Orthopedics 17:392–396

Kuo K N, Huang M J, Smith P 1997 Dynamic gait analysis in a long term follow-up of clubfoot surgery. Journal of Pediatric Orthopedics 6B:286

Lechner E D, McCarthy F C, Holden M K 1987 Gait patterns in patients with juvenile rheumatoid arthritis. Physical Therapy 67:1335–1341

Lee E H, Goh J C H, Bose K 1992 Value of gait analysis in the assessment of surgery in cerebral palsy. Archives of Physical Medicine and Rehabilitation 73:642–646

Lin C-J, Lai K-A, Kuan T-S, Chou Y L 2001 Correlating factors and clinical significance of flexible flatfoot in preschool children. Journal of Pediatric Orthopedics 21:378–382

Morton R 1999 New surgical interventions for cerebral palsy and the place of gait analysis. Developmental Medicine and Childhood Neurology 41(6):424–428

Nelson M E 1996 Rehabilitation concerns in myopathies. In: Braddom R L (ed.) Physical medicine and rehabilitation. WB Saunders, Philadelphia

Neptune R R, Kautz S A, Zajac F E 2001 Contributions of the individual ankle plantar flexors to support, forward progression and swing initiation during normal walking. Journal of Biomechanics 34:1387–1398

Perry J 1992 Gait analysis: normal and pathological function. McGraw-Hill, New York

Razeghi M, Batt M E 2002 Foot type classification: a critical review of current methods. Gait & Posture 15:282–291

Rose G K, Welton E A, Marshall T 1985 The diagnosis of flat foot in the child. Journal of Bone and Joint Surgery 67B:71–78

Rose J, Gamble J (eds) 1994 Human walking, 2nd edn. Williams and Wilkins, Baltimore

Roth E J, Harvey R L 1996 Rehabilitation of stroke syndromes. In: Braddom R L (ed.) Physical medicine and rehabilitation. WB Saunders, Philadelphia

Rudzki S J 1997 Injuries in Australian Army recruits. Part III: The accuracy of a pretraining orthopedic screen in predicting ultimate injury outcome. Military Medicine 162(7):481–483

Sarwark J F 1996 Spina bifida. Pediatric Clinics of North America 43(5):1151–1158

Schwartz R P, Heath A L 1933 Electrobasographic method of recording gait. Archives of Surgery 27:926–934

Smith M A 1992 Flat feet in children. British Medical Journal 301:1331–1332

Staheli L T 1999 Planovalgus foot deformity. Current status. Journal of the American Podiatry Medical Association 89(2):94–99

Suarez-Almazor M, Foster W 2001 Rheumatoid arthritis. Clinical Evidence 5:832–849

Sutherland D H, Olshen R A, Biden E N, Wyatt M P 1988 The development of mature walking. J B Lippincott, Philadelphia

Taylor K F, Bojescul J A, Howard R S et al 2001 Measurement of isolated subtalar range of motion: a cadaver study. Foot and Ankle International 22:426–432

Watelain E, Froger J, Barbier F et al 2003 Comparison of clinical gait analysis strategies by French neurologists, physiatrists and physiotherapists. Journal of Rehabilitation Medicine 35:8–14

Waters R L, Sie I H, Adkins R H 1995 Rehabilitation of the patient with a spinal cord injury. Orthopedic Clinics of North America 26(1):117–122

Watts H G 1994 Editorial. Gait laboratory analysis for preoperative decision making in spastic cerebral palsy: Is it all it's cracked up to be? Journal of Pediatric Orthopedics 14:703–704

Wild S, Roglic G, Green A et al 2004 Global prevalence of diabetes: estimates for the year 2000 and projections for 2030. Diabetes Care 27:1047–1053

Williams D S, McClay I S 2000 Measurements used to characterize the foot and the medial longitudinal arch: reliability and validity. Physical Therapy 80(9):864–871

Winter D A 1985 Concerning the scientific basis for the diagnosis of pathological gait and for rehabilitation protocols. Physiotherapy Canada 37(4):245–252

Winters T F, Gage J, Hicks R 1987 Gait patterns in spastic hemiplegia in children and young adults. Journal of Bone and Joint Surgery 69A:437–441

Woodburn J, Helliwell P S, Barker S 2002 Three-dimensional kinematics at the ankle joint complex in rheumatoid arthritis patients with painful valgus deformity of the rearfoot. Rheumatology 41(12):1406–1412

Woodburn J, Helliwell P S, Barker S 2003 Changes in 3D joint kinematics support the continuous use of orthoses in the management of painful rearfoot deformity in rheumatoid arthritis. Journal of Rheumatology 30(11):2356–2364

Young M J, Cavanagh P R, Thomas G et al 1992 The effect of callus removal on dynamic plantar foot pressures in diabetic patients. Diabetic Medicine 9:55–57

Zerbe K J 1985 "Your feet's too big": an inquiry into psychological and symbolic meanings of the foot. Psychoanalytical Reviews 72(2):301–314

Chapter 11

Loading

He who stumbles and does not fall mends his pace.

Spanish proverb

OBJECTIVES

- Know the methods used by the body for shock and impact absorption
- Know what happens during the first ankle rocker
- Understand the importance of stance phase knee flexion
- Awareness of how the normal loading response is impaired by common gait pathologies

The first task in the gait cycle is to ensure a safe landing of the leading foot, and smooth transfer of body weight from the trailing limb.

At initial contact, the ground reaction force rises rapidly as weight is transferred from the trailing to the leading limb. This force has two components. The first is an extremely brief high-frequency shock wave (the *heel-strike transient*), while the second is more long-lasting (about 100 ms, or 10% of the gait cycle).

SHOCK AND THE HEEL-STRIKE TRANSIENT

The heel-strike transient is a high-frequency shock wave in the ground reaction force (GRF) (Fig. 11.1) that occurs immediately following impact on the foot with the ground, and it is of such high frequency that it is often not recorded unless a high sampling rate is used with a well-mounted force platform. It is a consequence of the sudden deceleration of the foot and shank (remember that at this time most of the weight is being borne by the contralateral limb), and its size and shape are related to the stiffness properties of the heel (Whittle 1997). In barefoot walking, the heel fat pad is responsible for minimizing the force at heel-strike by increasing the contact time and hence reducing the peak deceleration (Tietze 1982, Ker et al 1989, Bennett & Ker 1990, Aerts et al 1995). When shoes are worn the materials used in the sole add further cushioning (Lafortune & Hennig 1992).

Whether this shock does any harm, e.g. leading to osteoarthritis at the ankle, knee (Lafortune et al 1996) or even spine (Wosk & Voloshin 1985), has been the subject of much speculation and debate (Radin et al 1972, 1980, Collins & Whittle 1989, Whittle 1999, Gill & O'Connor 2003), and as yet there is no clear evidence that it does. Nevertheless, people seem to feel more comfortable in shoes with shock-attenuating properties, giving rise to a huge industry in sports shoe design. It is worth noting that during running, transients may reach 2000 N (Nigg 1990).

There are two approaches to reducing shock: stiffness and viscosity. Low stiffness foams further reduce the acceleration at heel-strike (Noe

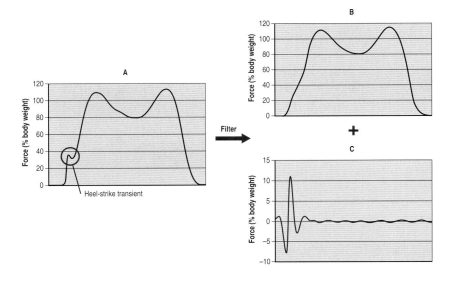

Figure 11.1 The heel-strike transient (C) can be separated from the GRF (A) by high-pass filtering (in this case at 10 Hz). It has a typical magnitude of about 10% body weight in normal gait. Often, because of low-pass filtering or inadequate sampling rate, only the low-frequency component (B) is recorded.

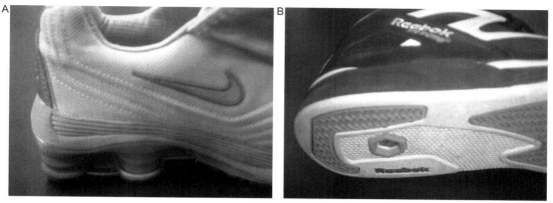

Figure 11.2 Innovation in sports shoe design: (A) Nike *Shox* with shock-absorbers and (B) Reebok *Pump* with *Hexalite* cushioning.

et al 1993), but have the disadvantage of making the shoe feel too compliant (soft and spongy). Viscoelastic materials are potentially better because they absorb the high-frequency shock (Voloshin & Wosk 1981) yet are stiff to low frequencies (just like a shock absorber on a car), and so feel firm and supportive to the wearer. With this aim in mind, the latest products incorporate air bubbles and pistons (Fig. 11.2).

ANKLE ACTION DURING LOADING

During loading, the ground reaction vector (GRV) is directed backwards, causing a plantarflexor external moment at the ankle and flexor moment at the knee. For equilibrium, the ankle dorsiflexors and knee extensors therefore need to be activated. This combination of muscle activity is called the *loading response* (Fig. 11.3).

THE ANKLE/FOOT DURING WEIGHT ACCEPTANCE

During this time (*first rocker*) the ankle plantarflexes from neutral (0°) to about 5° plantarflexion, pivoting about the calcaneus (Fig. 11.4) (Perry 1974).

The role of the foot during weight acceptance is to absorb impact power and adjust to any irregularity in the surface (*mobile adapter* function). Three mechanisms are principally responsible for this:

- The heel fat pad, which absorbs high-frequency shock
- Eccentric contraction of the dorsiflexors
- Pronation of the subtalar joint, which causes 'unlocking' of the transverse tarsal joint to make the foot into a compliant, flexible structure.

Figure 11.3 During weight acceptance (first 10% of the gait cycle until contralateral toe-off), the GRV is behind the ankle and knee joints, causing external plantarflexor and flexor moments, respectively. These moments are resisted by the dorsiflexors and knee extensors.

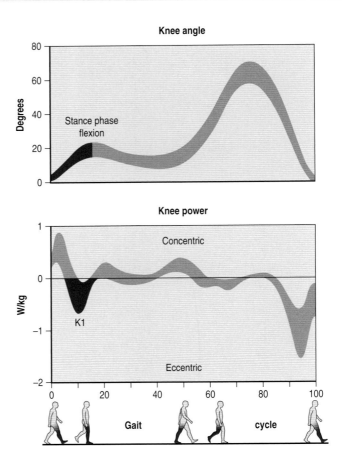

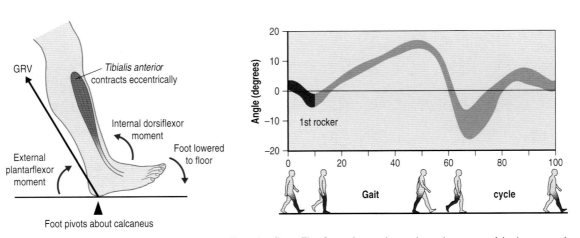

Figure 11.4 First rocker occurs when the heel strikes the floor. The foot pivots about the calcaneus, with the ground reaction passing posterior to the ankle joint. This causes an external plantarflexor moment, which is resisted by the *tibialis anterior*. Descent of the foot to the floor is controlled (slowed) by this eccentric activity of the dorsiflexors.

Breakdown of collagen fibrils may impair heel pad function in diabetes, resulting in increased shock (Shaw et al 1998, Hsu et al 2002). Eccentric contraction (an internal dorsiflexor moment while the foot is plantarflexing) of the *tibialis anterior* (aided by extensor *digitorum longus* and *peroneus tertius*) lowers the foot to the floor. Muscle activity is evident from EMG recordings, but the dorsiflexor moment is small so the amount of power absorption is consequently also minimal. It is responsible for preventing foot slap and providing a smooth transition into stance.

FIRST ROCKER DYSFUNCTION

Loss of dorsiflexor function (e.g. due to common peroneal nerve palsy or diabetic neuropathy) causes the foot to plantarflex uncontrollably, resulting in an audible 'foot slap' as it strikes the floor. There is increased loading time under the heel and metatarsal area, and reduced loading under the hallux (Giacomozzi et al 2002).

First rocker function can also be disrupted by plantarflexor spasticity (*equinus*). In this case the forefoot rather than the heel strikes the floor (Fig. 11.5). Since the ground reaction is anterior rather than posterior to

Figure 11.5 An equinus position of the foot causes a forefoot contact with abnormally high and premature plantarflexor moment.

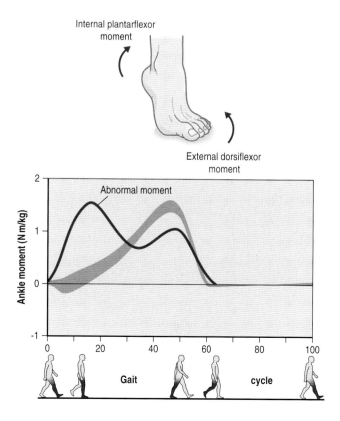

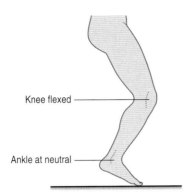

Figure 11.6 In pseudoequinus the ankle is normal but makes a forefoot contact because the knee is flexed.

the ankle, the ankle moment is plantarflexor rather than dorsiflexor. Moreover, the lever arm from the CoP to the ankle can be quite large, so the moment is often very high indeed. If the stretch reflex is hyperactive, forefoot landing can initiate a few beats of ankle *clonus* – phasic contraction of the plantarflexors, which can be seen in the ankle power curve.

In *false* or *pseudoequinus*, the ankle is normal (in the neutral position, i.e. 0°) but the knee is flexed at initial contact, so that there is forefoot or flat-foot contact (Fig. 11.6).

Overuse of the dorsiflexors has been thought to lead to medial tibial stress syndrome (MTSS) or 'shin splints', with pain along the postero-medial border of the tibia at the origin of the *posterior tibialis* muscle. The precise pathology is not clear and tibial stress fracture or microfracture, tibial periostitis, or distal deep posterior chronic compartment syndrome have all been postulated (Detmer 1986). A variety of shock-absorbing interventions have been suggested (shock-absorbent insoles, foam heel pads, heel cord stretching, alternative footwear, and surgical fasciotomy of the superficial posterior compartment). Despite the claim for compartment syndrome, the pressure in the posterior compartment was not found to be elevated (Mubarak et al 1982).

A recent review of 199 studies unfortunately found very little objective evidence to support such measures (Thacker et al 2002), and it now seems likely that the source of the pain is the *soleus* rather than *anterior tibialis* (Michael & Holder 1985, Beck & Osternig 1994). Another hypothesis is that hyperpronation causes increased stress on the *tibialis posterior*, and there seems to be some evidence that a hindfoot varus or hyper-pronatory foot type is related to the risk of MTSS (Sommer & Vallentyne 1995, Bennett et al 2001).

HEEL PAIN

Heel pain is a common complaint, usually as a result of plantar fasciitis (often called heel spur syndrome, although the presence of a spur is not necessary for diagnosis). It is also commonly treated with shock-absorbing heel pads (Fig. 11.7). Not surprisingly, heel pressures tend to be elevated in people with higher approach velocity (Morag & Cavanagh 1999).

FRONTAL PLANE

The foot must be correctly *prepositioned* immediately prior to initial contact. Due to the short distance between subtalar joint and heel (CoP), any inversion or eversion will tend to be accentuated by the ground reaction vector (Wright et al 2000) (Fig. 11.8).

Figure 11.7 Pre- and post-treatment plantar pressures following the successful reduction of force and pressure during heel-strike in a patient with heel pain (reproduced by permission of Tekscan Inc., South Boston, MA, USA).

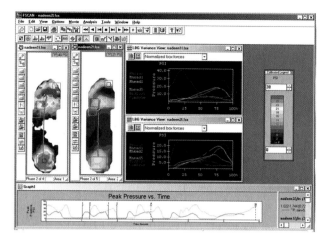

Figure 11.8 Ground reaction vector during loading tends to accentuate frontal plane malalignment.

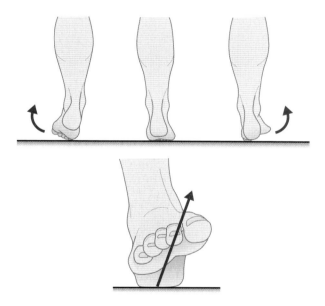

SHOE WEAR

Shoe wear is a useful guide to the type of loading. In runners, three major striking patterns have been described (Fig. 11.9). All three types wear the lateral heel area, but while overpronators tend to wear their shoes over the medial forefoot, supinators wear away the lateral forefoot.

Figure 11.9 Effect of running style on shoe-wear.

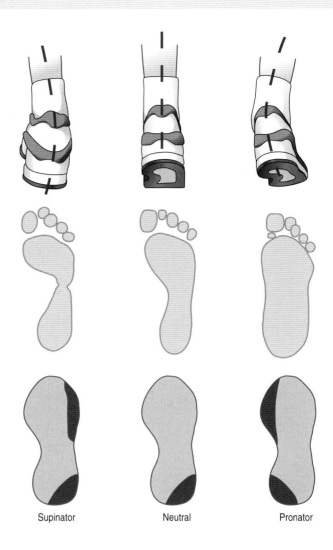

Supinator   Neutral   Pronator

Artificial loading response

All lower-limb amputees lack dorsiflexor musculature, so manufacturers of prosthetic feet have come up with a variety of mechanisms to provide some energy absorption. The simplest uses a solid ankle and cushioned heel (SACH foot), which compresses at initial contact to simulate the first rocker in controlling the lowering of the foot onto the floor. More complex designs (single and multi-axial feet) allow the rubber bumpers in the joint to absorb the impact, and respond to uneven terrain. It is also possible to incorporate a spring-damper (shock-absorber) mechanism into the foot or pylon.

Options for achieving impact absorption in prosthetic feet: the SACH foot absorbs impact in the heel cushion (Fig. 11.10), while in the multi-axial (College Park) feet rubber bumpers are used (Fig. 11.11); shock absorbers can also be incorporated into the foot (*Pathfinder*, Ohio Willow Wood, Mt Sterling, OH, USA) (Fig. 11.12).

Figure 11.10

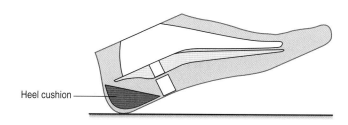

Heel cushion

Figure 11.11

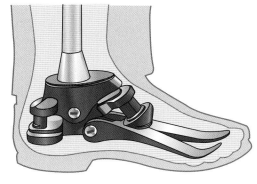

Figure 11.12 Courtesy of Ohio Willow Wood, Mt Sterling, OH, USA.

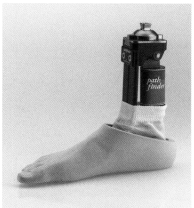

Doane N E, Holt L E 1983 A comparison of the SACH and single axis foot in the gait of unilateral below-knee amputees. Prosthetics and Orthotics International 7: 33–36

THE KNEE DURING LOADING

At initial contact, the knee is at or near full extension (0°), and on loading quickly flexes (stance phase flexion) to about 20°. This flexion is controlled by the knee extensors (quadriceps), which absorb power by their eccentric action. The loading response is typically impaired for two reasons:

1. Weak knee extensors (quadriceps)
2. Knee pain.

An absent loading response is characterized by the loss of stance phase flexion, i.e. fully extended knee throughout early stance (Kaufman et al 2001). Since there is no impact absorption at the knee, the gait has a jarring, staccato quality.

Loss of stance phase flexion may also be commonly seen in anyone with knee pain, which would be aggravated by the higher bone-on-bone forces generated by knee extensor activity. Instead of activating quadriceps, these patients use their hip extensors to pull the femur back and so lock the knee (Fig. 11.13).

Exercise training of the knee extensors in such patients is probably counter-productive, since they will reflexively inhibit the quadriceps to avoid pain – a *quadriceps-avoidance* strategy (Berchuk et al 1990). It could be argued that prevention of atrophy will be important should the knee pain be controlled or eliminated (e.g. by a replacement arthroplasty). Unfortunately, in most cases, once a quadriceps-sparing habit has been adopted it usually persists postoperatively. If exercise is prescribed, eccentric training is probably most appropriate since this most closely matches the functional role of the muscle (Winter 1995).

Figure 11.13 Abnormal loading response. The knee is locked and does not flex to absorb the impact.

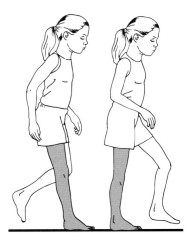

Walking on a flexed knee	Simulating the normal loading response in artificial knees has proved to be one of the most difficult challenges in prosthetics.

Above-knee amputees normally prevent the knee buckling at initial contact by hip extensor activity, which pulls the femur backwards and so locks the knee. Older, less active amputees, or those with a short stump, may have insufficient hip extensor strength, and require a weight-activated *stance-control* knee, which is locked by a brake mechanism when the limb is loaded. Unfortunately, such limbs are often *too* stable at toe-off, when the knee needs to flex quickly for swing initiation.

Polycentric designs, based on four-bar linkages, allow knee stability to be varied throughout the gait cycle, increasing stability at heel-strike and reducing it at toe-off (Fig. 11.14). It does this by creating a proximal instantaneous centre of rotation (ICR) that is posterior to the GRV when stability is required during loading, but anterior (unstable) during late stance to allow knee flexion to be initiated.

Moreover, polycentric knees can be voluntarily flexed while weight-bearing. For example, the Otto Bock 3R60 uses a polymeric spring to absorb impact as weight is transferred onto the prosthesis, allowing about 15° of stance flexion, and providing a more comfortable gait for the amputee.

Figure 11.14

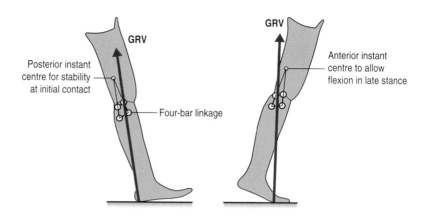

Blumentritt S, Scherer H W, Wellershaus U, Michael J W 1997 Design principles, biomechanical data and clinical experience with a polycentric knee offering controlled stance phase knee flexion: a preliminary report. Journal of Prosthetics and Orthotics 9(1):18–24

ANTERIOR CRUCIATE LIGAMENT (ACL) DEFICIENCY

Knee instability (*pivot shift* phenomenon, which is a feeling of the knee suddenly giving way or buckling) commonly results from ACL rupture, as the tibia slips forward on the femur. The ACL not only prevents anterior translation of the tibia on the femur, but also limits axial (internal/external) rotation (Markolf et al 1981). Loading is a particularly vulnerable time for such patients, especially if there is any axial stress (Markolf et al 1995), as occurs in *crossover cutting* movements.

 KEY POINTS

★ Weight acceptance is characterized by mechanisms for impact absorption

★ The ankle dorsiflexors act eccentrically to provide a controlled plantarflexion (1st rocker)

★ Subtalar pronation unlocks the transverse tarsal joints to increase foot compliance

★ An abnormal 1st rocker is typically seen in disorders with forefoot contact

★ The knee extensors act eccentrically to absorb impact by controlled stance phase flexion

★ Loss of stance phase flexion is seen in quadriceps weakness and knee pain

References

Aerts P, Ker R F, De Clerq D et al 1995 The mechanical properties of the human heel pad. Journal of Biomechanics 28:1299–1308

Beck B R, Osternig L R 1994 Medial tibial stress syndrome. The location of muscles in the leg in relation to symptoms. Journal of Bone and Joint Surgery 76A(7):1057–1061

Bennett J E, Reinking M F, Pluemer B et al 2001 Factors contributing to the development of medical tibial stress syndrome in high school runners. Canadian Journal of Orthopaedic and Sports Physical Therapy 31(9):504–510

Bennett M B, Ker R F 1990 The mechanical properties of the human subcalcaneal fat pad in compression. Journal of Anatomy 171:131–138

Berchuk M, Andriacchi T P, Bach B R 1990 Gait adaptations by patients who have a deficient anterior cruciate ligament. Journal of Bone and Joint Surgery 72A:871–877

Collins J J, Whittle M W 1989 Impulsive forces during walking and their clinical implications. Clinical Biomechanics 4:179–187

Detmer D E 1986 Chronic shin splints. Classification and management of medial tibial stress syndrome. Sports Medicine 3(6):436–446

Giacomozzi C, Caselli A, Macellari V et al 2002 Walking strategy in diabetic patients with peripheral neuropathy. Diabetes Care 25(8):1451–1457

Gill H S, O'Connor J J 2003 Heelstrike and the pathomechanics of osteoarthrosis: a simulation study. Journal of Biomechanics 36(11):1617–1624

Hsu T C, Lee Y S, Shau Y W 2002 Biomechanics of the heel pad for type 2 diabetic patients. Clinical Biomechanics 17(4):291–296

Kaufman K R, Hughes C, Morey B F et al 2001 Gait characteristics of patients with kenn osteaoarthritis. Journal of Biomechanics 34:907–915

Ker R F, Bennett M B, Alexander R McN, Kester R C 1989 Foot strike and the properties of the human heel pad. Engineering in Medicine 203:191–196

Lafortune M A, Hennig E M 1992 Cushioning properties of footwear during walking: accelerometer and force platform measurements. Clinical Biomechanics 7:181–184

Lafortune M A, Lake M J, Hennig E M 1996 Differential shock transmission response of the human body to impact severity and lower limb posture. Journal of Biomechanics 29(12):1531–1537

Markolf K L, Bargar W L, Shoemaker S C 1981 The role of joint load in knee stability. Journal of Bone and Joint Surgery 63A:570–585

Markolf K L, Burchfield D M, Shapiro M M et al 1995 Combined knee loading states that generate high anterior cruciate ligament forces. Journal of Orthopedic Research 13(6):930–935

Michael R H, Holder L E 1985 The soleus syndrome. A cause of medial tibial stress (shin splints). American Journal of Sports Medicine 13(2):87–94

Morag E, Cavanagh P R 1999 Structural and functional predictors of regional peak pressures under the foot during walking. Journal of Biomechanics 32(4):359–370

Mubarak S J, Gould R N, Lee Y F et al 1982 The medial tibial stress syndrome. A cause of shin splints. American Journal of Sports Medicine 10(4):201–205

Nigg B 1990 Biomechanics of running shoes. Shoes Trades Publ. Co., New York

Noe D A, Voto S J, Hoffmann M S et al 1993 Role of calcaneal heel pad and polymeric shock absorbers in attenuation of heel strike impact. Journal of Biomedical Engineering 15:23–26

Perry J 1974 Kinesiology of lower extremity bracing. Clinical Orthopedics and Related Research 102:20–31

Radin E L, Paul I L, Rose R M 1972 Role of mechanical factors in pathogenesis of primary osteoarthritis. Lancet i:519–521

Radin E L, Eyre D, Kelman J L, Schiller A L 1980 Effect of prolonged walking on concrete on the joints of sheep. Arthritis and Rheumatism 22:649

Shaw J E, van Schie C H, Carrington A L et al 1998 An analysis of dynamic forces transmitted through the foot in diabetic neuropathy. Diabetes Care 21:1955–1959

Sommer H M, Vallentyne S W 1995 Effect of foot posture on the incidence of medial tibial stress syndrome. Medicine and Science in Sports and Exercise 27(6):800–804

Thacker S B, Gilchrist J, Stroup D F, Kimsey C D 2002 The prevention of shin splints in sports: a systematic review of literature. Medicine and Science in Sports and Exercise 34(1):32–40

Tietze A 1982 Concerning the architectural structure of the connective tissue in the human sole. Foot & Ankle 2:252–259

Voloshin A, Wosk J 1981 Influence of artificial shock absorbers on human gait. Clinical Orthopedics and Related Research 160:52–56

Whittle M W 1997 Force platform measurement of the heelstrike transient in normal walking. Gait & Posture 5:173–174

Whittle M W 1999 Generation and attenuation of transient impulsive forces beneath the foot: a review. Gait & Posture 10:264–275

Winter D A 1995 Human balance and posture control during standing and walking. Gait & Posture 3:193–214

Wosk J, Voloshin A S 1985 Low back pain: conservative treatment with artifical shock absorbers. Archives of Physical Medicine and Rehabilitation 66:145–148

Wright I C, Neptune R R, van den Bogert A J, Nigg B M 2000 The influence of foot positioning on ankle sprains. Journal of Biomechanics 33:513–519

Chapter 12

Support and forward progression

OBJECTIVES

- Understand the importance of the plantarflexors in maintaining support during single limb stance
- Know the mechanism by which genu recurvatum deformity develops
- Understand the importance of hip abductor action to prevent Trendelenberg gait
- Appreciation of the significance of frontal plane knee moment in osteoarthritis
- Know the methods by which forward progression is achieved
- Understand the principles of operation of common walking aids

Following loading, the stance limb must be readied for support of the trunk during single limb support (SLS). Support during gait standing (Cerny 1984, Skinner et al 1985, Kerrigan et al 2000) follows the same basic principles as for quiet standing. During SLS (*2nd rocker*) the ankle plantarflexors generate a large moment that keeps the ground reaction force anterior to the knee joint, preventing its collapse – a mechanism known as the *plantarflexor-knee extensor (PF-KE) couple* (Fig. 12.1).

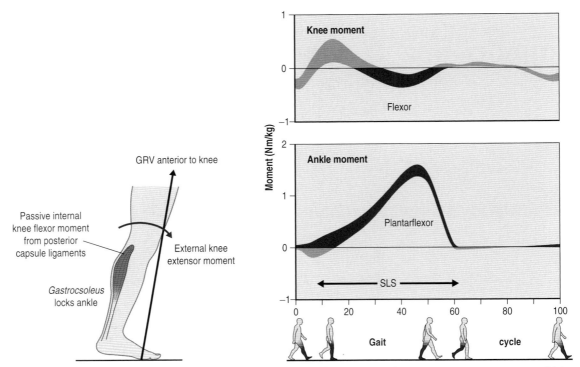

Figure 12.1 During single limb support (SLS), the plantarflexors (*gastrocsoleus*) generate a strong moment which locks the ankle joint. This places the GRV anterior to the knee joint, providing a passive external extensor moment which stabilizes the knee. Hyperextension is prevented by the posterior capsule ligaments, which are chiefly responsible for the internal knee flexor moment seen in the knee joint kinetics (right).

Hyperextension is checked by the gastrocnemius muscle and posterior capsule ligaments, which become taut as the knee extends. The internal knee moment measured by inverse dynamics is therefore flexor.

CLINICAL POINTER

Since the PF–KE couple is the major mechanism responsible for support (Pandy & Berme 1988, Kepple et al 1997, Anderson & Pandy 2003), weakness of the plantarflexors tends to result in collapse. This is particularly evident in the *crouch* gait of diplegic cerebral palsy (Fig. 12.2).

Crouch gait is a complex, *multi-level* disorder, characterized by collapse of all three joints (ankle dorsiflexion, knee and hip flexion). Although the main cause is a weak PF–KE couple, there is also often spasticity of the hamstrings and *iliopsoas* (especially *psoas*, which is polyarticular).

A Floor Reaction Orthosis (FRO) is commonly used to substitute the ankle stability normally provided by the plantarflexors (Saltiel 1969, Harrington et al 1984). The orthosis (sometimes called a Ground Reaction Orthosis, or GRO) is made in slight plantarflexion with an especially strong anterior shell in order to resist dorsiflexion (Fig. 12.3).

Figure 12.2 Crouch gait, in which the plantarflexor-knee extensor couple has failed due to weak plantarflexors, resulting in collapse of the ankle, knee and hip. Note that the GRV is posterior to the knee.

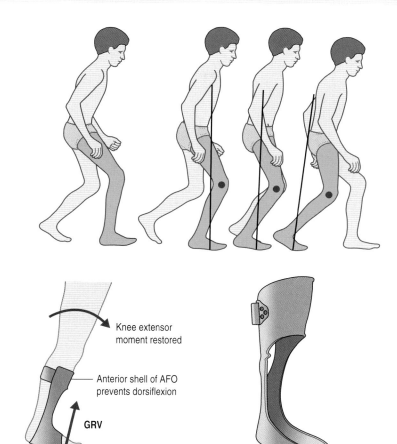

Figure 12.3 A floor or reaction AFO substitutes for the function of the ankle plantarflexors by preventing dorsiflexion and so forcing the GRV anterior to the knee to restore the external extensor moment.

Knee extensor moment restored

Anterior shell of AFO prevents dorsiflexion

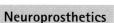

GRV

Neuroprosthetics

To securely lock the knee a Knee Ankle Foot Orthosis (also known as a long-leg brace) is usually prescribed. This consists of an AFO with metal uprights extending to a thigh shell. A knee joint is incorporated but this must be locked for standing and walking – it is only unlocked for sitting down. A pair of such braces (sometimes called Craig Scott braces) can facilitate rudimentary walking by people with complete paraplegia. In practice, such braces are rarely used, partly because the gait is very energy-intensive and tiring, but also because full-length bracing can be somewhat cumbersome and ugly.

An alternative scheme relies on the use of an AFO (FRO) to provide stability, since these braces are much more acceptable as they can be concealed inside the shoe. The FRO has a limitation, however, because the passive stabilization effect is lost whenever the GRV passes posterior to the knee. In normal gait, a rapid contraction of the quadriceps muscle is used to extend the knee and so restore stability, but in paraplegics the quadriceps is paralysed.

Figure 12.4

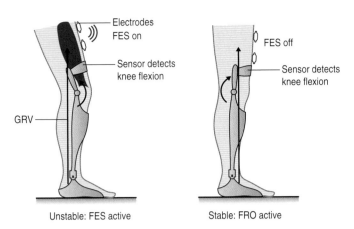

Unstable: FES active   Stable: FRO active

An ingenious solution to this problem utilizes Functional Electrical Stimulation (FES) of the quadriceps to activate the quadriceps via electrodes attached to the skin (Fig. 12.4). The resulting tetanic contraction is not as good as a normal physiological contraction, but it is sufficient to generate the required joint moment. Unfortunately, the muscle fatigues very quickly, so it can only be used for a brief burst, but in combination with the FRO knee stability can be sustained for long periods.

The unstable state is detected by a sensor in the suprapatellar strap – when pressure falls below a certain threshold, the system is programmed to trigger the stimulation until knee extension is restored and pressure under the strap returns. By this means the quadriceps can be rested and only activated to restore stability, in a similar manner to the way it functions naturally.

So far, such *neuroprostheses* have proven useful only in incomplete (unilateral, *Brown-Sequard* type) lesions, but implanted stimulators and sensors are currently undergoing clinical trials with the hope that they will also be useful for people with complete paraplegia.

Andrews B, Barnett R, Phillips G et al 1989 Rule-Base control of a hybrid FES orthosis for assisting paraplegic locomotion. Automedica 11:175–199
Granat M H, Ferguson A C B, Andrews B J, Delargy M 1993 The role of functional electrical stimulation in the rehabilitation of patients with incomplete spinal cord injury: observed benefits during gait studies. Paraplegia 31:207–215

Patients commonly compensate for an unstable knee by leaning forward in order to place the body centre of mass (CoM) (and therefore the ground reaction vector – GRV) anterior to the knee joint (Kerrigan et al 1996).

Some patients even press with a hand on the thigh (perhaps disguised in a trouser pocket) to push the knee into extension, and the repeated stretching of the posterior capsule ligaments can result in a *genu recurvatum* deformity (Fig. 12.5).

This gait and its resulting deformity used to be very common as a result of poliomyelitis, which thankfully is now rare due to mass vaccination, and spina bifida, which has been virtually eliminated by antenatal folate supplementation and early detection with ultrasound. It is still commonly seen, however, in many patients who have an overactive

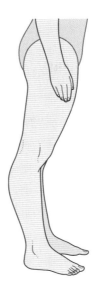

Figure 12.5   Genu recurvatum. Note that a small amount of recurvatum is normal in women.

plantarflexor-knee extensor couple due to equinus deformity (due to, e.g. stroke or cerebral palsy), and it can occur as a complication of FRO use. To prevent genu recurvatum and improve stability, a Knee Ankle Foot Orthosis (KAFO) must be prescribed to directly stabilize the knee and prevent hyperextension. An Anti-Recurvatum AFO, moulded in slight dorsiflexion with a heel lift, can also be used.

Support moment

Since collapse of the lower limb involves flexion of the hip and knee together with ankle dorsiflexion, the concept of *support moment* (M_S) has been proposed. This is a general measure of muscular support in the limb, calculated by summing the moments at each of the three joints (hip, h; knee, k; and ankle, a) (Winter 1980):

$$M_S = M_h + M_k + M_a$$

The advantage of the support moment is that unlike most other biomechanical measures, it integrates the activity at all three joints of the lower limb. It characterizes an overall support function or *synergy*, revealing that the body can be supported by an interchangeable combination of moments at any or all of the three joints. This could consist, for example, solely of knee action (quadriceps) or, in a patient with quadriceps paralysis, just the hip extensors and ankle plantarflexors. Note that a flexor (negative) moment at any joint needs to be subtracted rather than added to the total support moment.

The shape of the support moment (Fig. 12.6) resembles the ground reaction force. In fact, assuming that accelerations are minimal, which is usually the case during stance phase:

$$M_S = GRF \times k$$

Figure 12.6

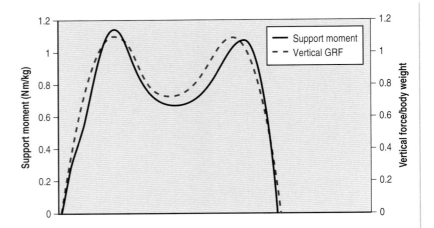

where *k* is the distance between the GRV and the knee joint: in other words, the required support moment increases with *k* (Hof 2000). This finding has important implications for pathologies such as the crouch gait of diplegic cerebral palsy, in which the knee is flexed throughout stance phase (Sutherland & Cooper 1978). Such gait patterns will require unusually high support moments.

Since it is a measure of the support *synergy*, variability in the support moment is lower than that of the contributing joint moments (Winter 1991).

Hof A L 2000 On the interpretation of the support moment. Gait & Posture 12:196–199
Sutherland D H, Cooper L 1978 The pathomechanics of crouch gait in spastic diplegia. Orthopedic Clinics of North America 9:143–154
Winter D A 1980 Overall principle of lower limb support during stance phase of gait. Journal of Biomechanics 13:923–927
Winter D A 1991 The biomechanics and motor control of human gait: normal, elderly and pathological. University of Waterloo Press, Ontario, Canada

SUPPORT IN THE AMPUTEE

As usual, a review of amputee gait offers further insights into normal gait. The alignment of a BK (below-knee) prosthesis determines the stability of the knee by moving the GRV with respect to the socket (Fig. 12.7). When the socket is moved posteriorly (i.e. foot moved anterior), the knee is effectively moved further posterior to the GRV and so stability is improved. Conversely, if the socket is attached anteriorly with respect to the foot, the knee will be moved more anterior and it will therefore be more difficult for the amputee to get the GRV into the stable zone in front of the knee (requiring increased internal extensor knee moment from the quadriceps).

The concept of heel and toe *levers* can be helpful in remembering these effects: as the socket moves backwards, the toe lever increases while heel lever decreases, and vice versa. Longer toe levers are associated with greater stability, longer heel levers with less stability.

If the prosthesis is aligned with insufficient stability (long heel lever), the knee may give way in late stance, resulting in a gait abnormality known as 'drop-off' (Fig. 12.8). Greater support is not always a good

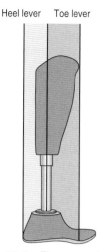

Heel lever   Toe lever

Figure 12.7 The concept of heel and toe levers is helpful in understanding support stability in the BK amputee. A longer heel lever tends to destabilize the limb, while a longer toe lever improves stability.

thing, however, because it can make the knee difficult to flex at toe-off, impairing the amputee's ability to initiate swing phase. The prosthetist therefore aims at an optimal alignment between these two extremes, depending on the fitness and activity level of the amputee. For example, stability is usually more important to elderly, sedentary amputees while young, fit amputees often prefer more control (reduced stability), since they have stronger residual musculature. The range of acceptable alignments is quite large for level gait, but alignment becomes more critical when the amputee is asked to walk up and down inclines (Sin et al 2001).

Angulation of the prosthetic foot and socket also affect stability (Table 12.1). Attaching the foot in slight plantarflexion increases the PF-KE couple and so improves stability, while attaching the socket in flexion improves control. In practice, the socket is normally set in about 12–14° of flexion. This has the important additional effect of placing body weight predominantly over the pressure-tolerant patellar tendon distally and muscle bulk posteriorly. The slight stretch of the quadriceps at heel-strike also improves stability and control, encouraging a smooth 'roll over' (amputees, of course, have no push-off) between midstance and heel-lift, and also helps prevent genu recurvatum.

The situation is more complicated in the AK (above-knee) amputee, but the same principles apply. Stability of the prosthetic knee is also influenced by relative length of heel and toe levers, and the joint itself can be attached more posterior (for improved stability) or anterior (for added control). The AK amputee has the added challenge of controlling a prosthetic knee unit. Those with good hip extensor strength can lock a *single-axis* knee by pulling the thigh back behind the GRV. For those with weak hip extensors, a weight-activated *stance-control* knee, which locks automatically on weight-bearing, is a better choice.

Figure 12.8 'Drop-off' in an amputee: the knee flexes suddenly and prematurely in late stance.

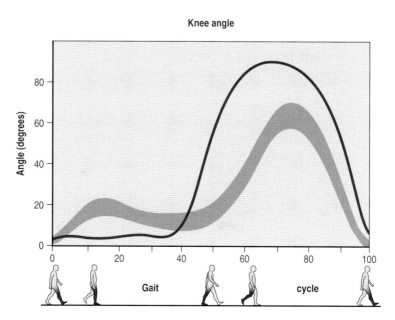

Knee angle

Angle (degrees)

Gait   cycle

Table 12.1   Effect of prosthetic alignment on support in the below-knee amputee

	Increased stability (reduced heel lever or increased toe lever)	Decreased stability (increased heel lever or reduced toe lever)
GRV with respect to knee	More anterior	More posterior
Knee moment during loading	Less extensor	More extensor
Socket translation with respect to foot	More posterior	More anterior
Ankle angle	Plantarflexed	Dorsiflexed
Socket angulation	More extended	More flexed
Activity level	Sedentary	Active
Potential problem for amputee	May have difficulty unlocking the knee for swing	'Drop off' (knee flexes too early before swing is initiated)

The dilemma facing the amputee in terms of achieving the ideal balance between support and control illustrates the challenge facing the intact locomotor system, which must also rapidly switch from maintenance of stability in single limb support to initiation of swing phase.

? MCQ 12.1

Which of these would result in a more stable prosthesis?
(a) Backward-set knee
(b) Dorsiflexed foot
(c) Anterior socket attachment
(d) Short toe lever

FRONTAL PLANE SUPPORT: TRENDELENBERG GAIT

As the swing limb is unloaded, the pelvis becomes unsupported on that side and would tend to list downwards. This would undo the clearance gained by shortening the limb, so it is prevented by a strong contraction of the contralateral hip abductors (principally *gluteus medius* and *minimus*).

In practice, the pelvis lists down by a couple of degrees, called *physiological Trendelenberg*, which is difficult to see with the naked eye. On the other hand, weakness of the hip abductors causes a much more obvious *pathological Trendelenberg* gait (Fig. 12.9), which resembles a duck waddle when viewed from behind.

Some compensation can be made for a Trendelenberg gait by leaning the trunk toward the weak side (*compensated Trendelenberg* or *Duchenne* sign). This has the effect of reducing the moment required of the hip abductors (Fig. 12.10).

The use of a walking stick or cane in the contralateral hand also helps reduce the load on the hip abductors (Brand & Crowninshield 1980, Mulley 1988, Vargo et al 1992, Neumann 1998). By unloading a proportion of body weight, the stick reduces the moment required to maintain

Figure 12.9 Trendelenberg gait. When the swing limb is unloaded there is a tendency for the pelvis to collapse on that side. To prevent this, the contralateral (stance) hip abductors contract to stabilize the pelvis. If they are weak the pelvis lists downward during swing phase, giving rise to waddling duck appearance.

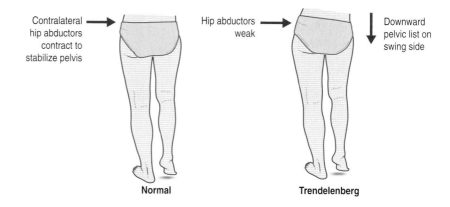

Contralateral hip abductors contract to stabilize pelvis

Hip abductors weak

Downward pelvic list on swing side

Normal　　　　　　**Trendelenberg**

pelvic stabilization (Fig. 12.11). Since less abductor muscle moment is needed, the bone-on-bone joint force through the joint is also decreased, so this strategy also ameliorates hip pain. Note, however, that the mechanism only works when the stick is held in the hand contralateral to the weak muscle or painful joint. Most people with knee pain also seem to find most relief when holding the stick in the contralateral hand, though the mechanism in this case is less clear (Vargo et al 1992).

ANTALGIC GAIT

Pain during gait usually manifests itself through compensatory (*antalgic*) strategies that the patient adopts in an effort to reduce the intensity and duration of the pain. Pain is almost invariably worse during weight-bearing, so the stance phase duration is usually shortened on the painful side, for which an asymmetrical arm swing is a useful flag. In addition, patients with hip pain will usually lean toward the affected side during stance phase. This reduces the hip abductor moment needed to support the contralateral hemipelvis, and so minimizes bone-on-bone force in the painful hip. Note that the resulting gait has a similar appearance to a compensated Trendelenberg (Duchenne) gait.

Patients with knee pain, as discussed in the previous chapter, generally adopt a quadriceps-sparing strategy, leaning forward to bring the GRV anterior to the knee in order to provide passive stabilization and so minimize knee extensor activity (Murray et al 1985). Pain over the forefoot (metatarsalgia), due to e.g. a callus, march fracture, or Morton's neuroma, inhibits push-off, and the patient will usually avoid forefoot loading by lifting the foot early and keeping the CoP posterior to the pain. It is difficult to avoid pain in the ankle, but once again muscle activity will be inhibited, with a loss of the normal rocker function.

An assessment of pain during gait can be made more objective by using a clinical scale, such as the Knee Pain Scale, which relates knee pain to activities of daily living (Rejeski et al 1995), or the Lequesne Algofunctional Index, a qualitative tool that measures pain during walking and other activities (Lequesne et al 1987).

Figure 12.10 Compensated Trendelenberg, or Duchenne sign. The trunk flexes to the contralateral side in swing (i.e. *away from* the swing side) in order to reduce the moment arm needed by the *gluteus medius.*

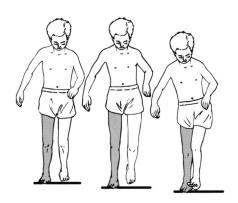

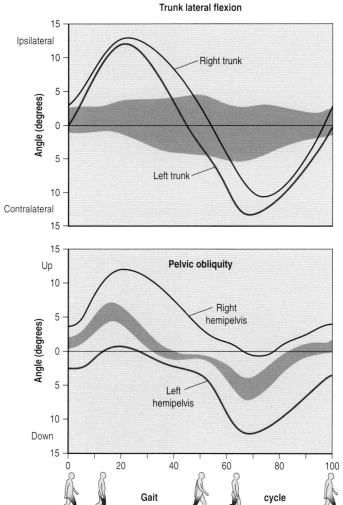

Figure 12.11   Effect of a walking stick on hip abductor force. The moment generated by the hip abductors is the product of the muscle force, M and distance to hip joint, d_M. This must equal the external moment generated by the weight of the HAT segment, W, acting at a distance d_W from the hip joint. When some force, F, is taken by the stick, the required muscle force is correspondingly reduced.

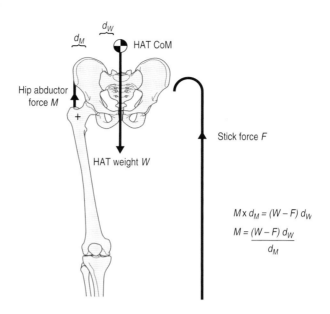

HAT CoM

Hip abductor force M

Stick force F

HAT weight W

$$M \times d_M = (W - F)\, d_W$$

$$M = \frac{(W - F)\, d_W}{d_M}$$

FRONTAL PLANE

At the knee, the ground reaction is medial, causing an external adductor moment (varus load) that compresses the medial compartment (i.e. medial *articular* centre of pressure), and is resisted by an internal abductor (valgus) moment generated by tension in the lateral collateral ligaments (Andriacchi et al 1984), reaching a peak between 40 and 50% cycle (Fig. 12.12). Not surprisingly, therefore, arthritis of the knee tends to be worse in the medial compartment, and commonly gives rise to a varus deformity (Kaufman et al 2001). Moreover, the varus load has been shown to correlate with disease severity and pain (Sharma et al 1998, Hurwitz et al 2000, 2002).

TRANSVERSE PLANE

FEMORAL ANTEVERSION

The foot can also be medially rotated during support (often called *in-toeing*, or a *pigeon toed gait*). The commonest cause of this is femoral anteversion. This is the angle that the head and neck of the femur make with the shaft, measured with respect to the frontal plane of the femur, defined by a line joining the condyles (Fig. 12.13).

At birth, the femoral neck is anteverted by 30°, resulting in an internally rotated limb. As the child walks and grows into adolescence, forces on the bone cause the angle to gradually fall to the normal adult value of 12°. If the forces are abnormal (e.g. in cerebral palsy) anteversion may persist and

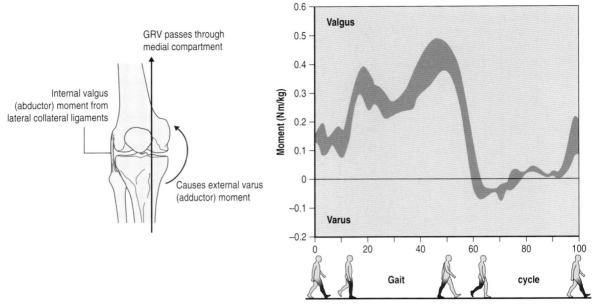

Figure 12.12 Internal frontal plane moment at the knee is valgus, indicating a varus external load through the medial compartment. The external moment is resisted by internal tension in the lateral collateral ligaments, which is what is measured by inverse dynamics in gait analysis.

results in an internally rotated foot. It is also possible (less commonly) for the angle to be decreased (retroverted), resulting in externally rotated foot.

To compensate, to bring the foot straight, the hip must be externally rotated, which can be observed in the kinematics. This in turn necessitates internal pelvic rotation on that side, giving rise to a *hip leading* gait. Note that anteversion alone cannot be detected by gait analysis because

Figure 12.13 Normal femur and femoral anteversion.

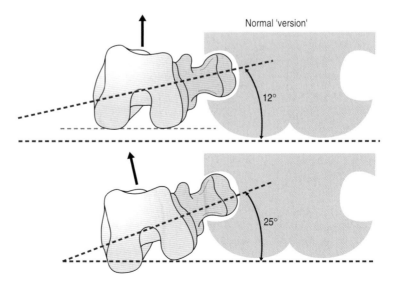

it is a bony deformity: motion analysis tracks the motion of bones, not their shape.

The foot also compensates. When it is internally rotated with respect to the line of progression, there is a tendency to supination. During swing phase there is a risk of collision with the contralateral limb, causing a trip. The usual compensation is to use the *peroneus brevis* to abduct the foot during swing.

TIBIAL (MALLEOLAR) TORSION

Tibial torsion is a twist in the tibia between condyles and malleoli. At birth there is no tibial torsion but it soon develops with weight-bearing, reaching a normal adult value of 18–25° external. Inadequate torsion results in in-toeing whereas excessive external tibial torsion is manifest as out-toeing (Stefko et al 1998). Note again that the amount of torsion cannot be seen in the gait kinematics, although it can be estimated in the static trial (as in the clinical examination) from the angle between markers on the malleoli (transmalleolar axis) compared to the knee axis.

It is worth noting that the final foot progression angle achieved should be the sum total of pelvic rotation + hip rotation + femoral anteversion + tibial torsion. Any discrepancy between the two numbers indicates error(s) in the individual measurements.

LEVER ARM DEFICIENCY

The PF-KE couple can be compromised if the foot is rotated out of the line of progression (Fig. 12.14). The normal foot progression angle is around 15° externally rotated. If the angle is increased, the lever arm of the plantarflexors in the sagittal plane is reduced, and the PF-KE couple effect impaired (Gage 1993, Liu et al 1995, Beyaert et al 2003).

Moreover, by acting laterally, the GRV places a valgus stress on both the foot and knee, which in time may result in a progressive planovalgus deformity of the foot and genu valgum of the knee. The main causes of lever arm dysfunction are talipes and other foot deformities.

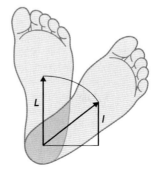

Figure 12.14 Lever arm dysfunction: the lever (moment) arm of the plantarflexors is maximum when the foot is orientated directly down the plane of progression (*L*). As the foot is externally (or internally) rotated, the lever arm is shortened (*l*), so reducing the moment generated for a given muscle force, and push-off power.

PLANTAR PRESSURE DURING SUPPORT

Calluses and ulceration occur most often at the site of maximum pressure (Stokes et al 1975), usually over the plantar surface of the metatarsal heads and on the plantar surface of the hallux (Fig. 12.15). When ulceration occurs on the side of the foot, it is most likely due to ill-fitting shoes and ischaemic pressure necrosis, and on the dorsum of the foot it is usually the result of trauma.

FORWARD PROGRESSION

Forward progression of the trunk or HAT (head-arms-trunk) segment over the leading limb also occurs during SLS. The energy required is derived from a number of sources (Fig. 12.16).

Firstly, although potential energy is at a maximum at this time (the body centre of mass is lowest), kinetic energy ($\frac{1}{2}mv^2 + \frac{1}{2}I\omega^2$) is at a maximum. This means that the velocity of the HAT is also at a maximum at this time, and hence also its momentum (mv). It thus has a tendency to progress over the new (leading) stance limb. Some of this energy (as discussed in chapter 10) comes from stored energy in the contralateral

Figure 12.15 Plantar pressure recording from a patient with diabetic neuropathy, showing areas of elevated pressure at risk for ulcer formation (Novel GmbH, Munich).

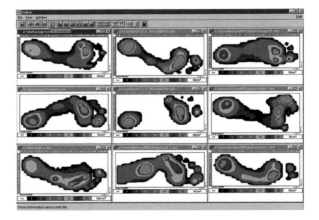

Figure 12.16 The contributors to forward progression. Push–from-behind power (H1) is generated by the hip extensors, while the *vasti* extend the knee. Meanwhile, some power is recovered from the decelerating contralateral swing limb.

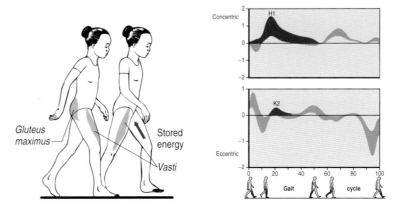

(swing) limb, which is transferred back to the trunk in late swing phase (Dillingham et al 1992).

Additional power is normally provided by the knee extensors (*vasti*) which extend the knee after it has flexed during loading response (K2). More importantly, the hip extensors (principally *gluteus maximus*) are also active during this time, generating a *push-from-behind* (H1) power burst (Winter 1991, Winter & Eng 1995).

Anything which disrupts the normal mechanism of forward progression will require the patient to compensate by increasing H1 power, and this is a very common finding in pathological gaits.

SWING-THROUGH AND SWING-TO GAIT

The normal gait pattern, in which the legs swing alternately back and forth, is not the only form of *reciprocal gait*. An alternative, *swing-through* gait is extremely important to people whose lower-limbs are paralysed as a result of, e.g. spinal cord injury or spina bifida, and to those with a healing fracture in one limb (Deathe et al 1993, Thys et al 1996). In such cases, progression is achieved by the upper-limbs through the use of crutches, which provide a shear force on the ground (Fig. 12.17).

Swing-through is effective, and can be very fast, but it is also very tiring due to the load placed on the upper-limbs. A related mechanism is also used by some patients using walking frames: *swing-to* gait, in which the feet are brought underneath the trunk rather than advanced ahead of it. In this case the frame is pushed forwards by the patient leaning on it (Fig. 12.18).

Figure 12.17 In swing-through gait, the crutch is used to apply a shear force to the ground, and pull the trunk forwards. In this case the shoulder extensors are being used for trunk progression. If paralysed, the lower-limbs are braced by KAFOs; if one leg is fractured, it is simply advanced unloaded along with the weight-bearing healthy side.

Figure 12.18 Swing-to gait with a walking frame. Progression is achieved by allowing the weight of the trunk to push the walker forwards. *Rollator* frames facilitate this action by having a wheel on the front.

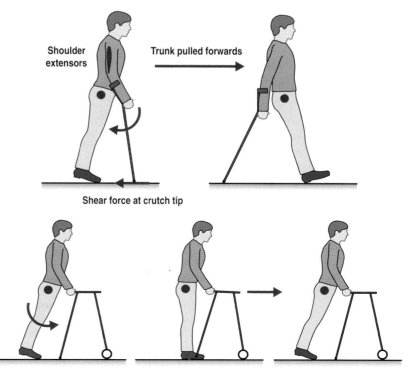

EFFECT OF SPEED

With increasing speed, there is a tendency for the trunk to progress too quickly over the stance limb. Consequently, the H2 power burst (eccentric iliopsoas), which is negligible at low speeds, gradually increases. This slows hip extension and controls the forward progression.

KEY POINTS

★ In normal gait, the plantarflexors provide a knee extensor moment during single limb support

★ Weakness of the plantarflexors tends to cause collapse of the ankle, knee and hip joints

★ Weakness of the contralateral hip abductors gives rise to a Trendelenberg gait

★ Frontal plane (internal valgus) knee moment reflects the severity of knee osteoarthritis

★ Forward progression is achieved by hip and knee extensors and energy return from the swing leg

★ In pathological gaits, walking aids facilitate support and forward progression

References

Anderson F C, Pandy M G 2003 Individual muscle contributions to support in normal walking. Gait & Posture 17(2):159–169

Andriacchi T P, Andersson G B J, Ortengren R, Mikosz R P 1984 A study of factors influencing muscle activity about the knee joint. Journal of Orthopedic Research 1:266–275

Beyaert C, Haumont T, Paysant J et al 2003 The effect of inturning of the foot on knee kinematics and kinetics in children with treated idiopathic clubfoot. Clinical Biomechanics 18(7):670–676

Brand R A, Crowninshield R D 1980 The effect of cane use on hip contact force. Clinical Orthopedics 147:181–184

Cerny K 1984 Pathomechanics of stance: clinical concepts for analysis. Physical Therapy 64:1851–1859

Deathe A B, Hayes K C, Winter D A 1993 The biomechanics of canes, crutches, and walkers. Critical Reviews in Physical and Rehabilitation Medicine 5:15–29

Dillingham T R, Lehmann J F, Price R 1992 Effect of lower limb on body propulsion. Archives of Physical Medicine and Rehabilitation 73:647–651

Gage J R 1993 Gait analysis: an essential tool in the treatment of cerebral palsy. Clinical Orthopaedics 288:126–134

Harrington E D, Lin R S, Gage J R 1984 Use of the anterior floor reaction orthosis in patients with cerebral palsy. Bulletin of Orthotics and Prosthetics 37:34–42

Hurwitz D E, Ryals A R, Block J A 2000 Knee pain and joint loading in subjects with osteoarthritis of the knee. Journal of Orthopedic Research 18(4):572–579

Hurwitz D E, Ryals A B, Case J P et al 2002 The knee adduction moment during gait in subjects with knee osteoarthritis is more closely correlated with static alignment than radiographic disease severity, toe out angle and pain. Journal of Orthopedic Research 20(1):101–107

Kaufman K R, Hughes C, Morrey B F et al 2001 Gait characteristics of patients with knee osteoarthritis. Journal of Biomechanics 34:907–915

Kepple T M, Siegel K L, Stanhope S J 1997 Relative contributions of the lower extremity joint moments to forward progression and support during stance. Gait & Posture 6:1–8

Kerrigan C, Deming L C, Molden M K 1996 Knee recurvatum in gait: a study of associated knee biomechanics. Archives of Physical Medicine and Rehabilitation 77:645–650

Kerrigan D C, Della Croce U, Marciello M, Riley P O 2000 A refined view of the determinants of gait: significance of heel rise. Archives of Physical Medicine and Rehabilitation 81:1077–1080

Lequesne M, Méry C, Samson M, Gérard P 1987 Indices of severity for osteoarthritis of the hip and knee. Scandinavian Journal of Rheumatology 65:85–89

Liu X C, Fabry G, Van Audekercke R et al 1995 The ground reaction force in the gait of intoeing children. Journal of Pediatric Orthopaedics B 4:80–85

Mulley G P 1988 Walking sticks. British Medical Journal 296:475–476

Murray M P, Gore D R, Sepic S B, Mollinger L A 1985 Antalgic maneuvers during walking in men with unilateral knee disability. Clinical Orthopedics 199:192–200

Neumann D A 1998 Hip abductor muscle activity as subjects with hip prostheses walk with different methods of using a cane. Physical Therapy 78:490–501

Pandy M G, Berme N 1988 Synthesis of human walking: a planar model for single support. Journal of Biomechanics 21:1053–1060

Rejeski W J, Ettinger W H, Shumaker S et al 1995 The evaluation of pain in patients with osteoarthritis: The knee pain scale. Journal of Rheumatology 22:1124–1129

Saltiel J 1969 A one-piece, laminated, knee locking, short leg brace. Bulletin of Orthotics and Prosthetics 23:68–75

Sharma L, Hurwitz D E, Thonar E J-M A et al 1998 Knee adduction moment, serum hyaluronan level and disease severity in medial tibiofemoral osteoarthritis. Arthritis and Rheumatism 41(7):1233–1240

Sin S W, Chow D H K, Cheng J C Y 2001 Significance of non-level walking on transtibial prosthesis fitting with particular reference to the effects of anterior-posterior alignment. Journal of Rehabilitation Research and Development 38(1):1–6

Skinner S R, Antonelli D, Perry J, Lester D K 1985 Functional demands on the stance limb in walking. Orthopedics 8:355–361

Stefko R M, de Swart R J, Dodgin D A et al 1998 Kinematic and kinetic analysis of distal derotational osteotomy of the leg in children with cerebral palsy. Journal of Pediatric Orthopedics 18(1):81–87

Stokes I A F, Farris I B, Hutton W C 1975 The neuropathic ulcer and loads on the foot in diabetic patients. Acta Orthopaedica Scandinavica 46:839–847

Thys H, Willems P A, Saels P 1996 Energy cost, mechanical work and muscular efficiency in swing-through gait with elbow crutches. Journal of Biomechanics 29(11):1473–1482

Vargo M M, Robinson L R, Nicholas J J 1992 Contralateral v. ipsilateral cane use -effects on muscles crossing the knee joint. American Journal of Physical Medicine and Rehabilitation 71:170–176

Winter D A 1991 The biomechanics and motor control of human gait: normal, elderly and pathological. University of Waterloo Press, Ontario, Canada

Winter D A, Eng P 1995 Kinetics: our window into the goals and strategies of the central nervous system. Behavioral Brain Research 67:111–120

Chapter 13

Propulsion and swing

It don't mean a thing if it ain't got that Swing!

Duke Ellington

In normal gait swing leg propulsion is generated by a combination of two concentric power bursts (Fig. 13.1):

- Ankle *push-off*
- Hip *pull-off*.

Of these, the former is most powerful, responsible for generating around 30% of the total energy generated in the gait cycle (Winter 1983). In order to swing the limb forward, there must first be sufficient *foot clearance* (Rose 1986). This requires unloading and shortening the limb, which is primarily accomplished by swing-phase knee flexion, though heel-rise of the contralateral (stance) limb also contributes (Kerrigan et al 2000a).

Somewhat surprisingly, in normal gait the toe clears the floor by only 13 mm. Moreover, the forward speed of the foot is at a maximum at this time (Fig. 13.2). This makes the achievement of clearance extremely critical if a trip is to be avoided (Winter 1992, Eng et al 1994).

Lower-limb length is most sensitive to knee angle, with flexion of approximately 60° being required to ensure clearance (Gage 1990). Knee flexion is highly dependent on the knee angular velocity at toe-off (Piazza & Delp 1996, Goldberg et al 2003), which is around 340 ± 70°/s at normal walking speeds (Fig. 13.3). Achieving sufficient knee flexion velocity is, in turn, dependent on push-off power, particularly from *gastrocnemius* activity (Gage 1991). There is also an inverse correlation between onset of heel-rise (normal = 50% cycle) and swing knee flexion, since delayed heel-rise is an indicator of impaired push-off (Kerrigan et al 1991).

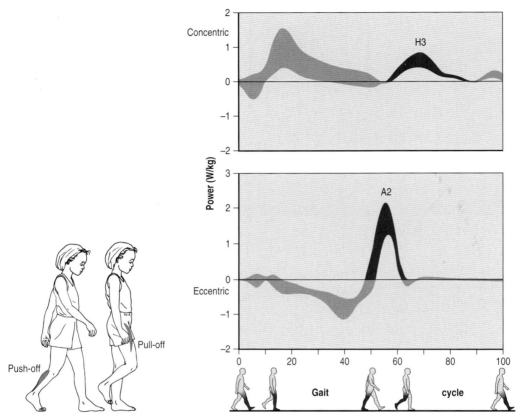

Figure 13.1 The two main contributors to swing initiation are ankle push-off (A2 power) and hip pull-off (H3 power).

As the knee flexes and lifts the foot, it is important that the foot does not drag on the floor (Fig. 13.4). This requires an adequate range of motion at the ankle and moderate dorsiflexor muscle strength so that the ankle can be held in neutral (right angle) position (0°).

As well as flaccid foot-drop caused by a lower-motor neuron lesion (e.g. peroneal neuropathy), the foot may also be held in a plantarflexed position due to spasticity (*dynamic equinus*) or tendoachilles contracture (*fixed equinus*). The usual treatment for these conditions is an Ankle Foot Orthosis (AFO), which prevents the foot from plantarflexing (Fig. 13.5). In a flaccid paralysis, a simple leaf-spring AFO is usually sufficient, whereas a spastic equinus will likely require a solid AFO, perhaps with a hinge to permit dorsiflexion.

Electrical stimulation can also be used, triggered by a footswitch under the sole of the foot (Liberson et al 1961).

Whatever the reason for clearance impairment, there are four fundamental ways that the patient can compensate (Sutherland & Davids 1993):

- Hip-hiking
- Circumduction
- Vaulting
- High-stepping (*steppage*) gait (hip hyperflexion).

Figure 13.2 The height and forward velocity of a marker placed on the 5th metatarsal head (mean ± 1 SD). During swing phase, there is only about 13 mm floor clearance at a time when the foot is travelling at maximum speed (data from Winter 1992).

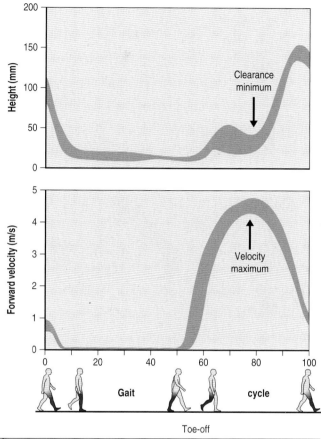

Figure 13.3 Knee angular velocity (dashed) at toe-off is a good predictor of peak swing phase knee flexion (data from Winter 1991).

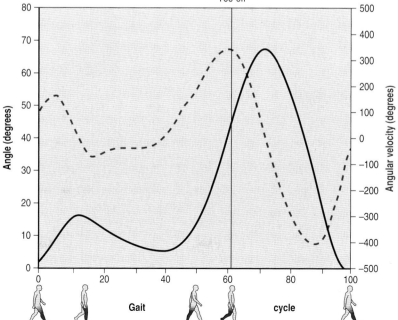

Figure 13.4 Reduced clearance caused by drop-foot.

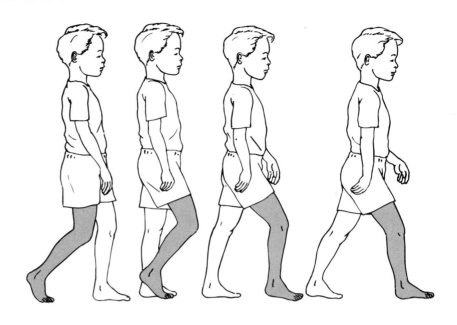

Figure 13.5 Types of AFO. The light leaf-spring is suitable for treating flaccid foot drop due to, e.g. peroneal neuropathy, whereas a solid design is needed when there is plantarflexor spasticity.

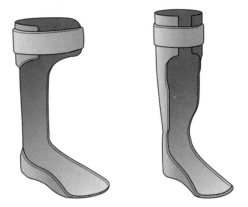

In hip-hiking, the hemipelvis on the swing side is lifted in mid-swing (principally by *quadratus lumborum*) to improve clearance (Fig. 13.6), while in circumduction, the swing hip is abducted such that the foot arcs round in a semicircle (Kerrigan et al 2000b). In vaulting, the contralateral plantarflexors are used to lift the body during early swing. Often a combination of these four methods will be used.

THE FOOT DURING PUSH–OFF

During push-off, the CoP progresses from the metatarsophalangeal joint (MTPJ) region to the hallux. In some conditions, toe amputation being a rather obvious example (Fig. 13.7), this roll-over is impaired.

Figure 13.6 Hip-hiking. The pelvis is pulled up during mid-swing to provide extra clearance. This of course means that the pelvis drops (lists downwards) on the stance side. Notice that this is the opposite of Trendelenberg gait.

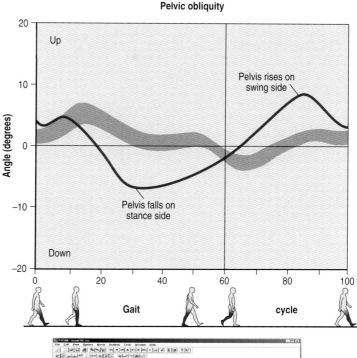

Figure 13.7 Plantar pressure study on a patient whose toes have been amputated on the right foot due to diabetic dysvascularity. Notice that not only does the CoP trajectory terminate over the MTPJ region on the amputated side, it also does so on the left. The patient has also developed a pressure ulcer under the 5th metatarsal head (reproduced by permission of Tekscan Inc., South Boston, MA, USA).

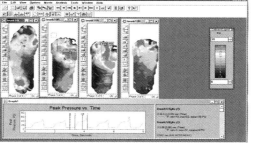

HALLUX LIMITUS

During push-off the foot needs to function as a rigid lever (Fig. 13.8). To do this, it must supinate and raise the longitudinal arch. One way that has been described is the *windlass mechanism* (Hicks 1954). Following heel-rise, the foot gradually lifts off the floor, with the toes lifting in sequence: fifth, fourth, third and second. Finally, the hallux dorsiflexes on the first metatarsal (Bojsen-Moller & Lamoreux 1979, Glasoe et al 1999).

As the first metatarsophalangeal joint dorsiflexes, it acts as a lever that winds the plantar fascia (aponeurosis) around the 'drum' of the first metatarsal head (Aquino & Payne 1999). This has the effect of shortening the distance between the hallux and the heel, so raising the arch, inverting the hindfoot, locking the mid-tarsal joint (Bojsen-Moller 1978, Roukis et al 1996, Vogler & Bojsen-Moller 2000) and externally rotating the leg (Aquino & Payne 2001). Inability of the first metatarsophalangeal joint (1MTPJ) to dorsiflex, called *hallux limitus*, prevents normal windlass function. The foot

Figure 13.8 The windlass effect: as the 1st MTPJ dorsiflexes, the plantar fascia is tightened, raising the longitudinal arch and causing the foot to convert to a rigid lever ready for push-off. While range of motion is around 42° (Nawoczenski et al 1999), the angle at which hindfoot inversion begins ranges between 4° (immediate onset) and 20° (delayed onset subgroup) and may indicate susceptibility to hyperpronation injuries (Kappel-Bargas et al 1998).

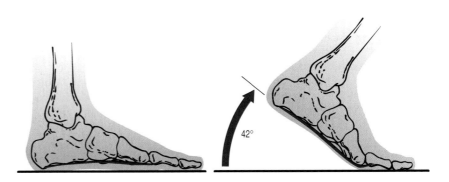

remains pronated and provides an unstable platform for push-off (Root et al 1997, Kappel-Bargess et al 1998). When flattened, the foot behaves more as a beam, with increased bending stress in the bones and ligamentous tension, whereas when converted to an arch, the bones are placed in compression with tension in the plantar fascia (Hicks 1955).

People seem to be divided into two subpopulations – an *immediate onset* group and those with a *delayed onset* windlass, in which a greater force (requiring more hallux extension) is needed to tense the plantar fascia to bring about hindfoot inversion (Clayton & Ries 1991). The relative deficiency of the windlass mechanism in this latter subtype may be more susceptible to over-use injury caused by hyperpronation (Kappel-Bargas et al 1998).

The aetiology of hallux limitus is often attributed to a hypermobile first ray (with impingement of the first metatarsal) or a severely arthritic joint (e.g. hallux valgus). Normal range of motion of the 1MTPJ is around 42° (Nawoczenski et al 1999), and progressive limitation classifies the hallux limitus according to Table 13.1.

Compensatory motions said to be associated with hallux limitus include early heel off, abductory twist, upper body sway, decreased thigh extension, internal tibial torsion, excessive pelvic tilts, circumduction, forward trunk flexion, diminished arm swing and early knee flexion (Dananberg 1993). Disorders associated with hallux rigidus include

Table 13.1 Grading of hallux limitus

Grade	Pathology
I (*functional* hallux limitus)	Less than 20° reduction in 1MTPJ dorsiflexion. Present only in weight-bearing, with little degenerative deformity. Associated with hyperpronation.
II	Bony hypertrophy and decrease in dorsiflexion even in non-weight-bearing.
III	Less than 10° 1MTPJ dorsiflexion. Further joint deterioration with arthrosis.
IV (hallux rigidus)	Loss of joint space. Bony ankylosis/fusion of 1MTPJ may occur.

shorter step length with reduced plantar flexion and power generation during push-off on the fused side (DeFrino et al 2002).

TRANSFER OF SHEAR FORCES

During push-off there is a considerable anterior shear force (equivalent to approximately 20% body weight). This force is transferred from the plantar skin through a series of septae, or lamellae, that attach via the plantar aponeurosis to the proximal phalanx (Fig. 13.9). The connective tissue is tightened as the toes dorsiflex, restraining the skin against the push-off shear force (Bojsen-Moller & Lamoreux 1979).

ANTALGIC PUSH–OFF

Peak pressures under the toes are generally reduced in rheumatoid arthritis (RA), with discrete islands of pressure appearing under the metatarsal heads, as the fat pad which normally cushions them migrates anteriorly (Soames & Carter 1981). There is also a tendency for the pressure to shift laterally to the 4th and 5th heads (Minns & Crawford 1984). This avoidance of medial weight-bearing may be an *antalgic* (pain avoidance) strategy in the presence of hallux abducto valgus deformity (common in RA), or due to failure of the normal windlass mechanism.

Figure 13.9   The skin of the ball of the foot is connected to the proximal phalanx by a series of fibrous septae, or lamellae, which tighten when the toe is dorsiflexed (Bojsen-Moller & Lamoreux 1979).

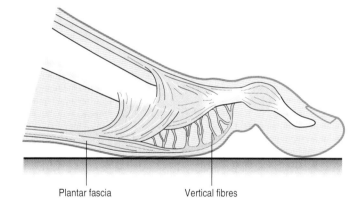

Plantar fascia   Vertical fibres

Artificial push-off

The windlass effect is emulated in a type of prosthetic foot called SAFE (Stationary Ankle Flexible Endoskeleton; Fig. 13.10). The plantar fascia is mimicked by Dacron fibres, which tighten as weight is transferred to the forefoot. This results in a smoother roll-over, but there is still no active push-off.

Figure   13.10

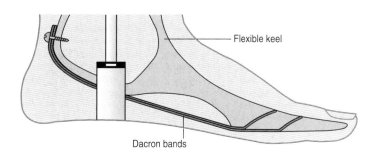

Flexible keel

Dacron bands

The large burst of power responsible for push-off is difficult to achieve in a prosthetic foot, because the plantarflexors are no longer functional. However, modern *energy-storing* feet are able to simulate it to some extent, by storing energy in a carbon fibre spring during weight-bearing in stance phase, and releasing it as the foot is unloaded for swing initiation. The peak power produced in this way can be around 15–20% of normal push-off, reducing the energy (as measured by oxygen consumption) expended by the amputee.

The use of energy-storing feet, such as the *Flex-foot*™ (Ossur, Reykjavik, Iceland; Fig. 13.11A), has been found to result in less vertical trunk motion than with conventional prosthetic feet, and they are certainly popular with amputees – particularly those who are very active. The same company also makes an energy-storing dynamic ankle foot orthosis (Fig. 13.11B).

Hafner B J, Sanders J E, Czerniecki J, Fergason J 2002 Energy storage and return prostheses: does patient perception correlate with biomechanical analysis? Clinical Biomechanics 17(5):325–344

Figure 13.11

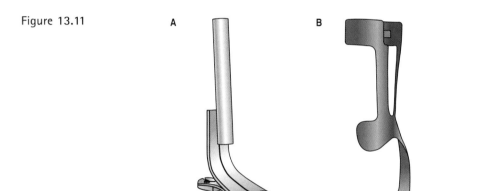

A   B

SWING TERMINATION

As the shank-foot swings forwards, the knee extends. To control this motion and prevent hyperextension (which would tend to damage the posterior capsule), the hamstrings muscles contract eccentrically (K4 power burst). At this time, energy is returned from the shank and thigh through the hip joint to the trunk (Caldwell & Forrester 1992), which aids forward progression (Fig. 13.12).

EFFECT OF SPEED

As speed or cadence increases, push-off and pull-off powers increase to throw the leg forwards more rapidly. As this occurs, there is a tendency for the heel to rise, which is controlled by the *rectus femoris* muscle, acting as a damper and transferring the energy into hip flexion (Gage 1991, Prilutsky et al 1998). Inappropriate (premature or excessive) activity of the rectus is responsible for the stiff-legged gait seen in spastic paresis

Figure 13.12 Swing of the shank-foot is terminated by the action of hamstrings, which slows (damps) knee extension. At this time a significant amount of power is returned to the trunk from the swing limb, which contributes to forward progression.

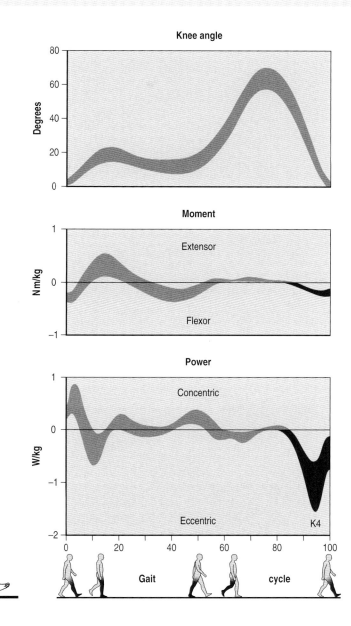

(Kerrigan et al 1991). In such patients, the rectus can be transferred to *sartorius* or *gracilis* to convert its action to a knee flexor (Gage et al 1987, Perry 1987, Nene et al 1993, Metaxiotis et al 2004), or at least reduce its knee extensor action (Riewald & Delp 1997, Asakawa et al 2002).

The hamstrings damper (K4 power) also increases with speed to control shank-foot speed in terminal swing. Premature activity often occurs in patients with spasticity (e.g. stroke, multiple sclerosis, cerebral palsy), in which the stretch reflex is overactive. Although this should aid knee flexion, in practice it often hinders it by restricting hip flexion, thereby limiting stride length (Kerrigan et al 1991, 2001).

FOOT PRE-POSITIONING

This action of hamstrings is important in lowering the forward speed of the foot (heel) ready for touchdown in a similar manner to an aircraft landing (Winter 1992, Mills & Barrett 2001). Anteroposterior heel contact velocity (A-P HCV) is an output variable with contributions from a number of kinematic variables, none of which appears to be significantly affected by age alone (Kerrigan et al 1998, Mills & Barrett 2001). Rather, it seems that the accumulation of small impairments in the control of each joint results in a rise in A-P HCV from around 1.1 m/s in young people to around 1.4 m/s in the elderly, and this may be a risk factor for slip-related falls (Gronquist et al 1989).

FRONTAL-PLANE CONTROL

For the leg to swing through, it needs to maintain a straight trajectory (Scott et al 1996). Hip adductor spasticity (common in cerebral palsy) may make the swinging limb contact the stance limb ('scissor' gait). Similarly, an internally rotated foot (as a result of femoral anteversion or internal tibial torsion) may also strike the stance limb as it swings through. Both problems will also interfere with foot pre-positioning ready for contact (Gage 1991).

Artificial swing-phase control

Perhaps the best way to understand the action of *rectus femoris* and hamstrings in swing is to examine what happens in the above-knee amputee. As the prosthesis is unloaded and swung forwards, there is a tendency for the knee to flex too much (excessive heel-rise) and then extend too quickly. In older prostheses, this was controlled by mechanical friction applied about the knee and adjusted to match the normal cadence of the opposite leg. However, the amputee was effectively limited to walking at a roughly constant cadence, with speeding up and slowing down very difficult.

Modern swing-phase hydraulic control units (e.g. the Hosmer Endurance hydraulic knee), which use silicone oil dampers, provide *cadence control*, allowing the amputee to vary walking speed. The most advanced knee units, e.g. Blatchford's *Intelligent Prosthesis* and Otto Bock's *C-leg*, now incorporate a microprocessor-controlled valve in the cylinder to enable the damping to be fine-tuned by the prosthetist while the amputee walks.

Wearing a Knee Ankle Foot Orthosis (KAFO) locks the knee in full extension, requiring compensatory hip-hiking and circumduction. An orthotic knee joint such as the Swing Phase Lock (SPL) by Basko Health Care (Netherlands) tackles the problem with a mechanism that locks and unlocks the knee depending on the angle of the knee. The device locks just prior to initial contact and unlocks at heel-off, to facilitate clearance and swing initiation.

Hicks R, Tashman S, Cary J M et al 1985 Swing phase control with knee friction in juvenile amputees. Journal of Orthopedic Research 3:198–201

KEY POINTS

★ Swing limb propulsion is normally generated by a combination of ankle push-off and hip pull-off

★ Foot clearance is facilitated by knee and hip flexion, while the ankle is returned to neutral

★ Compensations for inadequate clearance include hip-hiking, circumduction, vaulting, and steppage gait

★ Lever arm dysfunction may reduce the effectiveness of push-off

★ *Rectus femoris* and hamstrings act eccentrically to control the swing leg trajectory

★ Spasticity of these muscles commonly results in inadequate swing phase flexion and stiff knee gait

References

Aquino A, Payne C 1999 Function of the plantar fascia. The Foot 9:73–78

Aquino A, Payne C B 2001 Function of the windlass mechanism in pronated feet. Journal of the American Podiatry Medical Association 91(5):245–250

Asakawa D J, Blemker S, Gold G, Delp S L 2002 Motion of the rectus femoris after tendon transfer surgery. Journal of Biomechanics 35(8):1029–1037

Bojsen-Moller F 1978 Calcaneocuboid joint and stability of the longitudinal arch of the foot at high and low gear push-off. Journal of Anatomy 129(1):165–176

Bojsen-Moller F, Lamoreux L W 1979 Significance of free dorsiflexion of the toes in walking. Acta Orthopaedica Scandinavica 50:471–479

Caldwell G E, Forrester L W 1992 Estimates of mechanical work and energy transfers: demonstration of a rigid body power model of the recovery leg in gait. Medicine and Science in Sports and Exercise 24(12):1396–1412

Clayton M L, Ries M D 1991 Functional hallux rigidus in the rheumatoid foot. Clinical Orthopedics 271:233–238

Dananberg H J 1993 Gait style as an etiology to chronic postural pain. Part I. Functional hallux limitus. Journal of the American Podiatry Medical Association 83:433–441

DeFrino P F, Brodsky J W, Pollo F E et al 2002 First metatarsophalangeal arthrodesis: a clinical, pedobarographic and gait analysis study. Foot and Ankle International 23(6):496–502

Eng J J, Winter D A, Patla A E 1994 Strategies for recovery from a trip in early and late swing during human walking. Experimental Brain Research 102:339–349

Gage J R 1990 Surgical treatment of knee dysfunction in cerebral palsy. Clinical Orthopedics and Related Research 253:45–54

Gage J R 1991 Gait analysis and cerebral palsy. McKeith Press, Blackwell, Oxford, UK & Cambridge University Press, Boston/New York

Gage J R, Perry J, Hicks R R et al 1987 Rectus femoris transfer to improve knee function of children with cerebral palsy. Developmental Medicine and Child Neurology 29:159–166

Glasoe W M, Yack H J, Saltzman C L 1999 Anatomy and biomechanics of the first ray. Physical Therapy 79(9):854–859

Goldberg S R, Ounpuu S, Delp S L 2003 The importance of swing-phase initial conditions in stiff-knee gait. Journal of Biomechanics 36:1111–1116

Gronquist R, Roine J, Jarvinen E, Korhonen E 1989 An apparatus and a method for determining the slip resistance of shoes and floors by simulation of human foot motions. Ergonomics 32:979–995

Hicks J H 1954 The mechanics of the foot II: the plantar aponeurosis and the arch. Journal of Anatomy 88:25–31

Hicks J H 1955 The foot as a support. Acta Anatomica 25:34–45

Kappel-Bargas A, Woolf R D, Cornwall M W, McPoil T G 1998 The influence of the windlass mechanism on rearfoot motion during normal walking. Clinical Biomechanics 13:190–194

Kerrigan D C, Gronley J, Perry J 1991 Stiff-legged gait in spastic paresis: a study of quadriceps and hamstrings muscle activity. American Journal of Physical Medicine and Rehabilitation 70:294–300

Kerrigan D C, Todd M K, Della Croce U et al 1998 Biomechanical gait alterations independent of speed in the healthy elderly: evidence for specific limiting impairments. Archives of Physical Medicine and Rehabilitation 79:317–322

Kerrigan D C, Della Croce U, Marciello M, Riley P O 2000a Refined view of the determinants of gait: significance of heel rise. Archives of Physical Medicine and Rehabilitation 81:1077–1080

Kerrigan D C, Frates E P, Rogan S, Riley P O 2000b Hip hiking and circumduction: quantitative definitions. American Journal of Physical Medicine and Rehabilitation 70:247–252

Kerrigan D, Karvosky M, Riley P O 2001 Spastic paretic stiff-legged gait joint kinetics. American Journal of Physical Medicine and Rehabilitation 80:244–249

Liberson W T, Holmquest H J, Scott D, Dow A 1961 Functional electrotherapy: stimulation of the peroneal nerve synchronized with the swing phase of gait in hemiplegic patients. Archives of Physical Medicine and Rehabilitation 42:101–105

Metaxiotis D, Wolf S, Doederlein L 2004 Conversion of biarticular to monoarticular muscles as a component of multilevel surgery in spastic diplegia. Journal of Bone and Joint Surgery 86-B(1):102–109

Mills P M, Barrett R S 2001 Swing phase mechanics of healthy young and elderly men. Human Movement Science 20(4-5):427–446

Minns R J, Crawford A D 1984 Pressure under the forefoot in rheumatoid arthritis. Clinical Orthopedics 187:235–242

Nawoczenski D A, Baumhauer J F, Umberger B R 1999 Relationship between clinical measurements and motion of the first metatarsophalangeal joint during gait. Journal of Bone and Joint Surgery 81-A(3):370–376

Nene A V, Evans G A, Patrick J H 1993 Simultaneous multiple operations for spastic diplegia. Journal of Bone and Joint Surgery 75-B:488–494

Perry J 1987 Distal rectus femoral transfer. Developmental Medicine and Child Neurology 29:153–158

Piazza S J, Delp S L 1996 Influence of muscles on knee flexion during the swing phase of normal gait. Journal of Biomechanics 29:723–733

Prilutsky B I, Gregor R J, Ryan M M 1998 Coordination of two-joint rectus femoris and hamstrings during the swing phase of human walking and running. Experimental Brain Research 120:479–486

Riewald S A, Delp S L 1997 The action of the rectus femoris muscle following distal tendon transfer: does it generate knee flexion moment? Developmental Medicine and Child Neurology 39:99–105

Root M L, Orien E P, Weed J H 1977 Normal and abnormal function of the foot. Clinical Biomechanics Corporation, Los Angeles

Rose G K 1986 Orthotics: principles & practice. William Heinemann Medical Books, London.

Roukis T S, Scherer P R, Anderson C F 1996 Position of the first ray and motion of the first metatarsophalangeal joint. Journal of the American Podiatry Medical Association 86:538–546

Scott A C, Chambers C, Cain T E 1996 Adductor transfers in cerebral palsy: long-term results studied by gait analysis. Journal of Pediatric Orthopedics 16(6):741–746

Soames R W, Carter P G 1981 Barefoot walking: observations on normal and arthritic subjects. Journal of Anatomy 133:682

Stefanyshyn D J, Nigg B M 1997 Mechanical energy contribution of the metatarsophalyngeal joint to running and sprinting. Journal of Biomechanics 30(11/12):1081–1085

Sutherland D H, Davids J R 1993 Common gait abnormalities of the knee in cerebral palsy. Clinical Orthopedics and Related Research 288:139–147

Vogler H W, Bojsen-Moller F 2000 Tarsal functions, movement and stabilization mechanisms in foot, ankle and leg performance. Journal of the American Podiatry Medical Association 90:112

Winter D A 1983 Energy generation and absorption at the ankle and knee during fast, natural and slow cadences. Clinical Orthopedics and Related Research 197:147–154

Winter D A 1991 The biomechanics and motor control of human gait: normal, elderly and pathological. University of Waterloo Press, Ontario, Canada

Winter D A 1992 Foot trajectory in human gait: a precise and multifactorial motor control task. Physical Therapy 72:45–56

Chapter **14**

Observational gait analysis

I have two doctors, my left leg and my right.

George Trevelyan

OBJECTIVES

- Aware of the various methods in use for observational gait analysis
- Appreciate the reliability and accuracy limitations of various observational measures
- Know the ten pointers to making a rapid but comprehensive gait assessment in the clinic
- Aware of the common clinical terminology used in rehabilitation of gait disorders

While 3D instrumented gait analysis provides a 'gold standard' assessment of gait, observational gait analysis (OGA) is often the only form of gait assessment available in the clinical environment (Turnbull & Wall 1985, Patla et al 1987, Eastlack et al 1991, Malouin 1995). Nevertheless, many of the insights derived from biomechanical studies can be used to sharpen observation skills.

CHALLENGES OF OGA

Observation of a moving activity is difficult, because of the limited ability of the eye to discern rapid motion (the *flicker fusion rate* of the eye is about 16 Hz for most people, making it physically impossible to see events lasting less than 60 ms or so) and the complexity of many body segments moving simultaneously. Division of the cycle into sub-phases helps to focus the eye on individual tasks.

STRATEGIES

In general, diagnostic decisions in OGA fall into four categories:

1. Pattern recognition – the most rapid method, in which the movement is compared to similar gait pattern situations recalled from memory.
2. Hypothetico-deductive – in which hypotheses are generated and confirmed or refuted by further scrutiny.
3. Multiple branching – a variation of the hypothetico-deductive approach, in which a single hypothesis is generated and tested at a time. If it is rejected, a second hypothesis is generated, and so on.
4. Exhaustive – which requires a comprehensive and systematic evaluation of the motion of all body segments, and therefore tends to be more time-consuming and laborious.

In experienced practitioners, it appears that the vast majority (around 68%) of decision-making relies on pattern recognition, with some 28% using multiple branching, 3% hypothetico-deductive and very few (less than 1%) incorporating an exhaustive strategy (Jensen et al 1992, Ford et al 1995, Embrey et al 1996). Clearly, novice clinicians have less experience to draw upon for pattern recognition, and are therefore more likely to use the alternative strategies.

The chief constraints on OGA in the clinic are often time and the amount of information that can be processed, with most clinicians being typically able to consider only around six gait variables during each consultation (Goodkin & Diller 1973, Ford et al 1995). Traditional protocols for OGA (Bampton 1979, Perry 1989, 1992, Hughes & Bell 1994, Lord et al 1998) have encouraged an exhaustive approach (incorporating upwards of 30 or so variables), which is impractical for most practising clinicians. Some simplification is therefore desirable, relying on observation of discrete events and the presence or absence of typical gait deviations (Krebs et al 1985, Wade et al 1987, Fish & Nielsen 1993).

An explosion in a shingle factory

If a shadow is a two-dimensional projection of the three-dimensional world, then the three-dimensional world as we know it is the projection of the four-dimensional universe.

Marcel Duchamp

The Victorian chronographers' experiments in photographing human movement (Fig. 14.1) inspired a new generation of artists at the turn of

Figure 14.1   Photographs by Eadweard Muybridge (from the collection of the University of Pennsylvania Archives).

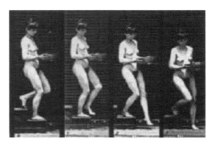

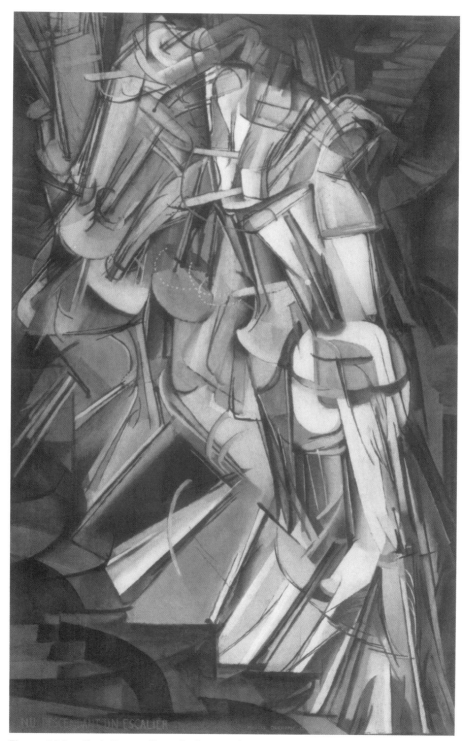

Figure 14.2 *Nude Descending a Staircase* © Succession Marcel Duchamp/ADAGP, Paris, and DACS, London 2005; reproduced with permission of the Philadelphia Museum of Art: The Louise and Walter Arensberg Collection, 1950.

the 20th century. *Nude Descending a Staircase* (Fig. 14.2) caused outrage at the New York Armory Show in 1913, with one critic calling it 'an explosion in a shingle factory', prompting the artist, Marcel Duchamp, to take it home in a taxi. Rodin was one of the original subscribers to Muybridge's book, and it inspired his famous statue, *Walking Man* (Fig. 14.3), a representation of St John the Baptist. Alberto Giacometti's gaunt version (Fig. 14.4) was a tribute to the people of Europe rising from the ashes of the Second World War. Movement was also a major concern of the Futurists, and Umberto Boccioni's bronze, *Unique Forms in the Continuity of Space*, now graces the Italian 20 Eurocent coin (Fig. 14.5) – an essential souvenir for all gait analysers; as is, of course, a video recording of John Cleese in Monty Python's *The Ministry of Silly Walks* television comedy (Fig. 14.6).

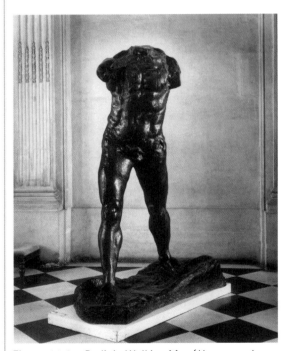

Figure 14.3 Rodin's *Walking Man* (*Homme qui marche*). S. 998, Auguste RODIN, bronze, 213.5 × 71.7 × 156.5 cm, photographed by Adam Rzepka; reproduced with permission from the Musée Rodin, Paris.

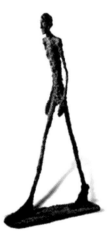

Figure 14.4 Giacometti's *Walking Man.* (© ADAGP, Paris and DACS, London 2005.)

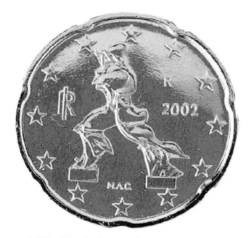

Figure 14.5   The Italian 20 Eurocent coin.

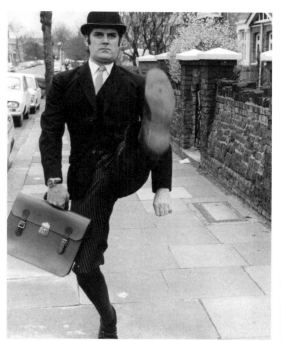

Figure 14.6   John Cleese, © BBC.

Henderson L D 1997 Marcel Duchamp's The King and Queen Surrounded by Swift Nudes (1912) and the Invisible World of Electrons. Weber Studies: An Interdisciplinary Humanities Journal 14:83–101

Given the sagittal emphasis of most observation gait protocols, it may be somewhat surprising to find that clinicians spend most (85%) of their time looking at the frontal plane (Ford et al 1995). This may simply reflect the lack of appropriate space for observation of gait available in many clinical facilities. OGA is often performed within the confined spaces of small consultation rooms or narrow corridors – conditions that are clearly inadequate for sagittal plane analysis. It may also simply reflect the greater difficulty in judging frontal plane angles (Fig. 14.7).

Videotape with slow-motion replay has been used to attempt to improve reliability (Eastlack et al 1991, Keenan & Bach 1996). The results, however, have generally been disappointing (Fig. 14.8).

CAUSE OR EFFECT?

While studying a gait it is important to try to distinguish between *primary* pathology and the *secondary* compensations made by the patient. The brain is highly adaptable and will very often learn the most appropriate bio-mechanical strategy for dealing with disruption in the normal locomotor system. It should not be surprising that the response to an abnormality generates a walking pattern that may be far from normal. Differentiating

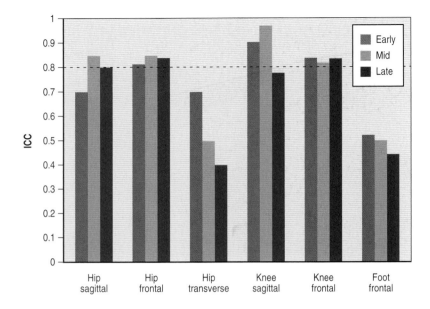

Figure 14.7 Intra-class correlation coefficient (ICC) for the inter-rater reliability of joint angles in each plane during early, mid and late stance. Values of at least 0.8 are usually regarded as indicating good reliability (data from Krebs et al 1985).

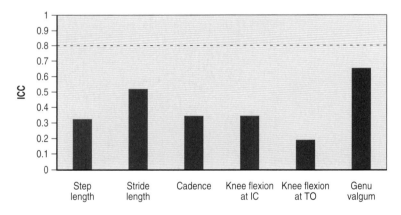

Figure 14.8 Reliability of various observational variables as assessed with slow motion video (data from Eastlack et al 1991).

between these two sources of abnormality is extremely difficult but essential if effective intervention is to occur (Moseley et al 1993).

THE TEN POINTERS

The approach to OGA described here is an attempt to build on these findings by developing a mode of assessment that is more appropriate to the clinical setting and therefore more likely to be routinely implemented. It is based on pattern recognition and multiple branching, and attempts to limit the amount of data and time needed for OGA. Ten pointers are suggested, which address the majority of gait abnormalities seen in practice, grouped around the three events and three tasks of gait (Table 14.1).

Table 14.1   Simplified OGA check sheet

Event or task	Ankle/foot	Knee	Hip/trunk
Initial contact	☐Neutral ☐Plantigrade ☐Forefoot	☐Extended ☐Flexed	
Loading response	☐Controlled plantarflexion ☐Foot slap	☐Flexion to 20° ☐Extended	
Support/progression	☐Dorsiflexion to 10° ☐Increased dorsiflexion ☐Plantarflexed	☐Extended ☐Jump knee ☐Recurvatum	☐Extension to 10° ☐Flexion ☐Trunk flexion
Toe-off	☐Plantarflexion to 20° ☐Foot supinated ☐Apropulsive ☐Contralateral step length	☐Extended ☐Flexed	
Swing	☐Clearance	☐Flexion to 60° ☐Stiff ☐Scissoring	☐Steppage ☐Trendelenberg

1. Step length asymmetry
2. Ankle at contact
3. Knee angle at contact
4. Stance phase knee flexion
5. Single-limb support
6. Ankle and foot during push-off
7. Swing phase knee flexion
8. Trunk angle
9. Frontal plane: Trendelenberg sign
10. Transverse plane: angle of patellae and feet, and arm posture.

Once the presence of these key gait deviations is detected, an assessment of the likely causes proceeds (Moseley et al 1993, Moore et al 1993).

1. STEP LENGTH ASYMMETRY

Step lengths are relatively easy to compare during successive double support phases (Fig. 14.9). Recall that stride length is equal to the sum of right and left step lengths, which should be equal. Also recall that stride length should be about 0.8 × height. There are four possible causes of a short step length (Winter 1985):

- Weak push-off
- Weak hip flexor activity in early swing
- Hyperactive hamstrings in late swing
- Limited contralateral extension.

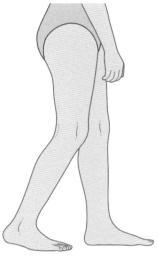

Figure 14.9   Short step length.

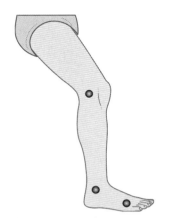

Figure 14.10   Flexed knee at contact. Note also the flat-footed contact (pseudoequinus).

? MCQ 14.1

A short right step length may indicate . . . ?
(a) Flexion contracture on the right
(b) Hyperactive hamstrings on the left
(c) Weak left hip flexors
(d) Weak right plantarflexors

2. ANKLE AT CONTACT

The ankle should be in neutral (0°) at initial contact, and the heel should touch down first. Flat-footed (Fig. 14.10) or forefoot contact is abnormal, with two possible causes:

- Drop-foot
- Flexed knee at contact (*pseudoequinus*): see pointer 4 below.

3. KNEE ANGLE AT CONTACT

The knee should normally be close to full extension at initial contact. Flexion at contact may indicate a knee flexion contracture, hamstrings spasticity or tightness due to a muscle sprain. Interestingly, the angle at contact does not seem to correlate with the popliteal angle measured on clinical examination (Õunpuu et al 1995).

4. STANCE PHASE KNEE FLEXION (LOADING RESPONSE)

The knee should flex to around 20° shortly after contact (stance phase flexion) in order to absorb the impact under eccentric control of the quadriceps (Fig. 14.11). An abnormal loading response, characterized by a fully extended knee throughout stance, is a common finding, indicating weak quadriceps and/or knee pain (Fig. 14.12). In *jump knee*, the knee is flexed at contact but then extends (Fig. 14.13).

Figure 14.11 Normal loading response. The knee is extended at contact, flexes to about 20° then extends again.

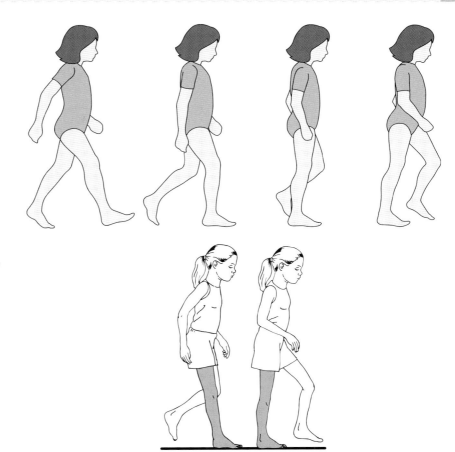

Figure 14.12 Absent loading response. The knee remains extended throughout stance.

? MCQ 14.2

What would you expect in a patient with osteoarthritis of the knee?
(a) Normal loading response
(b) Absent loading response
(c) Jump knee
(d) Flexed knee

5. SINGLE–LIMB SUPPORT

Assess how well the body is supported – does the knee collapse (e.g. *crouch* gait) or is it hyperextended (*genu recurvatum*)?

The heel should not rise before the contralateral limb swings past (around 30% gait cycle, or 50% stance). Premature heel-rise suggests some restriction of dorsiflexion due, for example, to calf spasticity and/or equinus deformity. It may also be *vaulting* – a compensation for reduced foot clearance on the contralateral side

6. ANKLE AND FOOT DURING PUSH-OFF

The ankle dorsiflexes to about 10° in late stance and then rapidly plantarflexes to about 15°. Although difficult, it is possible to make a reliable assessment of this important action (Patla et al 1997, McGinley et al 2003). The key factors to note are the total excursion of the joint (normal = 35°), and timing: to be effective the plantarflexion needs to occur while the

Figure 14.13 Jump knee: the knee is flexed at contact but then extends during stance phase.

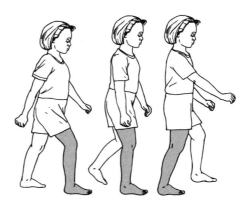

limb is still loaded (Fig. 14.14). The foot should supinate to provide firm leverage – persistent pronation results in an *apropulsive* gait.

7. SWING PHASE KNEE FLEXION

The knee should flex to around 60–70° during swing phase. Inadequate flexion indicates a failure of swing initiation in late stance. Sometimes the knee is stiff – hardly moving at all over the whole cycle (Fig. 14.15). Swing phase flexion may be excessive, indicating a *steppage* gait (Fig. 14.16).

8. TRUNK ANGLE

A forward lean of the trunk (Fig. 14.17) is a common compensation in many pathological gaits. Recall (see chapter 3) that muscle action opposes the ground reaction vector: if the vector is on the flexor side of the joint the extensors must act. Another way to look at this is to see the vector as *aiding* the muscle on the same side of the joint. So, flexing the trunk helps in two ways:

- By placing body weight ahead of the knee joint, it provides passive stability (against the posterior capsule ligaments), and relieves a weak quadriceps.
- It aids flexion of the hip (pull-off) by moving the ground reaction anterior to the hip.

Figure 14.14 Ankle push-off.

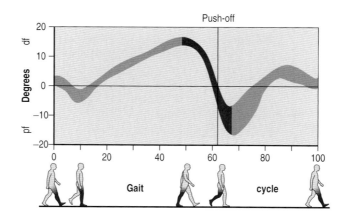

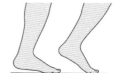

9. FRONTAL PLANE: TRENDELENBERG SIGN

Best observed from behind, this is characterized by a waddling motion, with the pelvis drooping down during swing (Fig. 14.18). It indicates contralateral hip abductor (*gluteus medius*) weakness and is a common finding in patients with e.g. hip pain, osteoarthritis, stroke and cerebral palsy.

Figure 14.15 Stiff knee gait – the knee is virtually fixed throughout. Note also the ankle equinus.

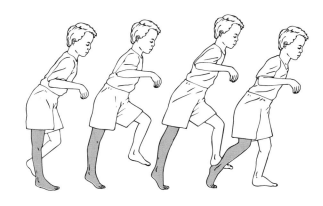

Figure 14.16 Fixed equinus. Note also the compensatory steppage gait (hip hyperflexion) to provide clearance.

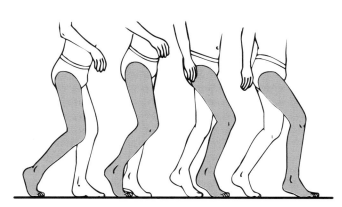

Figure 14.17 Forward trunk flexion.

A

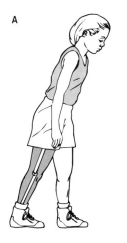

B

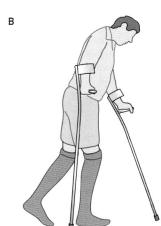

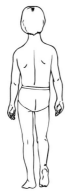

Figure 14.18 Trendelenberg gait, with pelvic list on the swing side, indicating contralateral hip abductor weakness.

Although they are both indicative of hip abductor weakness, a Trendelenberg *gait* should not be confused with a Trendelenberg *sign*, which is characterized by pelvic droop when standing on one leg, and weakness of hip abduction on side lying.

It is also important to distinguish a Trendelenberg gait from an antalgic (*coxalgic*) hip gait. Patients with hip pain often lean over the stance limb in order to reduce the bone-on-bone force across the hip. In this case the pelvis *rises* on the swing side.

The frontal plane view is also best for observing *equilibrium* (balance) – is there evidence of *ataxia* (a wide-based, staggering gait)?

Abnormalities of foot posture, such as *pes planus* or *cavus* should be noted. The angle that the rear foot makes with the floor (rear foot angle) can be estimated approximately (especially if slow-motion video is used). Maximum eversion during loading should be less than 15° (Cornwall & McPoil 2002).

10. TRANSVERSE PLANE: ANGLE OF PATELLAE AND FEET, AND ARM POSTURE

Looking from the front, observe the direction in which the patellae move. They should face forwards throughout the cycle. The feet should be turned outwards (abducted) about 15° – if they are turned in (*toeing-in* or 'pigeon-toe') this may also indicate femoral anteversion (Fig. 14.19), whereas excessive external rotation may indicate external tibial torsion. Whilst looking from the front, check also for any genu varus/valgus and hip adductor spasticity (*scissoring*).

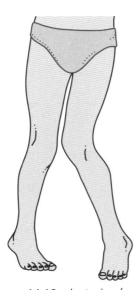

Figure 14.19 In-toeing (as indicated by the angle of the patellae and feet), characteristic of femoral anteversion and tibial torsion. Scissoring (hip adductor spasticity) is also apparent.

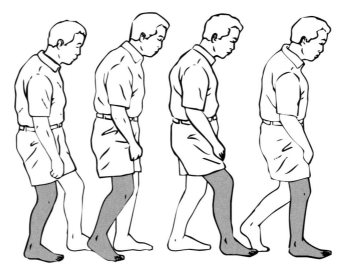

Figure 14.20 Characteristic posture in hemiplegia. The arm is motionless, held against the trunk with the fist clenched.

The upper-limbs are a good indicator of stance duration. A shortened stance time on one side suggests pain (antalgic gait). Note also the characteristic fixed, flexed posture of a hemiplegic upper-limb (Fig. 14.20), which provides a clue to problems in the ipsilateral lower-limb.

Readers should refer to the glossary for a list of common terms used to describe gait.

KEY POINTS

★ There is as yet no agreed approach to observational analysis and reliability is poor

★ Pattern recognition and multiple-branching strategies are most often used in clinical practice

★ Focus on key events (initial contact, toe-off) and functional tasks (loading, support, propulsion)

★ Try to distinguish between *primary* pathology and the *secondary* compensations

GLOSSARY

Some common clinical terms used to describe pathological gait.

Gait abnormality	Signs	Cause
Abducted gait	Hip held in abduction, leg circumducted	Clearance problem
Abductory twist	Forefoot abduction and heel adduction following heel-lift	Compensation for prolonged pronation/hallux limitus
Absent first rocker	Ankle fails to plantarflex during loading	Forefoot contact due to equinus deformity or drop foot.
Adducted	(Above-knee amputee) Lateral trunk flexion during mid-stance	Socket too flexed or posterior
Akathisia	Motor restlessness	May be side-effect of antipsychotic drugs
Akinesia	Paucity of movement	Parkinson's disease, supranuclear palsy
Antalgic	Shortened stance phase, unequal arm swing + other pain-avoiding compensations	Pain avoidance during weight-bearing
Anteversion	Excessive medial rotation of the femoral neck (normal is 20°)	Results in *in-toeing*, often compensated by ipsilateral internal pelvic rotation and external hip rotation

continued

Gait abnormality	Signs	Cause
Apraxia	Problem in sequencing and coordinating movements	Frontal lobe disorders
Apropulsive	Ineffective leverage during push-off	Inadequate supination – see *resupination*
Associated movements	Synergistic movements of the head, trunk and arms	Disruption seen in hemiparesis, spastic paresis, Parkinsonism, cerebellar ataxia
Astasia-abasia	Inability to stand and walk without support	Thalamic or midbrain stroke. May also be *psychogenic*
Ataxic	Staggering, unsteady, wide based	Cerebellar lesion or proprioceptive deficit; alcohol or drug intoxication
Athetosis, athetoid	Slow, writhing involuntary movements, often with speech problems	Extra-pyramidal cerebral palsy (e.g. kernicterus – now rare)
Atrophy	Muscle wasting	Chronic paralysis (especially lower-motor neuron) or disuse
Back knee	Loss of stance phase flexion; knee extended throughout stance (genu recurvatum)	Quadriceps weakness/knee pain
Blocq's disease/gait	See *astasia-abasia*	
Blount's tibia/disease	Bowing of the tibia resulting in a varus deformity	Dysplasia in posteromedial side of proximal epiphysis
Bow-legged	See *genu valgum*	
Calcaneal limp	Weight-bearing on the heel, increased dorsiflexion in late stance and weak push-off	*Gastrocnemius-soleus* weakness with good dorsiflexor strength
Cautious gait	See *senile gait*	
Cavovarus	See *talipes cavovarus*	
Cavus	High-arched foot	May be congenital or secondary (60%) to (dynamic) spasticity or iatrogenic (overlengthening of Achilles tendon)

Gait abnormality	Signs	Cause
Central cord syndrome	Form of paralysis in which arms are affected more than lower-limbs	Myelopathy (pressure on spinal cord) caused by cervical spondylosis (neck arthritis)
Cerebellar ataxia	Ataxia with steps of variable length and irregular rhythm (see *ataxic*)	Cerebellar tumour or stroke. Associated with intention tremor and nystagmus (no Rombergism)
Charcot's	Joint degeneration due to recurrent injury as a result of sensory loss	Diabetes, Friedreich's ataxia
Chorea, choreo-athetoid	Jerking motions	Basal ganglia degeneration (e.g. Huntington's chorea)
Chronic ankle instability	Momentary stumble with ankle inversion	May be secondary to hypermobility or tibial varum
Circumduction	Trunk and pelvic rotation	
Claudication	Calf pain on walking	Peripheral vascular disease
Claw toes	Dorsiflexed (extended) metatarsophalangeal joints with flexion of distal phalanges	Paralysis of intrinsic foot muscles; foot is stiff, with poor push-off
Clonus	Rhythmic contraction of a muscle in response to a sudden stretch	Spastic paralysis, especially of the ankle plantarflexors
Club foot	See *talipes*	
Compensated *gluteus medius*	Listing of the trunk toward the affected side at each step	*Gluteus medius* weakness
Compensated Trendelenberg	See *Duchenne*	
Coping response	Gait abnormality which is a secondary compensation for another problem	For example, circumduction, vaulting or hip-hiking to compensate for reduced clearance
Coxalgic	Trunk flexion and downward pelvic list to side of painful hip during stance (opposite of Trendelenberg)	Compensation to reduce bone-on-bone force generated by the hip abductors in a painful hip
Coxa vara	See *developmental dysplasia of the hip*	
Crepitus	Sound of bone rubbing on bone	Cartilage degradation, osteoarthritis (OA)

continued

Gait abnormality	Signs	Cause
Crouch gait	Dorsiflexed ankle with flexed knee and hip	Characteristic of diplegic cerebral palsy
DDH	See *developmental dysplasia of the hip*	
Delayed heel-rise	Delay in transferring weight to forefoot; normal heel-rise occurs around 44% cycle	Plantarflexor weakness. In the amputee, a sign of a posterior set foot, hip flexion contracture, or soft keel
Developmental dysplasia of the hip (DDH)	Formerly known as congenital dislocation of the hip (CDH), including acetabular dysplasia, subluxation and dislocation	Early (congenital) or late (after 6 months of age). Present in 2/1000 live births; associated with *metatarsus adductus* and *torticollis*
Diplegia, diplegic	Gait characterized by bilateral lower-limb spasticity, often with crouch gait and scissoring	Type of cerebral palsy characterized by weakness of legs and arms
Dorsal exostosis	Bony enlargement on dorsum or of 1st metatarsophalangeal joint	Similar to bunions without deviation of the hallux
Double bump	Pattern of pelvic kinematics with two periods of anterior tilt	Spastic *rectus femoris* pulls pelvis into anterior tilt
Double step	Length and/or timing of alternate strides is noticeably different	Hysterical conversion, malingering
Double tap	Noise heard as first heel then forefoot slaps floor	Proprioceptive disturbance – ataxia, sensory neuropathy
Drag-to	Feet are dragged (rather than lifted) toward the crutches	
Drop attack	Sudden fall without warning and without loss of consciousness, usually in elderly. Patient usually buckles at the knees and falls forwards	Transient ischaemic attacks, proximal weakness (e.g. quadriceps), neurodegenerative diseases (e.g. Parkinsonism), Ménière's disease. Most idiopathic
Drop-foot	Plantarflexion of foot during swing with reduced clearance	Dorsiflexor weakness due to peroneal neuropathy or plantarflexor spasticity
Drop-off	Hesitation and sudden drop of trunk during terminal stance in above-knee amputee	Knee instability caused by inadequate knee friction, anterior set knee, etc.
Duchenne	Trunk leans toward stance side	Compensated *Trendelenberg gait* (hip abductor weakness)
Duncan-Ely test	Knee rapidly flexed while patient is prone	Resistance to flexion suggests *rectus femoris* (but not *iliopsoas*) spasticity

Gait abnormality	Signs	Cause
Dysequilibrium	Unsteady gait with lengthened stance phase and step length	Balance problem (e.g. ataxia, vestibular disorder, frailty)
Dystrophic	See *myopathic*	
Early heel-rise	See *premature heel-rise*	
Egyptian foot	Hallux longer than 2nd toe (no clinical significance)	Present in 74% of people (cf. *Greek, squared foot*)
En bloc	Body turns as a whole (head remains in line with the body)	Parkinson's disease
Equilibrium reactions	Ability to maintain balance	
Equinovarus	See *talipes equinovarus*	
Equinus	Plantarflexed foot, causing a tip-toe gait with forefoot contact rather than a heel-strike	Plantarflexor spasticity with (static equinus) or without (dynamic) tendoachilles contracture
Erythema	Redness over joint	Inflammatory arthritis, sepsis, gout
Excessive heel-rise	Heel-rise in an AK amputee	Inadequate knee friction, extension assist too weak
Extensor synergy	Simultaneous ankle plantarflexion, knee and hip extension and hip adduction	Upper motor neuron lesion (e.g. stroke, cerebral palsy)
Fasciculations	Fine twitch of muscle	Denervation (e.g. motor neuron disease, post-polio syndrome)
Femoral anteversion	See *anteversion*	
Femoral retroversion	See *retroversion*	
Festinating	Gait characterized by short steps of rapid cadence, giving the appearance of falling forwards	Parkinson's disease. Also seen in phenothiazine, carbon monoxide and manganese poisoning
Flail foot	Floppy ankle (sagittal plane and coronal plane instability)	Flaccid (lower motor neuron) paralysis, e.g. spina bifida, poliomyelitis, peroneal muscle atrophy, Charcot–Marie–Tooth

continued

Gait abnormality	Signs	Cause
Flat foot contact	Contact with heel and forefoot	Calf spasticity
Flessum	See *genu recurvatum*	
Flexed knee	Inadequate knee extension	Knee flexion contracture (e.g. polio), weak plantarflexors, prolonged hamstrings activity preventing knee extension
Flexor synergy	Simultaneous flexion of hip, knee and ankle dorsiflexion	Upper motor neuron lesion (e.g. stroke, cerebral palsy)
Foot-drag	Dragging of foot during swing	Foot-drop or equinus
Foot-drop	See *drop-foot*	
Foot pain		Midstance pain indicates corns, calluses, fallen transverse arch, rigid pes planus, subtalar arthritis; push-off, metatarsalgia
Foot progression	Angle made by foot with plane of progression	Normal is around 15° external. See *in-toeing, toeing out*
Foot slap	Sudden, often audible plantarflexion of foot at contact	Weak dorsiflexors, heel cushion too soft in amputee
Forefoot abduction	Forefoot deviates laterally	May compensate for the in-toeing caused by femoral anteversion
Forefoot contact	Initial contact with the toes or forefoot	Equinus or drop-foot
Forefoot valgus	Forefoot everted relative to the rearfoot. Requires subtalar inversion to make foot plantigrade	Congenital deformity, perhaps due to abnormal forces *in utero*
Forefoot varus	Forefoot inverted relative to the rearfoot. Requires subtalar eversion to make foot plantigrade	Congenital deformity, perhaps due to abnormal forces *in utero*
Forward power	Total muscle activity responsible for forward progression	Ankle plantarflexors, hip flexors and extensors + knee extensors
Four-point	Reciprocating gait with two crutches or other walking aid (left crutch, right foot, right crutch, left foot, etc.)	Slow, but safe, and requires less energy than swing-through gait
Freezing	See *ignition failure*	Parkinson's, often precipitated by stress
Frontal ataxia	See *apraxia*	
Frontal gait disorder	Stiff upright stance, difficulty initiating gait, short steps and exaggerated arm movements, with freezing episodes but no rest tremor or bradykinesia	Arteriosclerotic Parkinsonism (Binswanger's disease)

Gait abnormality	Signs	Cause
Functional hallux limitus	See *hallux limitus*	
Genu recurvatum	Knee hyperextension during stance	Weak quadriceps, plantarflexion contracture (excessive plantarflexor–knee extensor couple)
Genu valgum (valgus)	Abduction deformity of the knee	Common in chronic rheumatoid arthritis. Note that there is a physiological genu valgum of about 3°, so 10° of valgus implies 7° of deformity
Genu varum (varus)	Adduction deformity of the knee	Note that there is a physiological genu valgum of about 3°, so 6° of varus implies 9° of deformity. About 70% of body weight passes through medial knee compartment in single support, increasing to 90% with a 4–6° varus (Hsu et al 1990)
Gluteal	See *Trendelenberg*	
Gluteus maximus lurch	Shoulders and head thrown backwards during stance phase on affected side	Weak hip extensors (rare)
Gluteus medius	See *Trendelenberg*	
Greek foot	Hallux shorter than 2nd toe (no clinical significance)	Present in 18% of the population (cf. *Egyptian, squared* foot)
Haglund's deformity	Bump on the back of the heel	Irritation from repeated trauma to calcaneus from, e.g. shoes, rear foot varus

continued

Gait abnormality	Signs	Cause
Hallux limitus	Restricted dorsiflexion of the first metatarsophalangeal joint during push-off (normal is about 70°). A *functional hallux limitus* is present only when weight-bearing	Associated with hyperpronation and apropulsive gait
Hallux rigidus	Severe form of hallux limitus with less than 5° of hallux dorsiflexion	Osteoarthritis
Hallux (abducto) valgus	Bunion deformity of 1st metatarsophalangeal joint	Unknown, though hyperpronation and high-heeled footwear have been postulated as a cause
Hammer toe	Flexible or rigid flexion deformity of proximal interphalangeal joint	Thought to be related to footwear. Common in flat feet and rheumatoid arthritis
Heel-rise	Earlier than 30% cycle. Normal = 44%. See also *early heel-rise*	
Heel-strike pain	Pain on heel-strike	Plantar fasciitis/bursitis
Heel-toe	Normal gait, with heel-strike and toe-off. See *forefoot contact*	Normal, healthy gait
Helicopod	Feet describe semi-circles	Hysterical conversion
Hemiballismus	Sudden violent jerking	Basal ganglia disorder (rare)
Hemiplegic	Unilateral equinovarus and extended hip and knee, shoulder abduction and internal rotation, forearm pronation and wrist and finger flexion, with reduced arm swing. Usually with circumduction and forward trunk flexion	Stroke, cerebral palsy or other contralateral upper motor neuron lesion, with extensor spasticity, pelvic retraction
High-level gait disorder	See *senile gait*	
High-stepping	See *steppage*	
Hip dysplasia	See *developmental dysplasia of the hip*	
Hip extensor gait	See *gluteus maximus lurch*	
Hip flexion deformity	Contracture of the *iliopsoas* muscle/ tendon revealed by inadequate stance hip extension	May be primary (due to spasticity) or secondary (to prolonged sitting)

In the Hallux limitus row, an illustration of a foot shows a curved arrow and the label **70°**.

Gait abnormality	Signs	Cause
Hip-hiking	Ipsilateral elevation of the iliac crest by *quadratus lumborum*	Compensation to increase clearance
Hip-leading	Transverse rotation of the pelvis (internal on the affected side)	Compensation for femoral anteversion
Hitching	See *hip-hiking*	
Hollow foot	See *claw toes*	
Hyperpronation	See *pronated*	
Hypertrophy	Increased muscle girth	Secondary to increased usage
Hypokinesia	See *akinesia*	
Hysterical gait	Bizarre gait pattern not due to a physical cause, e.g. helicopod or stuttering, intermittent double-step gait	Hysterical conversion neurosis
Ignition failure	Inability to initiate locomotion	Parkinsonism, frontal lobe lesions
Iliotibial band syndrome	Lateral knee pain relieved by stiff knee gait	Overuse injury casued by friction over lateral femoral condyle
Intermittent claudication	See *claudication*	
In-toeing	Foot appears turned in (adducted)	Bony torsion deformity (femoral anteversion, tibial torsion)
Jump knee	Knee flexion at contact followed by rapid extension (giving appearance of jumping)	Characteristic of diplegic cerebral palsy
Knee snap	Sudden and delayed knee flexion at toe-off in above-knee amputee	Over-stable prosthetic knee joint
Knock-knee	See *genu varum*	
Kyphosis	Increased thoracic curvature	Type 1 (Sheuermann's disease) Type 2 (thoracolumbar)

continued

Gait abnormality	Signs	Cause
Lateral thrust	Outward motion of the knee immediately after initial contact	Late complication of osteoarthritis, genu varum, anterior cruciate ligament (ACL) deficiency or meniscectomy
Lateral tibial torsion	See *tibial torsion*	
Lateropulsion	Sensation of being pushed to the side, sometimes causing a fall	Wallenberg's syndrome (lateral medullary stroke)
Leg length discrepancy (LLD) Real Apparent	Shortening of one lower-limb. Can be *real (true)* or *apparent* (due to pelvic obliquity or hip instability). Discrepancies less than 2 cm are usually regarded as being normal. Can cause pain and functional scoliosis if not treated. Measure from anterior superior iliac spine to medial malleolus	Congenital coxa vara, fractures (esp. growth plate injury), hemiatrophy, hemihypertrophy, hemimelias, bone dysplasia, vascular, scoliosis, neurological, Wilms' tumour (excluded by kidney ultrasound)
Legg–Calve–Perthes disease	See *Perthes disease*	
Lever arm dysfunction	Over-abduction of the foot (externally rotated foot progression angle) causing impaired push-off	Bony torsion (femoral anteversion, tibial torsion) and/or foot deformities
Line of progression	Line between the footsteps in the direction of travel	
Lordosis	Increased lumbar curvature	Increased in pregnancy and obesity; decreased with lumbar spondylosis
Magnetic gait	Hesitation and shuffling on the spot	Parkinson's disease
March fracture	Metatarsal stress fracture	Repetitive strain injury
Marche à petit pas	See *festinating*	
Mass movement	Spasticity at more than one joint, e.g. *extensor synergy, flexor synergy*	Upper motor neuron lesion (e.g. stroke, cerebral palsy)
Maximus gait	See *gluteus maximus*	
Medial tibial torsion	See *tibial torsion*	
Metatarsal break	Shoe crease indicating metatarsophalangeal joint functioing	Important in supination and windlass function
Metatarsalgia	Pain over the forefoot	Morton's neuroma, march fracture
Metatarsus adductovarus	Adduction and inversion at Lisfranc's joint	Forefoot component of *talipes equinovarus*

Gait abnormality	Signs	Cause
Metatarsus adductus	Medial deviation of the forefoot. Common (1/1000 live births) congenital foot deformity	Intrauterine positioning. Flexible types generally resolve spontaneously. Surgery needed for inflexible types. May be sign of *developmental dysplasia of the hip*
Metatarsus primus elevatus	1st metatarsal dorsiflexed compared to the others	
Metatarsus primus varus	Oblique 1st metatarsal	Thought to casue juvenile hallux valgus in girls
Metatarsus varus	See *metatarsus adductus*	
Midfoot break	Subtalar joint pronation compensating for limitation in dorsiflexion	Equinus deformity
Military gait	Short steps and exaggerated arm movement	Parkinsonism
Morton's foot	Short 1st metatarsal with overpronation	
Mycoclonus	Sudden shock-like muscle contraction (positive myoclonus) or inhibition of a contraction (negative myoclonus)	Multiple sclerosis, brainstem strokes
Myopathic	Exaggerated waddling of alternating lateral trunk flexion. See *Duchenne*	Bilateral hip abductor weakness characteristic of proximal myopathy, e.g. muscular dystrophy, spinal muscular atrophy
Neck hyperextension		Akinetic-rigid syndromes, e.g. progressive supranuclear palsy
Osgood–Schlatter disease	Pain and oedema over tibial tubercle in adolescents	Benign, self-limiting traction apophysitis
Out-toeing	See *toeing out*	
Paraplegic/paraparetic gait	Bilateral stiff knees, hip flexion and ankle equinus, usually with circumduction and foot-drag	Spinal cord injury, transverse myelitis
Patella alta	Abnormally elevated patella	Associated with chondromalacia patellae and knee flexion contractures in cerebral palsy

continued

Gait abnormality	Signs	Cause
Patella baja/infera	Abnormally low patella	Associated with *Osgood–Schlatter disease* and ruptured quadriceps tendon
Patterned walking	*Mass movement*, in which the ankle, knee and hip joints move simultaneously in either flexion or extension	Upper motor neuron lesion (e.g. stroke, cerebral palsy)
Perthes disease	Hip pain with coxalgic gait in adolescent	Idiopathic avascular necrosis of femoral head
Pes cavus	See *cavus*	
Pes planus	Flat foot	
Pes valgus	Eversion deformity of foot	Common in spastic diplegia
Pes varus	Inversion deformity of foot	Common in spastic hemiplegia
Phelps test	Hip abducted and knee flexed then extended	Hip adduction suggests *gracilis* (but not other adductor) spasticity
Pistoning	Stump moves inside prosthetic socket during swing phase	Ineffective socket suspension
Planovalgus/varus	Flat foot with valgus or varus deformity	
Plantigrade	Foot flat	
Point gait	At least one foot and one crutch on ground at any given time. See *two-point, three-point, four-point*	
Popliteal angle	Maximum knee extension angle (normally full extension)	Reduced due to hamstrings spasticity
Postural reflexes	Tested by gently pushing the patient backwards or forwards	Impaired in sensory ataxia
Premature heel-rise	Lift-off of heel before 50% stance (30% cycle)	Limitation of dorsiflexion, calf spasticity, equinus deformity, *vaulting* for reduced clearance
Pronated	Flat flexible foot	
Propulsive	See *festinating*	
Protraction	Internal rotation, esp. of shoulder	
Psychogenic gait disorder	Bizarre staggering gait with jerking and thrashing of the arms. See also *astasia-abasia*	Hysterical conversion neurosis, in which psychological problems are somatized into physical symptoms (rare)
Pump bump	See *Haglund's deformity*	

Gait abnormality	Signs	Cause
Puppet-on-a-string	Irregular dancing gait	Huntington's chorea
Push-off	Time between heel-lift and toe-off	Plantarflexor power generation for swing leg propulsion
Push-off pain	Sharp pain on push-off	Corns between toes, metatarsal callosities, metatarsalgia, hallux problems
Q-angle	Angle between line drawn from ASIS to central patella and line from central patella to tibial tubercle	Normal = 14° in males, 17° in females. Increased in femoral anteversion, genu valgum, external tibial torsion, weak *vastus medialis*
Quadriceps-sparing	Lack of knee flexion during loading, trunk tends to lurch forward	Quadriceps weakness
Quadriplegia, quadriplegic	Spastic disorder involving all four limbs	Type of cerebral palsy
Rearfoot angle	Angle between the calcaneus and midline of the calf	Maximum normal eversion is around 8–15° during loading
Rearfoot valgus	Subtalar eversion	Puts stress on medial side of the ankle complex
Rearfoot varus	Subtalar inversion	Associated with tibial varum and recurrent ankle sprain
Reciprocating	Gait in which the legs are swung forwards alternately	
Recurvatum	See *genu recurvatum*	
Reel foot	See *talipes*	
Resupination	Delayed supination, with medial roll-off during push-off	
Retraction	External rotation, esp. pelvis	Common in hemiplegia
Retrocalcaneal bursitis	See *Haglund's deformity*	
Retroversion	Backward deviation of femoral neck	Acetabulum faces posteriorly
Roll-over	See *push-off*	
Rombergism	Instability when eyes are closed	See *spinal ataxia*
Rotation of foot at heel-strike	Amputee problem	Prosthetic heel cushion too hard
Scissoring	Adduction of a leg such that it crosses in front of the other	Adductor spasticity, esp. diplegic cerebral palsy

continued

Gait abnormality	Signs	Cause
Scoliosis	Twisting deformity of the spine, characterized by a rib hump and pelvic obliquity	Early (before 5 years) and late (after 5 years) onset. May be idiopathic or secondary to a neuropathic or myopathy cause
Secondary abnormality	See *coping response*	
Senile gait	Unsteady, cautious gait, with 'walking on ice' appearance. Patient frequently reaches out for furniture or other objects for support	Seen in the elderly as compensation for arthritis or frequent previous falls
Sensory ataxia	Slow and deliberate steps, slapping or steppage (especially in the dark), Rombergism	Sensory loss due to peripheral neuropathy, tabes dorsalis
Short leg gait	Head bobs down during stance phase of the short leg	Leg length discrepancy
Shuffling	See *festinating*	
Silverskiöld test	Knee is flexed to 90° then extended while foot is held in dorsiflexion and varus	Plantarflexion on knee extension suggests *gastrocnemius* (but not *soleus*) spasticity
Slipped upper femoral epyphysis	Proximal femoral epiphysis separates from the femur	Idiopathic
Slipping clutch phenomenon	See *magnetic gait*	
Snapping hip	Click felt over lateral hip	See *Iliotibial band syndrome*
Space phobia	Patient walks timidly around the periphery of the room	See *senile gait*
Spastic diplegia	See *diplegia*	
Spastic gait	Stiff, foot-dragging gait	Stroke, cerebral palsy, multiple sclerosis
Spinal ataxia	Ataxia caused by proprioceptive deficit (see *ataxic*)	Lesions in dorsal tracts: tabes dorsalis, B vitamin deficiencies
Spinal stenosis	Forward flexed wide-based gait with leg pain/parasthesia, especially walking downhill	Narrowing of spinal canal due to degenerative changes

Gait abnormality	Signs	Cause
Spring foot	See premature heel-rise	
Squared foot	Hallux and 2nd toe equal length (no clinical significance)	Present in 8% of people (cf. *Egyptian*, *Greek*)
Steppage	Increased hip and knee flexion to compensate for reduced clearance	Dorsiflexor weakness (peroneal neuropathy, multiple sclerosis, cauda equina lesions), or plantarflexor spasticity (due to stroke, cerebral palsy and other upper motor neuron lesions)
Stiff-knee	Inadequate knee flexion in swing phase	Intense and prolonged rectus action or compensation for knee pain
Stuttering	Hesitancy or stuttering	Hysterical conversion, schizophrenia, head injury
Subcortical dysequilibrium	See *astasia-abasia*	
Substitutive recurvatum	Progressive decrease in plantarflexion during late stance	
Supinated	High-arched, rigid foot	
Swaying	See *cerebellar ataxia*	
Swing-through	Crutches are advanced and then the legs are swung past them	
Swing-to	Crutches are advanced and the legs are swung to the same point	
Tabetic	Ataxic, high-stepping gait	Characteristic of tabes dorsalis
Talipes calcaneocavus	Deformity in which foot is dorsiflexed with a high arch	
Talipes calcaneovalgus	Deformity in which heel is turned out and foot is dorsiflexed	

continued

Gait abnormality	Signs	Cause
Talipes cavovarus	High-arched foot with heel turned in	Typical deformity of peripheral neuropathies such as Charcot–Marie–Tooth disease
Talipes cavus	See *cavus*	
Talipes equinovalgus	Heel turned out (valgus) and the foot plantarflexed (equinus). Often seen in spastic diplegia	Spastic peroneals (esp. brevis), ligamentous laxity and contracted tendoachilles
Talipes equinovarus	Typical clubfoot deformity, in which the heel is turned in (varus) and the foot plantarflexed (equinus). Associated with supination, adduction, and a high arch (cavus)	Spasticity of *tibialis posterior* ± *anterior*
Talipes equinus	See *equinus*	
Talipes planovalgus	See *talipes valgus*	
Talipes valgus	Heel turned outward, resulting in a lowering of the longitudinal arch	May be congenital or spasmodic as a result of peroneal spasticity

Gait abnormality	Signs	Cause
Talipes varus	Heel turned in	*Tibialis posterior* spasticity
Tandem walk	Request patient to walk heel-to-toe along a straight line	Tests of lateral stability (impaired in cerebellar ataxia)
Three-point	Use of a crutch or other walking aid (first both crutches with weaker leg, then stronger one, etc.)	Unloads affected leg – useful for fractures, amputations or pain. Requires good balance and coordination
Tibial torsion	Rotational deformity of tibia, usually internal rotation. Associated with genu varum	External torsion often a compensation for femoral anteversion. 90% correct in first year. Surgery may be needed
Tibial valga/valgum	Lateral curvature of tibial shaft in the frontal plane	
Tibial vara/varum	Lateral bowing of tibia ('bandy legs'). See also *Blount's tibia*	Usually bilateral, cf. *genu varum*
Titubation	Head tremor	Cerebellar ataxia, Parkinsonism
Toe-drag	See *foot-drag*	
Toe-rise test	Ability to stand on tip-toes	Demonstrates plantarflexor strength/ weakness
Toe-walking	Walking on a plantarflexed ankle, with forefoot contact	May be idiopathic or due to plantarflexor spasticity/equinus
Toeing in	See *in-toeing*	
Toeing out		Pes valgus, talipes calcaneovalgus, congenital planovalgus, lateral tibial torsion
Too many malleoli sign	Medial prominence of talonavicular joint giving the appearance of a second medial malleolus just below the actual one	Excessive pronation

continued

Gait abnormality	Signs	Cause
Too many toes sign	More than two toes lateral to the heel visible, as seen from behind	Excessive forefoot abduction, hyperpronation
Torsional deformity	Twist in long bone	Abnormal forces during growth
Torsion dystonia	Focal dystonia, with twisting movements of an arm or leg	Inherited, begins in childhood and results in severe disability
Torsional malalignment	Abnormal joint axis direction	Torsional deformity
Torticollis	Focal dystonia, with head twisted to one side	May be congenital or acquired, due to shortening of the sternocleidomastoid muscle
Trendelenberg gait	Pelvic droop in midswing	Contralateral hip abductor weakness
Trendelenberg lurch	See *Duchenne*	
Triplegia	Spastic disorder involving three limbs, usually arms and one leg	Type of cerebral palsy (rare)
Tripod gait	See *drag-to*	
Trunk flexion	Forward lean of the trunk	Compensation for weak knee extensors: ground reaction provides a passive extensor moment
Two-point	Right foot and left crutch (or cane) advanced together, and then left foot and right crutch	Provides stability. Faster than 4-point gait. Reduces weight bearing bilaterally. Useful for bilateral weakness or poor coordination (e.g. ataxia)
Uncompensated *gluteus medius*	Pelvis on the opposite side dips (cf. *compensated gluteus medius*)	Moderate weakness of the *gluteus medius* muscle
Unequal arm swing	See *antalgic*	
Unequal cadence	See *antalgic*	
Vaulting	Contralateral plantarflexion to compensate for reduced clearance	
Vertical talus	Rigid rockerbottom flat foot causing painful apropulsive gait	Congenital (uncommon)
Vestibular ataxia	*Dysequilibrium* with staggering towards the affected side	Labyrinthine lesions (Ménière's disease, acoustic neuroma)
Waddling	See *Trendelenberg*	
Walking on ice	See *senile gait*	
Whip	Sudden medial or lateral motion of foot just before contact in transfemoral amputee	Malrotation of prosthetic knee joint axis

Gait abnormality	Signs	Cause
Wide-based	Increased base of support	Dysequilibrium, ataxia, outset foot in amputee
Windswept hips	Abduction of one hip with contralateral adduction contracture	Complication of *developmental dysplasia of the hip*
Wry neck	See *torticollis*	

References

Bampton S 1979 A guide to the visual examination of pathological gait. Temple University Rehabilitation Research and Training Center, Moss Rehabilitation Hospital, Philadelphia

Cornwall M W, McPoil T G 2002 Motion of the calcaneus, navicular, and first metatarsal during the stance phase of walking. Journal of the American Podiatry Medical Association 92(2):67–76

Eastlack M, Arvidson J, Snyder-Mackler L et al 1991 Interrater reliability of videotaped observational gait analysis assessments. Physical Therapy 71(6):465–472

Embrey D G, Guthrie M R, White O R, Dietz J 1996 Clinical decision making by experienced and inexperienced pediatric physical therapists for children with diplegic cerebral palsy. Physical Therapy 76:20–33

Fish D J, Nielsen J-P 1993 Clinical assessment of human gait. Journal of Prosthetics and Orthotics 5(2):39–48

Ford N, Poole B, Bach T 1995 Interobserver reliability of observational gait analysis in transtibial prosthesis alignment. Prosthetics and Orthotics Australia 11(1):27–31

Goodkin R, Diller L 1973 Reliability among physical therapists in diagnosis and treatment of gait deviations in hemiplegics. Perception and Motor Skills 37:727–734

Hsu R W W, Himeno S, Coventry M B, Chao E Y S 1990 Normal axial alignment of the lower extremity and load bearing distribution at the knee. Clinical Orthopedics and Related Research 255:215–227

Hughes K, Bell F 1994 Visual assessment of hemiplegic gait following stroke: pilot study. Archives of Physical Medicine and Rehabilitation 75: 1100–1107

Jensen G M, Shepard K F, Gwyer J, Hack L M 1992 Attribute dimensions that distinguish master and novice physical therapy clinicians in orthopedic settings. Physical Therapy 72:711–722

Keenan A, Bach T 1996 Video assessment of rearfoot movements during walking: a reliability study. Archives of Physical Medicine and Rehabilitation 77:651–655

Krebs D, Edelstein J, Fishman S 1985 Reliability of observational kinematic gait analysis. Physical Therapy 65(7):1027–1033

Lord S E, Halligan P, Wade D 1998 Visual Gait Analysis: the development of a clinical assessment procedure and scale. Clinical Rehabilitation 12:107–119

Malouin F 1995 Observational gait analysis. In: Craik R, Oatis C (eds) Gait analysis: theory and application. Mosby, Baltimore

McGinley J L, Goldie P A, Greenwood K M, Olney S J 2003 Accuracy and reliability of observational gait analysis data: judgments of push-off in gait after stroke. Physical Therapy 83(2):146–160

Moore S, Schurr K, Wales A et al 1993 Observation and analysis of hemiplegic gait: swing phase. Australian Journal of Physiotherapy 39(4):271–278

Moseley A, Wales A, Herbert R et al 1993 Observation and analysis of hemiplegic gait: stance phase. Australian Journal of Physiotherapy 39(4):259–267

Õunpuu S, Davis R, Walsh H 1995 Sagittal plane pelvic motion relationship to standing pelvic tilt and clinical measures. Developmental Medicine and Child Neurology 37:25

Patla A, Proctor J, Morson B 1987 Observations on aspects of visual gait assessment: a questionnaire study. Physiotherapy Canada 39(5):311–316

Perry J 1989 Observational gait analysis handbook. The Pathokinesiology Service and The Physical Therapy Department of Rancho Los Amigos Medical Center. The Professional Staff Association, California

Perry J 1992 Gait analysis: normal and pathological function. McGraw-Hill, New York

Turnbull G I, Wall J C 1985 The development of a system for the clinical assessment of gait following a stroke. Physiotherapy 71(7):294–298

Wade D T, Wood V A, Heller A et al 1987 Walking after stroke : measure and recovery over the first 3 months. Scandinavian Journal of Rehabilitation Medicine 19:25–30

Winter D A 1985 Concerning the scientific basis for the diagnosis of pathological gait and for rehabilitation protocols. Physiotherapy Canada 37(4):245–252

Afterword

Gait analysis in the clinic

Many clinicians do not have access to a full gait laboratory, so the question arises: what can be done with limited technology and time? The following is a list of suggestions in ascending order of cost and sophistication.

1. An area that is large enough to observe gait, especially in the sagittal plane (at least 6 m long by 3 m wide).
2. A measured walkway length for computation of TSPs.
3. A stopwatch for recording walk times and pulse rates for PCI measurements.
4. A video camcorder, or computer with frame grabber.
5. Software for 2D analysis.
6. A plantar pressure recording system.
7. A force platform and video vector display unit.
8. A four- or eight-channel surface electromyography amplifier.
9. A 3D motion analysis system.
10. A breath-by-breath gas analysis system.

Gait analysis should similarly be looked upon as a step-wise investigation:

1. Observational gait analysis.
2. Measurement of walking speed, cadence and calculation of stride length at natural and fast speeds.
3. Measurement of PCI.
4. Measurement of key angles at key events from 2D video:
   - Ankle at contact
   - Hindfoot angle during loading

- Knee at contact
- Knee in late stance
- Ankle plantarflexion during push-off
- Knee flexion in swing.
5. Plantar pressures.
6. A qualitative assessment of ankle and knee joint moments using the ground reaction vector.
7. 3D kinematics.
8. Dynamic electromyography.
9. Joint moments and powers by inverse dynamics.
10. Oxygen consumption and cost measurement.

It should be noted, however, that the more advanced the equipment the more time will be required to maintain and support it. These days, familiarization with computer software, upgrading and debugging can unfortunately be extremely time-consuming. Steps 7–10 (and possibly 4–6) will usually require the assistance of one or two technical support personnel if the clinician is to have any time left for treating patients!

The need for good record keeping, with a computerized database, cannot be overemphasized, and much can be learnt from the analysis of outcomes of previous cases. By setting an objective goal (whether this be, e.g. stride length, joint range of motion, PCI, push-off power, or simply pain level on a visual analogue scale), a judgement can be made about treatment success. If this is not done, there is a temptation to set the goal retrospectively and it will be difficult to evaluate progress.

KEEP UP TO DATE!

In these internet days, there is no excuse for not following new developments. Here are a few suggestions:

- Clinical Gait Analysis website (>1200 subscribers): *http://www.univie. ac.at/cga* Join the email list at the bottom of the homepage.
- Biomechanics list (>5000 subscribers): *http://listserv.surfnet.nl/scripts/ wa.exe?A0=biomch-l.html* Search more than 10 years of archives
- PubMed (>14 million biomedical journal articles): *http://www.ncbi. nlm.nih.gov/PubMed* Search the National Library of Medicine from the 1950s up to the present day
- Gait and Posture (one of the most respected and comprehensive journals on gait analysis: *http://www1.elsevier.com/cdweb/journals/09666362/ viewer.htt?viewtype=journal*

CONFERENCES TO ATTEND

- Annual Meeting of the Gait and Clinical Movement Analysis Society (GCMAS); rotates around US gait laboratories. *http://www.gcmas.org*

- Annual Scientific Meeting of the European Society of Movement Analysis for Adults and Children (ESMAC); rotates around European gait laboratories. *http://www.esmac.org*
- International Symposium on the 3-D Analysis of Human Movement, a Technical Group of the International Society for Biomechanics (ISB), providing a forum for discussion of issues that relate to the measurement of human movement in three dimensions. *http://pe.usf.edu/3D-HumanMovement*
- International Society for Postural and Gait Research (ISPGR), a forum for scientists and clinicians who are interested in all aspects of the control of posture, balance and gait. *http://www.ispgr.org*

Appendix: Answers to multiple-choice questions

CHAPTER 1

1.1 (c)
Stance = (DS + 100)/2
    = (30 + 100)/2
    = 65%

1.2 (d)
Speed = Distance/Time
Time = Distance/Speed
    = 30/1.5
    = 20 s

1.3 (c)
Cadence in strides/s = (Cadence in steps/min)/120
          = 80/120
          = 0.67 strides/s

1.4 (b)
Stride Length = (120 × Speed)/Cadence
      = (120 × 1)/120
      = 1 m

1.5 (d)
Stride Length = (120 × Speed)/Cadence
Cadence = (120 × Speed)/Stride length
    = (120 × 0.8)/1.2
    = 80 steps/min
Stride time = 120/Cadence
     = 120/80
     = 1.5 s

1.6 (a)

- Double support time falls as speed increases.
- Double support increases as base of support falls.
- Shoes increase base of support.

So, the longest double support would be expected from walking barefoot at the slowest speed.

1.7 (b)

Normal stance = 60%, so 55% is shortened stance. Ataxia and other balance problems tend to result in **increased** stance duration

Children have **longer** stance times compared to adults. Stance is **shortened** due to pain (antalgic gait).

1.8 (c)

SLR = shorter/longer step length
$$= 30/50$$
$$= 0.6$$

CHAPTER 2

2.1 (a)

The foot (and pelvis) are segments; all the others are joints.

2.2 (c)

Optimal cutoff = 6 × stride frequency
Stride frequency = 160/120
$$= 1.33 \text{ strides/s}$$
So optimal cutoff = 6 × 1.33
$$= 8 \text{ Hz}$$

2.3 (a)

Joint angle = proximal segment angle − distal segment angle
$$= 120° − 30°$$
$$= 90°$$
But we need to subtract 90° to transform the angle to the clinical convention of ankle angle, so Joint angle = 0° (*neutral* or *plantigrade*).

2.4 (c)

A lower cutoff frequency results in over-smoothed data. There will be less noise, but the peaks will be decreased in amplitude.

CHAPTER 3

3.1 (b)

Attaching the sacral marker to S3 instead of S2 would result in a posterior tilt artefact. There would be no obliquity introduced because this is defined by the ASIS markers. The hip joint centre will move inferiorly, but this will not affect the flexion angle recorded.

CHAPTER 4

4.1   (c)
If the GRF passes through the joint axis, the moment arm is zero.
Moment = $80 \times 10 \times 0 = 0$ N m

4.2   (c)
Half body weight passes through each foot. Taking the GRF moment arm as 5 cm, the tendon moment arm as 4 cm, and using $g = 10$ m/s^2:
Tendon Force = Ankle Moment/Tendon Moment Arm
$$= (mgd/2) \div 0.04$$
$$= (60 \times 10 \times 0.05)2 \div 0.04$$
$$= 15/0.04$$
$$= 375 \text{ N}$$

4.3   (d)
Tendon Force = Ankle Moment/Tendon Moment Arm
Ankle Moment = $mgd/2 = (60 \times 10 \times 0.07)/2$
So
Tendon Force = $(60 \times 10 \times 0.07)/(2 \times 0.04)$
$$= 525 \text{ N}$$

4.4   (b)
Tendon Force = Ankle Moment/Tendon Moment Arm
$$= (mgd/2) \div 0.05$$
$$= (80 \times 10 \times 0.01)/(2 \times 0.05)$$
$$= 80 \text{ N}$$

4.5   (d)
Active muscle is on the opposite side of the joint to the GRF. The GRF is anterior, so the active muscle must be posterior, i.e. the *gluteus maximus* (external moment is flexor, internal moment is extensor).

CHAPTER 5

5.1   (a)
F = $mg + ma$
$$= (70 \times 10) + (70 \times 2)$$
$$= 700 + 140$$
$$= 840$$
Scales assume $F = mg$, so will read $m = F/g$.
$m = 840/10$
$$= 84 \text{ kg}$$

5.2   (c)
Total GRV = $\sqrt{(400^2 + 300^2)}$
$$= 500 \text{ N}$$

CHAPTER 6

6.1 (a)
Pressure = ρgh, where $\rho = 13.6 \times 10^3$ kg/m^3, $g = 9.81$ m/s^2, and $h = 100$ mm $= 0.1$ m
Pressure = $13.6 \times 1000 \times 9.81 \times 0.1$ Pa
$\qquad$ = 13,300 Pa
$\qquad$ = 13 kPa (2 s.f.)

CHAPTER 7

7.1 (a)
Active muscle is on the opposite side of the joint to the GRF. So muscle posterior to the ankle (plantarflexors) and anterior to knee (*vasti*) must be active.

7.2 (a)
In walking up a slope, shear is directed anteriorly, directing the GRV forwards, with increasingly plantarflexor ankle moment, flexor knee and extensor hip moments.

7.3 (c)
Muscle tension, T = Joint Moment/Lever Arm
$\qquad$ = 25/0.05
$\qquad$ = 500 N

CHAPTER 8

8.1 (a)
Psoas takes origin from the lumbar vertebrae, crossing the intervertebral joints and the hip joint before inserting on the femur.

8.2 (c)
Polio affects motor neuron cell bodies in the ventral horns.

8.3 (a)
Postural muscles need good blood flow for aerobic (oxidative) metabolism.

8.4 (c)
CMRR = $20 \log_{10}$ (Differential Gain/Common Gain)
Differential Gain/Common Gain = $10^{(CMRR/20)} = 10^5$
So,
Common Gain = Differential Gain/10^5
$\qquad$ = 1000/10^5
$\qquad$ = 10^{-2}
i.e. 1/100 or 0.01.

CHAPTER 9

9.1   (b)
The CoM falls during double support, and rises during single support.

9.2   (c)
Internal rotation and knee flexion will both tend to shorten the limb. Pelvic list would need to occur during double support. Contralateral internal pelvic rotation is equivalent to ipsilateral external pelvic rotation, which is what is needed at initial contact to lengthen the limb.

9.3   (c)
$$a_{vertical} = (F_{vertical} - Mg)/M$$
$$= (1000 - 75 \times 10) \div 75$$
$$= 3.33 \text{ m/s}^2$$

CHAPTER 10

10.1   (d)
Power = Force × Velocity
$$= 100 \times 2$$
$$= 200 \text{ W}$$

10.2   (b)
Power = Moment × Angular Velocity
$$P = 10 \times (1/0.5)$$
$$= 20 \text{ W}$$

10.3   (d)
The shank is rotating forward, i.e. the ankle is dorsiflexing.
The moment is plantarflexor, so contraction is eccentric (power absorption).
Power Absorbed = Moment × Angular Velocity
$$= 50 \times 2$$
$$= 100 \text{ W}$$
Power Transfer to Foot = Moment × Angular Velocity
$$= 150 \times 0$$
$$= 0 \text{ W}$$

PART II PRACTICE: INTRODUCTION

B1   (b)
0.2% of 60 million = $(0.2/100) \times 60,000,000$
$$= 120,000$$

CHAPTER 12

12.1 (a)
A backward-set knee moves the GRV more anterior.

CHAPTER 14

14.1 (d)
Flexion contracture on the right, hyperactive hamstrings on the left and weak left hip flexors would all cause short step on the **left**. Weak right plantarflexors would result in reduced push-off and short **right** step.

14.2 (b)
Knee pain and quadriceps atrophy cause the patient to use passive knee stabilization using the GRV, i.e. absent loading response (extended knee during loading).

Index

Page numbers in italic refer to illustrations, boxes and tables